Thieme Dissector

Upper Limb and Thorax

Volume I

Thieme

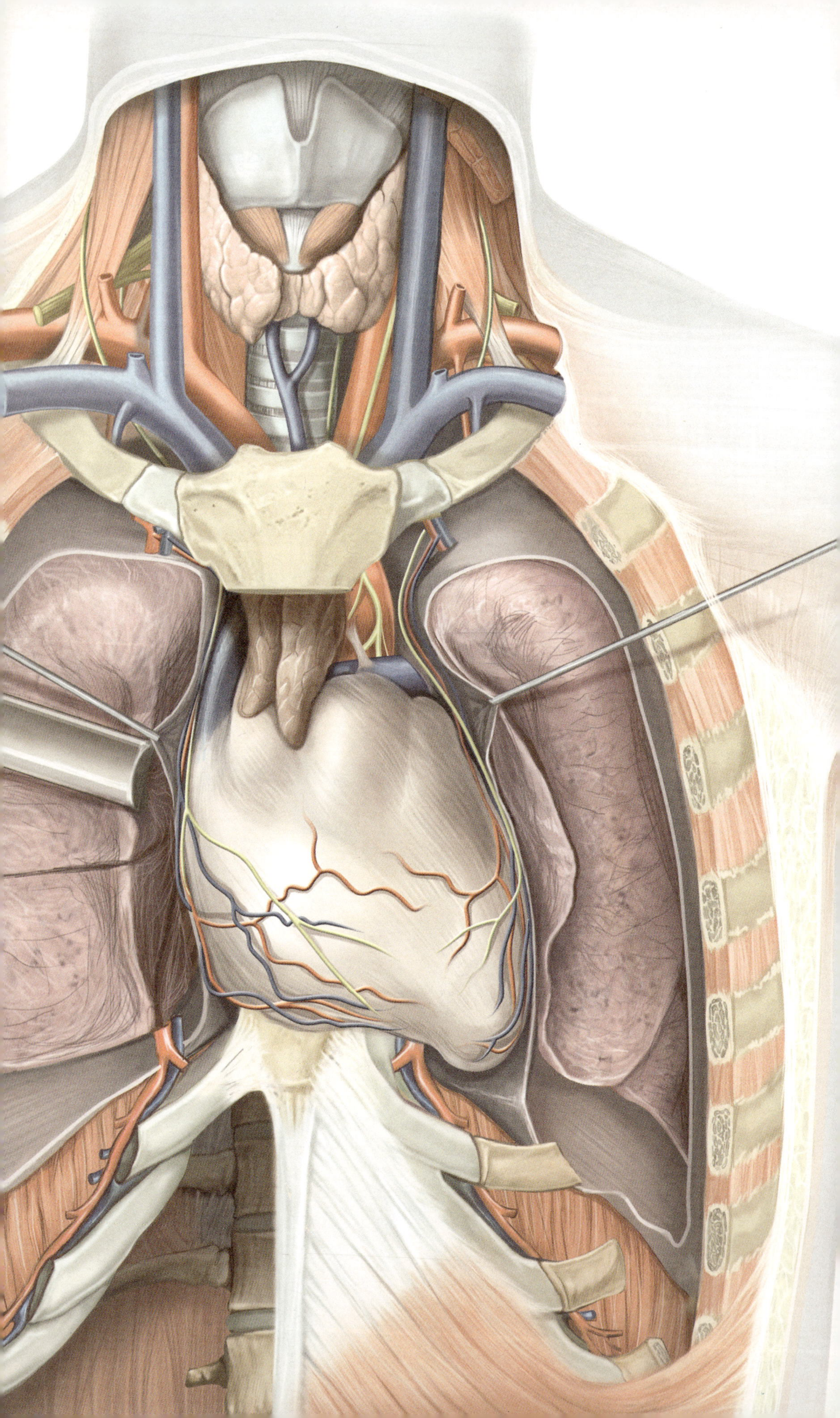

Thieme Dissector

Upper Limb and Thorax

Volume I

Vishram Singh, MBBS, MS, PhD (hc), MICPS, FASI, FIMSA,
Professor and Head,
Department of Anatomy,
Santosh Medical College;
Member of the Academic Council and Core Committee PhD Course,
Santosh University,
Ghaziabad, Delhi NCR, India;
Editor-in-Chief,
Journal of the Anatomical Society of India

G. P. Pal, MBBS, MS, DSc, FASI, FAMS, FNASc, FASc, Bhatnagar Laureate,
Director/Dean,
Modern Institute of Medical Sciences,
Indore, Madhya Pradesh, India

S. D. Gangane, MBBS, MS, FAIMS,
Professor and Head,
Department of Anatomy,
Terna Medical College,
Navi Mumbai, Maharashtra, India

159 illustrations

Thieme
Delhi • Stuttgart • New York • Rio de Janeiro

Publishing Director: Dr. Sonu Singh
Development Editor: Dr. Nidhi Srivastava
Head, Editorial Services: Rachna Sinha
Project Manager: Rupnarayan Das
Sales and Marketing Director: Arun Kumar Majji
Chief Executive Officer: Ajit Kohli

Thieme Medical and Scientific Publishers Private Limited.
A - 12, Second Floor, Sector - 2, Noida - 201 301,
Uttar Pradesh, India, +911204556600
Email: customerservice@thieme.in
www.thieme.in

All illustrations in this volume were created by Markus Voll and Karl Wesker (except Figs. 1 on page xxviii; 8 on page xxxv; 22 on page xlii; 23 on page xliii; 2.1 on page 10; 2.7 on page 15; 3.1 on page 28; 3.2 on page 29; 9.2 on page 86; 11.1 inset on page 108) for the *Atlas of Anatomy* which is based on the work of Michael Schuenke, Erik Schulte, and Udo Schumacher and is edited by Anne M. Gilroy, Brian R. MacPherson, and Lawrence M. Ross.

Cover design: Thieme Publishing Group
Typesetting by Cerebrum Cross Media Services

Printed in India by Replika Press Pvt Ltd

First Reprint, 2015
Second Reprint, 2016
Third Reprint, 2017

Thieme Dissector (Volume I): Upper Limb and Thorax

ISBN: 978-93-82076-79-7
eISBN: 978-93-85062-35-3

Contributor to Volume I

Shabana M. Borate, MBBS, MS,
Associate Professor,
Department of Anatomy,
Grant Government Medical College and
Sir J. J. Group of Hospitals,
Mumbai, Maharashtra, India

Contents

Video Contents

Use the **scratch-off code** as provided at the beginning of the book to access the real dissection videos. Visit WinkingSkull.com and follow these instructions to get started.
If you do not already have a free WinkingSkull.com account, visit www.winkingskull.com

1. Click on "Register" and complete the registration form.
2. Enter the scratch-off code from the access code panel given on the inside front cover of this book.

If you already have a WinkingSkull.com account,

1. Click on "Log in" to enter "Email or User name" and "Password".
2. Click on "Account" and then "Register a Code".
3. Enter the scratch-off code from the access code panel.

This will give you access to 60+ instructional dissection videos.

Chapter 2
https://www.winkingskull.com/dissector/V1/video.aspx?vid=73
Posterior Compartment of Leg
Review: Structures posterior to the medial malleolus

https://www.winkingskull.com/dissector/V1/video.aspx?vid=242
Pectoral Region (Anterior Shoulder)
Review: The deltopectoral triangle

https://www.winkingskull.com/dissector/V1/video.aspx?vid=81
Pectoral Region (Anterior Shoulder)
Show me how: Reflect the pectoralis major

https://www.winkingskull.com/dissector/V1/video.aspx?vid=243
Pectoral Region (Anterior Shoulder)
Review: The pectoral region

https://www.winkingskull.com/dissector/V1/video.aspx?vid=247
Axilla
Review: Walls of the axilla

https://www.winkingskull.com/dissector/V1/video.aspx?vid=131
Axilla
Show me how: Remove the axillary vein and its tributaries

https://www.winkingskull.com/dissector/V1/video.aspx?vid=246
Axilla
Review: Axillary artery

https://www.winkingskull.com/dissector/V1/video.aspx?vid=245
Axilla
Review: Brachial plexus - Divisions and cords

Chapter 4
https://www.winkingskull.com/dissector/V1/video.aspx?vid=84
Posterior Shoulder and Arm
Show me how: Reflect the deltoid

https://www.winkingskull.com/dissector/V1/video.aspx?vid=248
Posterior Shoulder and Arm
Review: The quadrangular space

https://www.winkingskull.com/dissector/V1/video.aspx?vid=251
Posterior Shoulder and Arm
Review: Neurovasculature of the supraspinous fossa

https://www.winkingskull.com/dissector/V1/video.aspx?vid=133
Posterior Shoulder and Arm
Show me how: Reflect the infraspinatus

https://www.winkingskull.com/dissector/V1/video.aspx?vid=252
Posterior Shoulder and Arm
Review: Neurovasculature of the infraspinous fossa

Chapter 5
https://www.winkingskull.com/dissector/V1/video.aspx?vid=254
Anterior Arm and Cubital Fossa
Review: Muscles of the anterior arm

https://www.winkingskull.com/dissector/V1/video.aspx?vid=256
Anterior Arm and Cubital Fossa
Review: Nerves of the arm

https://www.winkingskull.com/dissector/V1/video.aspx?vid=255
Anterior Arm and Cubital Fossa
Review: The brachial artery and branches in the arm

https://www.winkingskull.com/dissector/V1/video.aspx?vid=257
Anterior Arm and Cubital Fossa
Review: Superficial vessels of the cubital fossa

https://www.winkingskull.com/dissector/V1/video.aspx?vid=258
Anterior Arm and Cubital Fossa
Review: Boundaries of the cubital fossa

https://www.winkingskull.com/dissector/V1/video.aspx?vid=259
Anterior Arm and Cubital Fossa
Review: Contents of the cubital fossa

Chapter 6
https://www.winkingskull.com/dissector/V1/video.aspx?vid=253
Posterior Shoulder and Arm
Review: Muscles of the posterior arm

Chapter 7
https://www.winkingskull.com/dissector/V1/video.aspx?vid=260
Anterior Compartment of the Forearm
Review: Superficial muscles of the anterior forearm

https://www.winkingskull.com/dissector/V1/video.aspx?vid=262
Anterior Compartment of the Forearm
Review: Vasculature of the anterior forearm

https://www.winkingskull.com/dissector/V1/video.aspx?vid=87
Palm of the Hand
Show me how: Reflect the flexor retinaculum

https://www.winkingskull.com/dissector/V1/video.aspx?vid=271
Palm of the Hand
Review: Contents of carpal tunnel

https://www.winkingskull.com/dissector/V1/video.aspx?vid=270
Palm of the Hand
Review: The hypothenar compartment

Chapter 8
https://www.winkingskull.com/dissector/V1/video.aspx?vid=263
Posterior Compartment of the Forearm and Dorsum of the Hand
Review: Superficial muscles of the posterior forearm

https://www.winkingskull.com/dissector/V1/video.aspx?vid=266
Posterior Compartment of the Forearm and Dorsum of the Hand
Review: Extensor digitorum and the extensor hood

https://www.winkingskull.com/dissector/V1/video.aspx?vid=264
Posterior Compartment of the Forearm and Dorsum of the Hand
Review: Deep muscles and neurovasculature of posterior forearm

https://www.winkingskull.com/dissector/V1/video.aspx?vid=265
Posterior Compartment of the Forearm and Dorsum of the Hand
Review: The anatomic snuffbox

Chapter 13
https://www.winkingskull.com/dissector/V1/video.aspx?vid=233
Muscles of the Anterior Thoracic Wall
Review: Muscles of the anterior thoracic wall

Chapter 14
https://www.winkingskull.com/dissector/V1/video.aspx?vid=275
Pleural Cavities and Mediastinum
Review: Divisions of the pleura

https://www.winkingskull.com/dissector/V1/video.aspx?vid=202
Lungs
Show me how: Remove the lungs

https://www.winkingskull.com/dissector/V1/video.aspx?vid=277
Lungs
Review: Surface anatomy of the lungs

https://www.winkingskull.com/dissector/V1/video.aspx?vid=279
Lungs
Review: Anatomy of the left lung

https://www.winkingskull.com/dissector/V1/video.aspx?vid=281
Lungs
Review: Hilum of the right lung

https://www.winkingskull.com/dissector/V1/video.aspx?vid=280
Lungs
Review: Hilum of the left lung

https://www.winkingskull.com/dissector/V1/video.aspx?vid=282
Lungs
Review: Impressions on the right lung

https://www.winkingskull.com/dissector/V1/video.aspx?vid=89
Lungs
Show me how: Dissect a bronchopulmonary segment

https://www.winkingskull.com/dissector/V1/video.aspx?vid=285
Pericardial Sac
Review: The heart in situ

https://www.winkingskull.com/dissector/V1/video.aspx?vid=204
Pericardial Sac
Show me how: Locate the oblique pericardial sinus

https://www.winkingskull.com/dissector/V1/video.aspx?vid=203
Pericardial Sac
Show me how: Locate the transverse pericardial sinus

https://www.winkingskull.com/dissector/V1/video.aspx?vid=204
Pericardial Sac
Show me how: Locate the oblique pericardial sinus

https://www.winkingskull.com/dissector/V1/video.aspx?vid=286
External Heart
Review: Sternocostal surface structures of the heart

https://www.winkingskull.com/dissector/V1/video.aspx?vid=287
External Heart
Review: Inferior and diaphragmatic surface structures of the heart

https://www.winkingskull.com/dissector/V1/video.aspx?vid=92
External Heart
Show me how: Dissect the right coronary artery
https://www.winkingskull.com/dissector/V1/video.aspx?vid=288
External Heart
Review: Course of the right coronary artery

https://www.winkingskull.com/dissector/V1/video.aspx?vid=205
External Heart
Show me how: Dissect the left coronary artery

https://www.winkingskull.com/dissector/V1/video.aspx?vid=289
External Heart
Review: Course of the left coronary artery

https://www.winkingskull.com/dissector/V1/video.aspx?vid=93
Chambers of the Heart
Show me how: Cut the right atrium

https://www.winkingskull.com/dissector/V1/video.aspx?vid=291
Chambers of the Heart
Review: The right atrium

https://www.winkingskull.com/dissector/V1/video.aspx?vid=94
Chambers of the Heart
Show me how: Cut the right ventricle

https://www.winkingskull.com/dissector/V1/video.aspx?vid=292
Chambers of the Heart
Review: The right ventricle

https://www.winkingskull.com/dissector/V1/video.aspx?vid=207
Chambers of the Heart
Show me how: Cut the left ventricle

https://www.winkingskull.com/dissector/V1/video.aspx?vid=294
Chambers of the Heart
Review: The left ventricle

https://www.winkingskull.com/dissector/V1/video.aspx?vid=293
Chambers of the Heart
Review: The left atrium

https://www.winkingskull.com/dissector/V1/video.aspx?vid=296
Superior Mediastinum
Review: Structures of the superior mediastinum

https://www.winkingskull.com/dissector/V1/video.aspx?vid=297
Superior Mediastinum
Review: The major branches of the aortic arch

https://www.winkingskull.com/dissector/V1/video.aspx?vid=298
Superior Mediastinum
Review: The right and left recurrent laryngeal nerves

https://www.winkingskull.com/dissector/V1/video.aspx?vid=208
Posterior Mediastinum
Show me how: Remove the pericardial sac

https://www.winkingskull.com/dissector/V1/video.aspx?vid=299
Posterior Mediastinum
Review: Posterior mediastinum - Vagus nerves, thoracic duct, and the trachea

https://www.winkingskull.com/dissector/V1/video.aspx?vid=300
Posterior Mediastinum
Review: Veins of the posterior thoracic wall

https://www.winkingskull.com/dissector/V1/video.aspx?vid=301
Posterior Mediastinum
Review: Autonomic structures and neurovasculature of the posterior thoracic wall

Note from the Author

There was a long-felt need of a good dissection manual for first-year undergraduate medical students undertaking the anatomy course. Anatomy is the foundation of all medical subjects, and hence, its thorough knowledge is essential for all students aspiring to become good doctors, especially in surgical fields.

The best *modus operandi* to learn anatomy is through dissection. Recently, due to information explosion in the medical field, the health sciences curricula have markedly reduced the time allocation for studying and teaching anatomy; yet it is realized by all that the gross structure of the human body, including its three-dimensional conceptualization, must be understood thoroughly before proceeding further to learn medicine.

Therefore, we have made a sincere effort to meet all the needs of the students in creating this 3-volume set of dissection manuals. They not only delineate instructions for students to perform perfect dissection but also provide gross anatomy descriptions, supplemented by clinical correlations of gross structures studied during dissection. The textual descriptions are complemented by numerous coloured illustrations that will help students recognize significant structures with more precision. To further enhance understanding, the content of the volumes is organized in sections like (a) Learning Objectives, (b) Surface Landmarks, (c) Dissection and Identification, (d) Description of Gross Anatomy and (e) Clinical Notes. Laced with all these features, we hope that these volumes will be useful not only for medical and dental students but also for teachers of anatomy. The value of these volumes is further enhanced by providing videos at relevant places.

As educators of anatomy, we have tried our best to make these manuals easy for learning. We highly appreciate the contribution of Prof. Poonam Kharb and Mr. D. Krishna Chaitanya in Vol. II and Prof. Shabana M. Borate in Vol. I. For further improvements, we would sincerely welcome comments and suggestions from all students and teachers.

Vishram Singh

Note from the Author

The medical curriculum in India requires basic anatomy, along with some other basic subjects, to be taught to students in the first year of the course. This often leads to an information overload for them. For some students, the situation is made even more difficult due to linguistic limitations and late admissions. As a result, there has long been a pressing need for comprehensive teaching resources that create thorough understanding of these courses in a short time span. Specifically for anatomy, one cannot stress enough on the value of a complete and detailed dissection manual that explains basic concepts in a simple and lucid manner, without duplication of facts or unnecessary complexities.

In Volume III, every care has been taken to describe all steps involved in the dissection of the head, neck and brain in a stepwise manner that is easy to understand for the beginners. Several high-quality illustrations have been used to explain each step. They help show the dissections with a great amount of detailing and clarity. To make the discourse interesting, relevant clinical conditions have also been presented under separate sections called "Clinical Notes".

Producing a book with hundreds of illustrations is a joint effort by the author and the publisher in a true sense.

I strongly believe that this book will be an invaluable learning resource for students and teachers of anatomy in medical and dental courses.

G. P. Pal

Note from the Author

Dissection of a cadaver is integral to understanding the human anatomy. It gives an unmatched, first-hand experience of exploring the structure of organs as well as knowing their relationship with each other. *Thieme Dissector* has been designed as a set of three volumes to provide students a complete account of the dissection of human body.

Anatomy is one of the basic sciences under the faculty of medicine. Being basic means it forms a base, a foundation, and it goes without saying that a strong building requires a strong foundation. Thus, a thorough knowledge of anatomy is highly desirable to develop surgical skills in many fields, such as General Surgery, Orthopaedics, Obstetrics and Gynecology, ENT, Ophthalmology, Plastic Surgery, Neurosurgery, and so on.

The first volume of the set deals with upper limb and thorax; the second with abdomen and lower limb and the third with head, neck and brain. The "Introduction" of this volume contains general information about the preservation of a cadaver, the instruments required for dissection, and anatomical terms, followed by a discussion on the basic tissues of the body. This is followed by 10 chapters on upper limb and 5 chapters on thorax. Each chapter begins with a set of "Learning Objectives", followed by an introduction on the topic, the dissection steps with description of the relevant structures set in special coloured boxes, and clinical notes.

To further facilitate the understanding of the subject, students have also been provided access to over 200 real dissection videos across the chapters. The links to these videos have been placed at relevant places. I am confident that this extremely useful approach adopted in these volumes will help enrich students' learning process tremendously.

I am grateful to Dr Shabana Boate, Associate Professor of Anatomy at Grant Medical College, Mumbai, and Dr Sachin Yadav, postgraduate student from the department, for their support and untiring efforts in the preparation of this volume. It would not have been possible to present this volume to you without their contribution.

I am fortunate to be associated through this project with two most reputed and eminent persons in the field of anatomy: Dr Vishram Singh and Dr G. P. Pal. I express my heartfelt gratitude to them for their support during the writing of this volume.

In spite of all the care taken in the preparation of this volume, I would like to apologize for any errors that might have remained. I will highly appreciate receiving valuable feedback and suggestions from readers to improve the next edition of this work.

S. D. Gangane

About the Authors

Vishram Singh

(Editor-in-Chief and Author, Volume II, Abdomen and Lower Limb)

Vishram Singh, MBBS, MS, PhD (hc), MICPS, FASI, FIMSA, is Professor and Head, Department of Anatomy, Santosh Medical College; and in-charge of Medical Education Unit and member of the Academic Council and Core Committee PhD Course at Santosh University, Ghaziabad, Delhi NCR, India.

A renowned anatomist, Prof. Singh has taught undergraduate and postgraduate students at sev-eral colleges and institutes, such as King George Medical College, Lucknow; All India Institute of Medical Sciences, New Delhi; and Al Arab Medical University, Benghazi, Libya. He has more than 40 years of experience in teaching, research and clinical practice. He has various bestselling titles to his credit, such as *Textbook of Clinical Neuroanatomy, Textbook of Anatomy,* and *Textbook of Clinical Embryology*.

Prof. Singh has received various recognitions and awards for his contributions in the field of anatomy. He has been elected Vice President of the Anatomical Society of India many times. He is currently Editor-in-Chief, *Journal of Anatomical Society of India* (JASI).

G. P. Pal

(Author, Volume III, Head, Neck and Brain)

G. P. Pal, MBBS, MS, DSc, FASI, FAMS, FNASc, FASc, Bhatnagar Laureate, is currently the Director/Dean of Modern Institute of Medical Sciences, Indore, Madhya Pradesh, India. An eminent anatomist with a teaching experience of four decades, Prof. Pal has earlier served as the Head of Department of Anatomy at M.P. Shah Government Medical College, Jamnagar, Gujarat and was the visiting Associate Professor at The Medical College of Pennsylvania, Philadelphia, United States. He has to his credit numerous pub-lications in journals of international repute. He has received several national awards and honours for his research works. He has been elected the fellow of various leading academies of sciences in India. His research work is cited in more than 50 standard textbooks throughout the world. Prof. Pal has authored many well-received books such as *Textbook of Histology, Illustrated Textbook of Neuroanatomy, Medical Genetics, Genetics in Dentistry, General Anatomy, Human Osteology, Basics of Medical Genetics* and *Medical Genetics for Dental Students*. He has also co-authored Prof. Inderbir Singh's *Human Embryology*.

S. D. Gangane

(Author, Volume I, Upper Limb and Thorax)

S. D. Gangane, MBBS, MS, FAIMS is currently serving as Professor and Head, Department of Anatomy at Terna Medical College, Nerul, Navi Mumbai. He has been Professor and Head, Department of Anatomy and Genetic Division at Grant Medical College, Mumbai and Sir J. J. Group of Hospitals, Mumbai. This is a unique Anatomy Department offering services to patients having genetic disorders. Prof. Gangane has authored a bestselling book titled *Human Genetics* which has been widely accepted by faculty and both undergraduate and postgraduate students.

Prof. Gangane has over four decades of teaching experience and has been guiding students for MD Anatomy, and MSc and PhD in Applied Biology courses at Mumbai University. He has also been a guide for the MD Anatomy and PhD Genetics courses at Maharashtra University of Health Sciences (the State Health University). He has published several articles in national and international journals and is also a co-author of the recently published *Textbook of Pathology and Genetics for Nurses*. In addition, he has been on the national advisory board and the executive editorial board for a few journals, including *Indian Journal of Anatomy* and *National Journal of Medical Sciences*.

Prof. Gangane has also worked as an Officer of Special Duty (OSD) for the Government of Maharashtra under the Directorate of Medical Education and Research. He is a member of the advisory panel for the South Asian region of the international publishing house, Lippincott Williams and Wilkins. He is the founder Trustee of "Sandnya Sanwardhan Sanstha", an organization that takes care of mentally challenged children by imparting vocational training and enabling them to lead better lives.

Dedication

To my students, past and present.

Vishram Singh

To my grandson, Yatharth.

G. P. Pal

Upper Limb and Thorax

Introduction to Dissection

Anatomy is one of the basic subjects in medical education. It deals with the structure of human body. A sound knowledge of this subject provides better understanding of the clinical subjects. The subject of anatomy is best studied by dissection. It will be appropriate to say that dissection forms an integral part of teaching or learning anatomy. It gives you an opportunity to explore, observe and learn about structures/organs. The experience that you gain in the dissection room is unmatched. It cannot be compared to learning through books, illustrations, CDs and DVDs that are available to learn the subject. Dissecting a cadaver improves your skill of handling the tissues and instruments that you will be trying later when you start practising on living subjects. It gives you an understanding about the relationship of various structures to each other and helps you know what is normal and what is anomalous. It offers an anatomical basis of tests that you may do, various signs and symptoms that you encounter in a patient, variations that you may see in some subjects and overall better understanding of many disease processes. It is well said that *the cadaver is the best teacher of anatomy*. Once it is accepted, it is our duty to treat the cadaver with the same respect and dignity which is offered to a living patient.

Preservation of the Cadavers

It is done by embalming the cadaver with the embalming fluid which contains a strong fixative. Subsequently, the cadaver is submersed in the preservative fluid. When the cadaver is partly dissected, proper care should be taken by wrapping it so that it is kept moist, or else the cadaver will dessicate and once the part is dry it cannot be restored. Therefore, expose only the part which is to be dissected. Ideally, all the parts of the body should be periodically inspected and moistened during the dissecting session.

Anatomical Terms

It is essential to get familiar with many anatomical terms which are repeatedly used to describe structures, organs, parts, etc. Some of them are given in the following paragraphs.

Anatomical Position

It is the position of the structure or an organ in the body with the person standing erect, feet approximated (together), toes pointing forward, arms by the side of the body, palms facing forward and the gaze at horizon (**Fig. 1**).

All the descriptions in anatomy are provided assuming the body is in anatomical position, though the cadaver is lying horizontally on the dissection table. Its relationship with the neighbouring structures is essential when you study the structure; remember that the description applies assuming the structure is in anatomical position. The frequently used terms can be put into two groups: the terms of positions and the terms of movements.

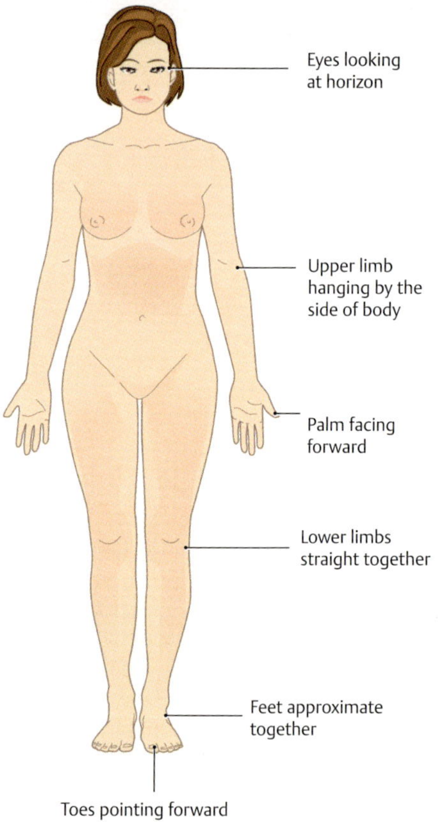

Fig. 1 Anatomical position.

Terms of Positions (Fig. 2)

1. *Anterior*: It means nearer to the front of the body.
2. *Posterior*: It means nearer to the back.
3. *Ventral* and *dorsal* are used in the case of trunk instead of anterior and posterior, respectively.
4. In the hand, *palmar* means anterior and *dorsum* means posterior. In the foot, the terms used are *dorsum* for the upper side and *plantar* for the sole of the foot.
5. *Median*: It means in the middle.
6. *Medial*: It means nearer the median plane.
7. *Median plane*: It is an imaginary plane bisecting the body into nearly two equal halves.
8. *Lateral*: It means away from the median plane; for example, there are two forearm bones, the radius is on the lateral side and the ulna is on the medial side. In the bones of the leg, the tibia is on the medial side and the fibula is on the lateral side.
9. *Superficial*: It means nearer to the skin of surface.
10. *Deep/profundus*: It means deeper (as compared to superficial) from the surface.
11. *Proximal* (nearer to): It indicates relative position of the structure.
12. *Distal* (further from): For example, elbow is distal to the shoulder but proximal to the wrist.
13. *Superior/cephalic*: The term refers to the position of the part which is nearer to the head.
14. *Inferior/caudal*: It means nearer to the feet.

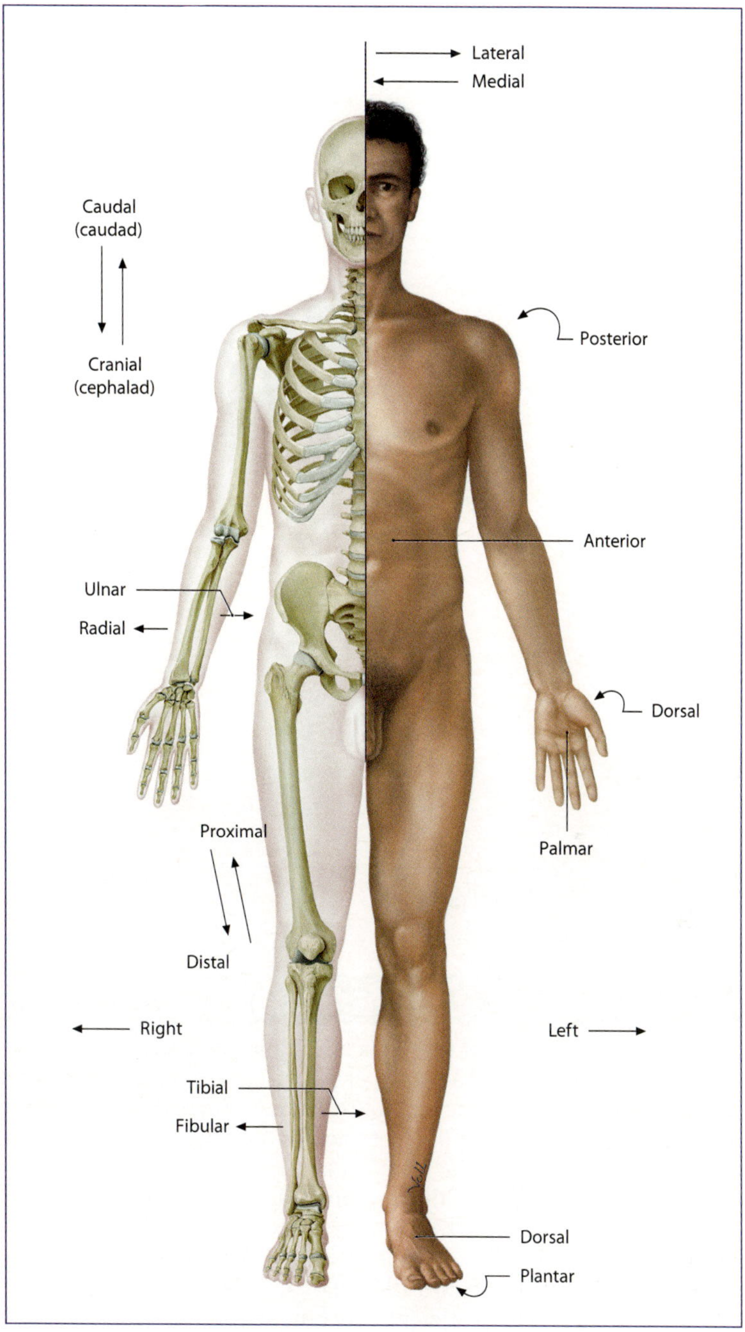

Fig. 2 A diagram illustrating the use of anatomical terms.

Anatomical Planes

There are four imaginary planes (**Fig. 3**) that pass through the body in anatomical position:

1. *Median/sagittal plane*: A vertical plane which passes through the centre of the body and, dividing it into two equal halves.
2. *Paramedian/parasagittal plane*: Any vertical plane which is parallel to the median plane.
3. *Coronal plane*: Any vertical plane perpendicular to the median plane.
4. *Transverse/horizontal plane*: Any plane at right angle to coronal and sagittal planes.

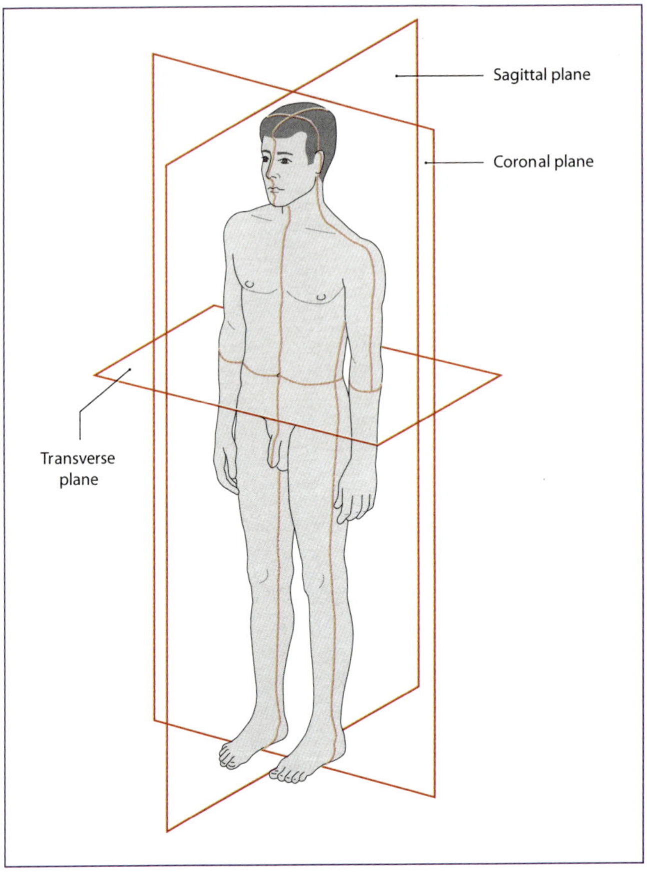

Fig. 3 Anatomical planes.

Terms of Movements

1. *Flexion*: It means forward bending of the trunk and folding of limbs.
2. *Extension*: In case of the trunk, it is backward or posterior bending and in limbs it is straightening.
3. *Dorsiflexion*: It is the movement of the foot towards the dorsum. It occurs at the ankle joint.
4. *Plantar flexion*: It is the movement of the foot towards the sole. It also occurs at the ankle joint.
5. *Adduction*: The movement towards the median plane.
6. *Abduction*: The movement away from the median plane.
7. *Lateral flexion*: It is movement of the trunk in the coronal plane.
8. *Pronation and supination*: These are movements involving the forearm and occur at the radioulnar joints (joints between the forearm bones, the radius and ulna). In anatomical position, the forearm is supinated and the palm faces forward. In pronation, the palm faces backwards/posteriorly.
9. *Inversion and eversion*: These movements involve the foot and occur at the subtalar and calcano-cuboid joints (joints of the tarsal bones, the bones of the foot). In inversion, the medial border of the foot is raised so that the sole faces medially. In eversion, the lateral border of the foot is raised and the sole of the foot faces laterally.
10. *Rotation*: The term signifies the movement where the part of the body is turned around its own longitudinal axis. In the limbs, it can be *medial* or *lateral rotation* at a particular joint, for example, the shoulder joint.

Structures That Are Encountered in Dissection

The body surface is covered by the skin, beneath which lies the superficial fascia and still deeper lies the deep fascia. The *skin* consists of the outer, avascular stratified keratinized epithelium, the *epidermis*, and inner vascular dense fibrous tissue, the *dermis*. Dermis has protrusions into the epidermis. This increases the area of contact between them; thus, the two are firmly bound together.

Superficial fascia: It consists of fat-filled fibrous mesh, connecting the dermis (of the skin) with the deep fascia. In the region of the scalp, palms of the hands, soles of the feet and the back of the neck, the superficial fascia is dense. Hence, in these places the skin is firmly bounded to the underlying deep fascia. In other parts of the body, the superficial fascia is loose and elastic so that the skin can move freely.

The amount of fat in the superficial fascia varies. It is scanty in the nipple and areola of the breast and absent in some parts of the external genital organs. The subcutaneous fat is responsible for the rounded contours of the body and differs in its distribution in males and females. The superficial fascia contains the cutaneous blood vessels, lymphatics and nerves.

Blood Vessels

The blood vessels comprise arteries and veins (**Fig. 4**). The arteries convey blood (oxygenated) from the heart to the tissues under high pressure. The arteries can be categorized as follows: (a) *Large* or *elastic arteries*, for example, the aorta, resist high internal pressure and their elastic recoil smoothens the intermittent systolic pumping action of the heart producing a continuous flow of blood. (b) The medium-sized arteries are also called *muscular* or *distributing arteries*. Their lumen is controlled through the sympathetic nerves, which determines the volume of blood to be distributed through them. (c) As the arteries branch and rebranch into finer vessels, the muscular tissue increases and the elastic elements reduce. The smallest among them, having diameter of less than 0.1 mm, are called *arterioles*. They then end up into capillaries.

Anastomosis found in many tissues form tubular loops through which some smaller arteries unite with each other. The anastomoses are found around joints, for example the cubital anastomosis around the elbow joint. Anastomosis also occurs at the base of the brain, in the gastrointestinal tract and at other

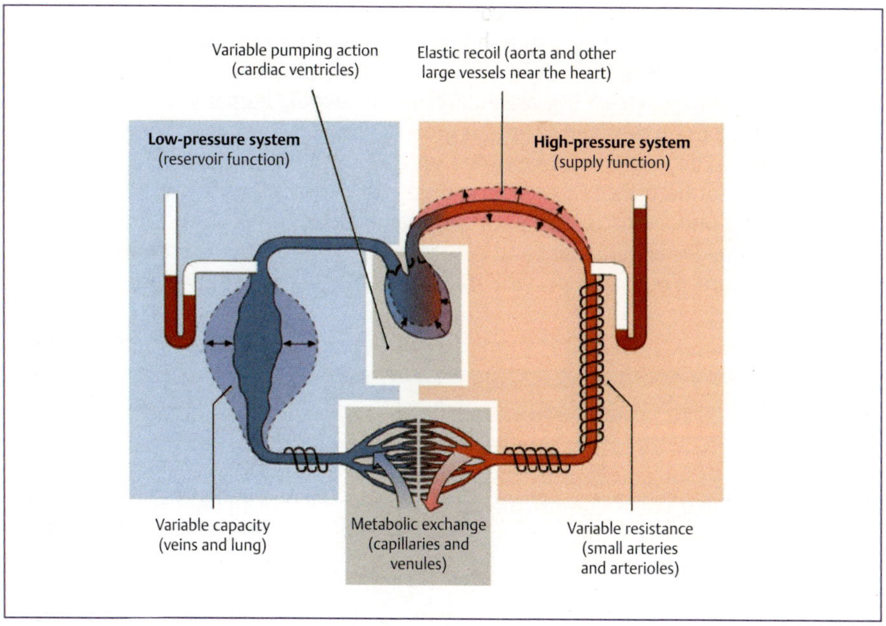

Fig. 4 Basic functional diagram of the circulatory system (no distinction is made between the systemic and pulmonary systems in the diagram).

sites as well. The importance of anastomosis is that it maintains the circulation when *one of the arteries is blocked*. Under these circumstances, the anastomosing channels enlarge to a considerable extent to establish *collateral circulation*. In some tissues, the extent of anastomosis between the adjacent arteries is scanty and hence blockage of such an artery results in death of the tissue supplied by it. Such arteries are called *end arteries*. This situation occurs in the brain, eyes, kidneys, lungs, etc.

Capillaries: The arterioles discharge blood through the microscopic tubes called *capillaries* into the tributaries of the veins. The capillary has a single layer of flat endothelial cells forming its wall. Through this thin wall, substances can be exchanged between the blood and tissues.

Arteriovenous anastomosis: In this, the capillaries do not exist and there is direct communication between the smaller arteries and veins. Such anastomoses exist in many exposed parts of the body, for example, the skin. A considerable amount of blood flows when this anastomosis opens. The increased blood flow permits greater transfer of heat without raising the metabolic rate of the tissue. This promotes heat loss from the skin.

Veins: The blood delivered to the tissue/organ through the arteries and capillaries is collected by the veins. The flow of blood in the veins is sluggish. This is because in each inspiration, there is a fall in intrathoracic pressure helping to draw air as well as venous blood into thorax and compression of veins by the surrounding muscles. Even a light compression can retard the blood flow in the veins because of low pressure within them. However, to prevent the backward flow of blood, veins are provided with *valves*. The position of these valves can be observed in the superficial veins of the forearm as localized swellings when the veins are distended with blood by compression at the elbow.

Venae comitantes: This refers to the veins that accompany deep arteries. This helps in maintaining the temperature of the venous blood as it returns to the heart. The surrounding muscles serve as pumps to direct the flow of blood through the veins. Once these deep veins are emptied by muscular contraction, they get filled again by the communications (perforators) between deep and superficial veins.

Lymphatics and Lymph Nodes

Lymph nodes are firm gland-like structures serving as filters for the *lymph*. Lymph is a clear fluid that flows through the lymph vessels. Lymphatics/lymph vessels are fine tubes (**Fig. 5**). They are more in number in tissues closer to the epithelial surfaces, for example the skin, the lining of the gastrointestinal tract and respiratory epithelium. They are absent in the central nervous system. Lymph passes into the tissue through the capillary walls. It provides a medium of exchange of substances between the blood and tissues. It is drained by the lymph vessels. More lymph is produced in the active tissues and the inflamed tissues. In fact, the lymph capillaries collect lymph from the tissues and form plexus. They unite to form larger lymph vessels. The larger lymph vessels carry lymph to the lymph node. They are called *afferent vessels*. From the hilum of the lymph node, an efferent vessel carries it further. Lymph nodes vary in size. They produce lymphocytes. They are enlarged and become palpable when inflammation occurs in the areas/tissues they drain or when a tumour growth occurs in the tissue. They are particularly large in the groin and axilla. They are often associated with veins. They decrease in size in old age. Though the lymph vessels cannot be traced in cadaveric dissection except the largest one, that is, the *thoracic duct*, they are clinically important as they permit spread of infection or cancerous growth (tumours). In *infection*, the regional nodes are enlarged and become tender. In *tumour/cancerous* growth, the regional nodes become stony hard. Thus, they provide important information to the clinician about the disease process.

Nerves

The nerve cell along with its processes is called *neuron*. The cell body is called *soma*, the short processes are dendrites and a single long process is called axon.

Nerves are pale-looking cords comprising large number of thin filaments called *nerve fibres*. The nerve fibre is a process (axon) of the nerve cell (neuron) (**Fig. 6**). Each nerve fibre is surrounded by the *endoneurium*, a fibrous sheath. A collection of these fibres forms a fascicle/bundle which is surrounded by a sheath of cells and fibres. It is called the *perineurium* (**Fig. 7**). Many such fascicles form the nerve which is surrounded by a sheath called the *epineurium*. These fibrous tissue coverings confer considerable tensile strength to the delicate nerve fibres. The large nerve fibre is enclosed in a sheath cell (*Schwann cell*) which forms a series of concentric layers of discontinuous, laminated, fatty sheath around the fibre. This is the *myelin sheath*. The thin nerve fibre is simply enclosed in sheath cells which do not form concentric layers. They are called the *unmyelinated nerve fibres* (**Fig. 7**).

The nerve fibres transmit nerve impulses from the central nervous system to the various parts/tissues of the body or from these structures to the central nervous system. Among these fibres, those that carry impulses from the central nervous system to the peripheral structures are called the *efferent fibres*. Some of them pass to the muscles. They are called the *motor nerve fibres*. The fibres which carry impulses to the central nervous system are called the *afferent nerve fibres/sensory nerve fibres*. They carry sensory impulses, for example, sensations of pain, touch and temperature from the skin and other tissues to the central nervous system.

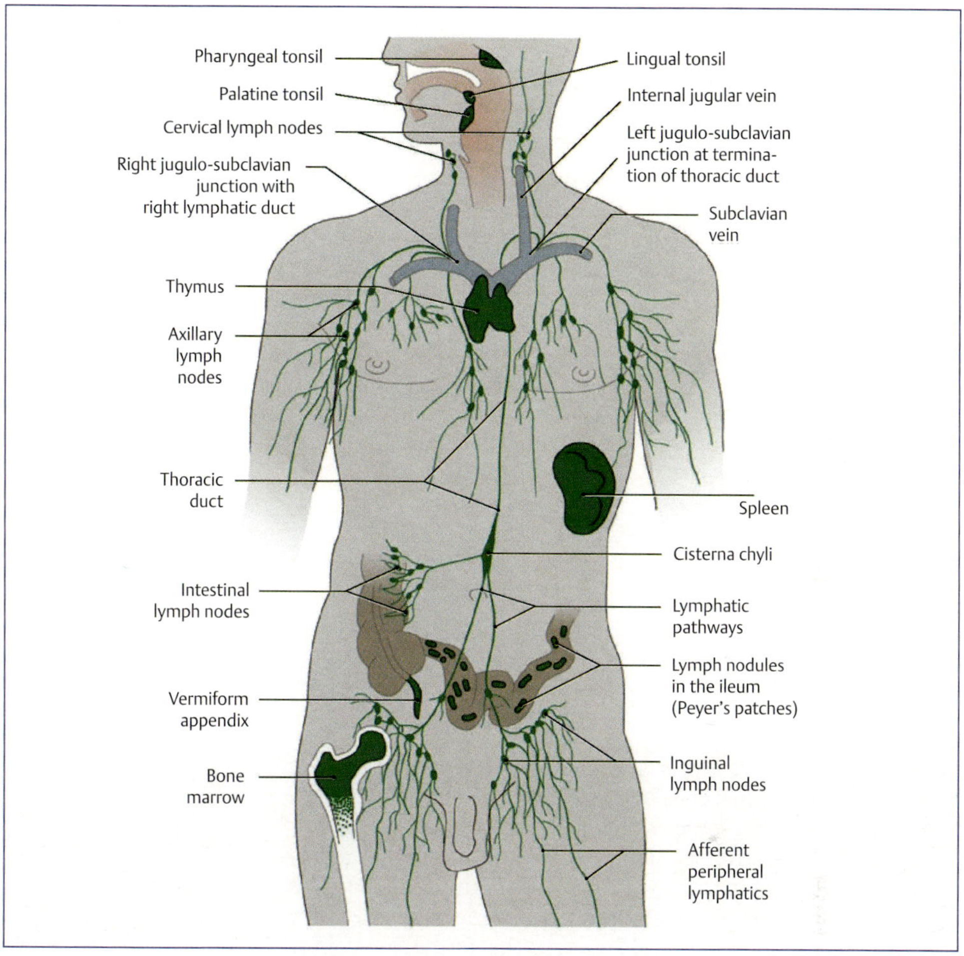

Fig. 5 Lymphatic system (lymphatics and lymph nodes).

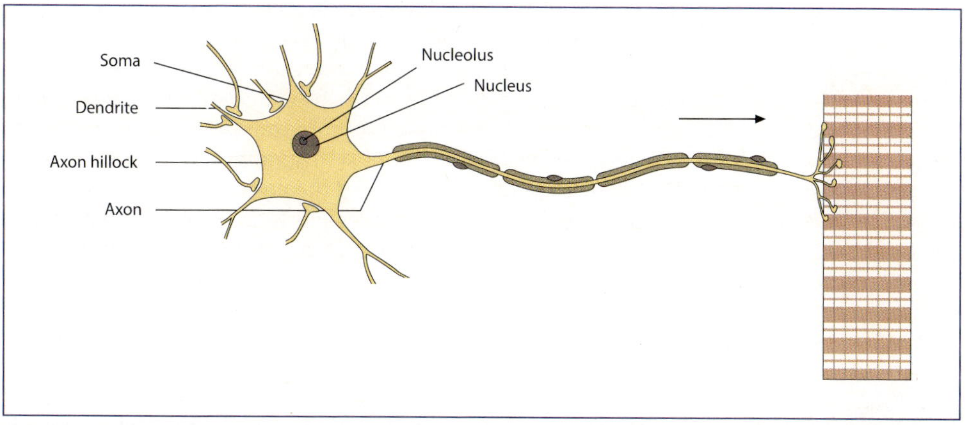

Fig. 6 Typical neuron.

The nerves are broadly classified into (a) *cranial nerves* which are attached to the brain and (b) *spinal nerves* which arise from the spinal cord.

Spinal nerves: There are 31 pairs of the spinal nerves. These are cervical (8), thoracic (12), lumbar (5), sacral (5) and coccygeal (1). They emerge through the intervertebral foramina. All of them emerge caudal to the corresponding vertebra *except* the cervical nerves which emerge cranial to the corresponding vertebra. The first seven cervical nerves are cranial to the corresponding vertebra and the eighth cervical

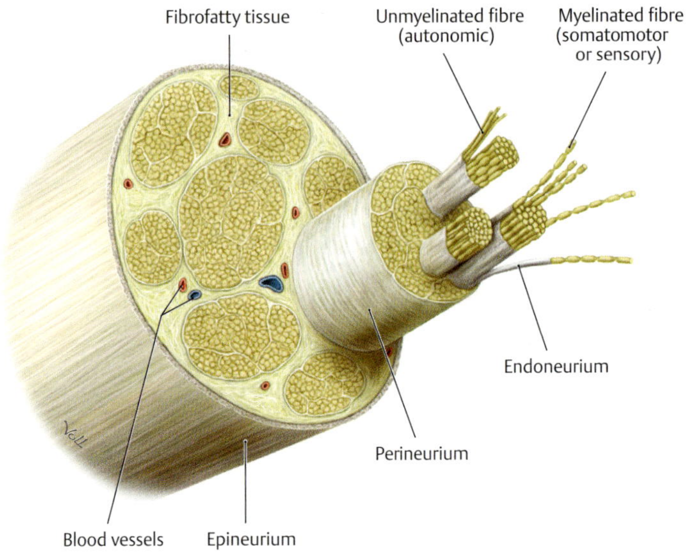

Fig. 7 Structure of a peripheral nerve.

nerve passes below the seventh cervical, that is, between it and the first thoracic vertebra. Each spinal nerve is attached to the spinal cord by two roots, the *ventral* and *dorsal* (**Fig. 8**).

Ventral root consists of efferent fibres that arise from the nerve cells in the spinal cord. The *dorsal root* is a bundle of afferent fibres. Along the dorsal root, there is a collection of nerve cells that forms a swelling called the *dorsal root ganglion*. The fibres of the dorsal root are derived from these cells as their central processes while the peripheral process enters the spinal nerve. The two roots unite at the dorsal root ganglion in the intervertebral foramen. This forms the main trunk of the spinal nerve which is short and has a mixture of both the afferent and efferent fibres. It then divides into a *ventral ramus* and a *dorsal ramus*.

The dorsal ramus is smaller and it passes backwards in the muscles of the back (erector spinae). It then divides into *medial* and *lateral branches* which supply the muscle and also the overlying skin. These cutaneous branches are placed in a row on each side of the midline on the back.

The larger ventral ramus runs laterally. In the thoracic region, the ventral rami run along the lower border of the corresponding ribs and form the intercostal and subcostal nerves. Each of them supplies the muscles (intercostal muscles) and gives an *anterior* and *lateral cutaneous branch* supplying the strip of the skin designated as *dermatome*. *Dermatome* is the strip of skin supplied by a single spinal nerve (**Fig. 8**). The muscle mass supplied by a single spinal nerve is called the *myotome*.

The ventral rami in the cervical, lumbar, sacral and coccygeal regions form the nerve plexuses, that is, the cervical and brachial plexuses that later supply the upper limb. The ventral rami of the lumbar and sacral regions contribute to form the plexuses which supply the lower limb. Each ventral ramus receives a slender *grey ramus communicans* from the corresponding ganglion of the sympathetic chain/trunk.

The sympathetic chain/trunk is formed by the ganglia arranged in a vertical row and connected by nerve fibres. They extend from the base of the skull to the coccyx. They run on each side of the vertebral column. The nerve fibres in the grey ramus arise from the nerve cells (neurons) of the sympathetic ganglia. These are the *postganglionic fibres*; they pass into the ventral ramus to be distributed through its branches. Through the ventral ramus, some fibres enter the dorsal ramus and are distributed through its branches. These sympathetic nerve fibres supply the muscular element in the wall of blood vessels, arrectores pilorum (associated with the hair follicle) and sweat glands.

In the thoracic and upper lumbar (L1–L3), ventral roots and the rami have myelinated fibres which pass from the ventral ramus to the sympathetic ganglion. These are the *preganglionic fibres* and they constitute *white rami communicans*. These fibres run longitudinally. Through them, the central nervous system controls the activity of the sympathetic nerve cells in the sympathetic chain. Thus, the central nervous system can control the amount of blood flowing through various tissues, the secretions of the sweat glands, gooseflesh by action on arrectores pilorum, etc.

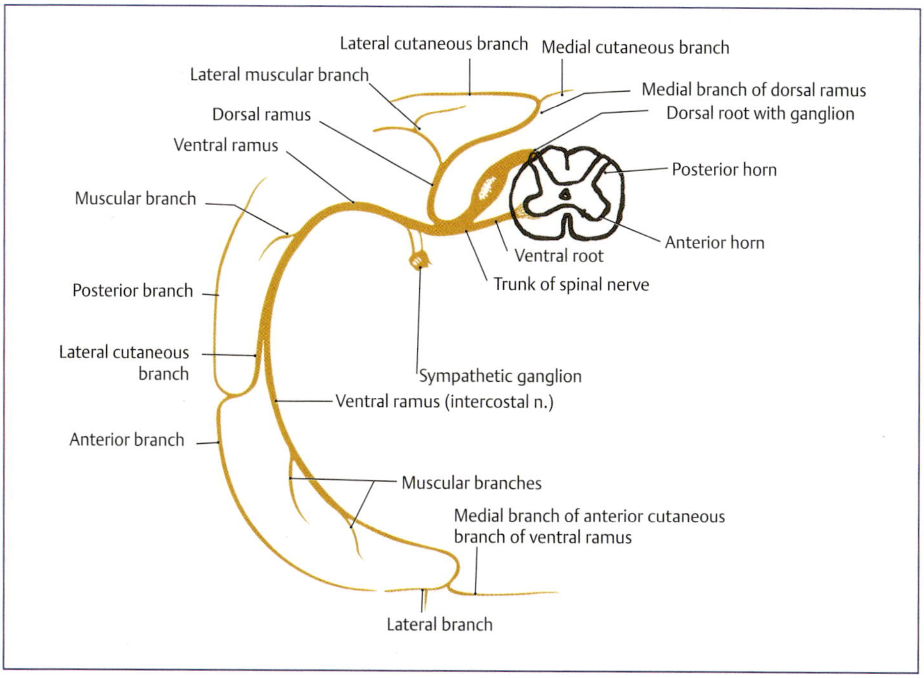

Fig. 8 Typical spinal nerve.

Note that the cutaneous nerve supplying the skin is not only entirely sensory but also has sympathetic efferent fibres in it. Likewise, a branch given to a muscle is not entirely motor but contains sensory and sympathetic fibres. Therefore, a nerve injury not only results in paralysis of the muscle but also leads to the loss of sensation, sweating, goose flesh and control of blood vessels.

Apart from the grey rami communicans, the sympathetic trunk sends postganglionic fibres which pass along the arteries of the limbs, head and neck and also the body wall. The postganglionic sympathetic fibres also supply the viscera (internal organs) through the *periarterial plexus* of nerve fibres.

The *parasympathetic nervous system* supplies the viscera and the eye. This system comprises the peripheral ganglia located in or close to the viscera which they supply. It innervates glands and the smooth muscles of the gastrointestinal tract. This is done by releasing acetylcholine from the terminals of the *cholinergic nerve fibres*. Similarly, the sympathetic postganglionic fibres are called the *adrenergic fibres*.

The parasympathetic nervous system has the craniosacral outflow, whereas the sympathetic system has the *thoracolumbar outflow*. They together form the *autonomic nervous system*.

Deep Fascia

It is formed by a dense, unyielding membrane that separates the superficial fascia from the deeper structures. It envelops the muscles and sends in *intermuscular septa* between adjacent muscles. It ensheathes vessels and nerves which lie between the muscles. The intermuscular septa are attached to the bone. The *retinacula* occurring around the wrist and ankle joints are merely the thickened bands of the deep fascia. They help in holding the tendons in position and also serve as pulleys altering the direction of muscle pull, adding to the efficacy of the muscular contraction. When the muscles contract within the deep fascial sheaths, they compress the veins within and this helps in venous return. It is for this reason that if there is severe muscle wasting or damage to the deep fascia, it results in sluggish venous return, giving rise to *oedema*. It is believed that if any forces are applied to the fascia, it responds by laying down collagen fibres parallel to the forces. This gives rise to *aponeurosis, retinacula* and *ligaments*.

Ligaments

They are thick, inelastic bands of the white fibrous tissue connecting the bones at the joints. Structurally, they are similar to the tendons, both being formed by collagen fibres.

Muscles

The muscles produce movement when they contract (shorten). Each muscle has at least two attachments. When we consider shortening or contracting a muscle, one end is fixed while the other moves. The fixed end is called the *origin* and the moving end is called the *insertion*. However, these terms are deceptive; for example, muscles that are used to pull downwards on a rope can also be used to climb up the rope. Hence, instead of using origin and insertion, one can use the terms as *proximal* and *distal attachments*.

When the muscles shorten/contract to approximate its two attachments, it is *concentric action*. When the tension developed by the muscle is equal to the load against which it is acting, then it helps in fixing the part of the body. This is called *isometric contraction*, for example holding an arm outstretched. If the tension developed in a muscle is less than the load acting against it, then the muscle will lengthen, thus paying out slowly. This is called *eccentric action*. This controls the speed and force of the movement, for example lowering the arm to the side from its outstretched position.

In order to test all the three actions of the muscle (described earlier), put your left hand on the lateral side of the right shoulder (on the right deltoid muscle). Now start abducting the right arm till it becomes horizontal, and simultaneously feel the contracting deltoid. This is *concentric action* of the muscle. Now note that as long as you hold the arm in this horizontal position (fixing the part), the deltoid remains in the state of contraction. This is the *isometric contraction*. Now start lowering the arm to the side and note that the deltoid is still in contraction till the movement stops. This is the *eccentric action* of the muscle.

The muscle has a fleshy part called the *muscle belly*. It consists of *muscle fibres*. It attaches to the bone through the fibrous inelastic cord, the *tendon*, or through the thin wide sheet called the *aponeurosis*. Some of these tendons have bone developed within them. Such bones are called the *sesamoid bones*, for example, the tendon of flexor pollicis brevis (muscle of the thumb) or quadriceps femoris muscle having patella, the largest sesamoid bone in the body.

The muscular contraction generates power. To have greater power, the muscle is provided with more number of muscle fibres and they may have more diameter. The number of fibres may be increased by placing them obliquely, thus packing shorter but more number of fibres in the same space. This is achieved by having either bipennate or multipennate character; for example, bipennate are dorsal interossei, while multipennate muscles are deltoid and subscapularis (**Fig. 9**). Depending upon this, the muscles may have intramuscular tendinous septa in multipennate muscle. Though the obliquity reduces the power of the muscle fibre, total proportionate power generated is much more. Thus, in places where powerful muscle is required in relatively smaller space the muscle is multipennate. The contractile elements in the muscle are myofibrils. The muscles are clustered around the joint. Their action on joint depends upon their position relative to the joint. They may act concentrically, isometrically or eccentrically on the joint.

The muscles are often grouped according to their action, such as flexors, extensors, adductors and abductors. However, it may be noted that this may not hold true always, for example deltoid muscle at shoulder joint. Its anterior fibres are flexors and medial rotators; middle (acromial) fibres are abductors, while the posterior fibres are extensors and lateral rotators of the shoulder joint.

Synovial Sheaths and Bursae

These are located in places where the muscle, tendon or skin slides over the bone or fascia. A synovial bursa minimizes the friction between them. Bursa is an enclosed sac lined by synovial membrane. The membrane secretes small amount of fluid in the sac. If there is irritation or infection, the bursa is swollen and becomes tender. It is called bursitis. The movement of the part then becomes painful (**Fig. 10**).

The synovial sheaths enclose tendons of the muscles having considerable range of movement, for example tendons of digital flexors (in fingers).

Bone

It is a specialized connective tissue with numerous functions such as support, movement, protection and haemopoiesis. Morphologically bones are classified as follows:

1. Long bones (e.g., humerus, femur)
2. Miniature long bones (e.g., metacarpals, metatarsals)
3. Short bones (e.g., carpals and tarsals)
4. Flat bones (e.g., bones of vault of skull)

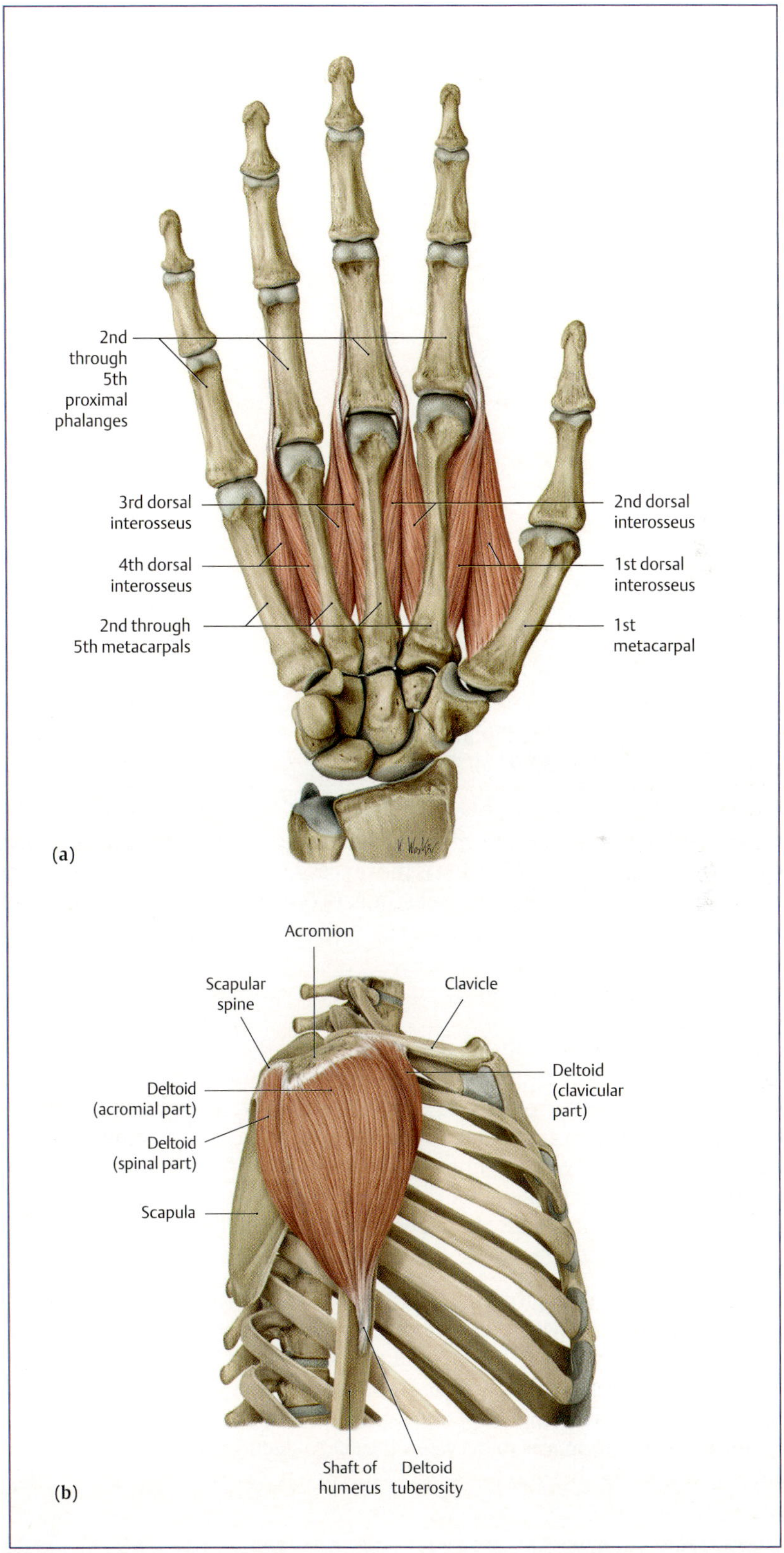

Fig. 9 **(a)** Bipennate muscle (e.g., dorsal interossei.). **(b)** Multipennate muscle (e.g., deltoid).

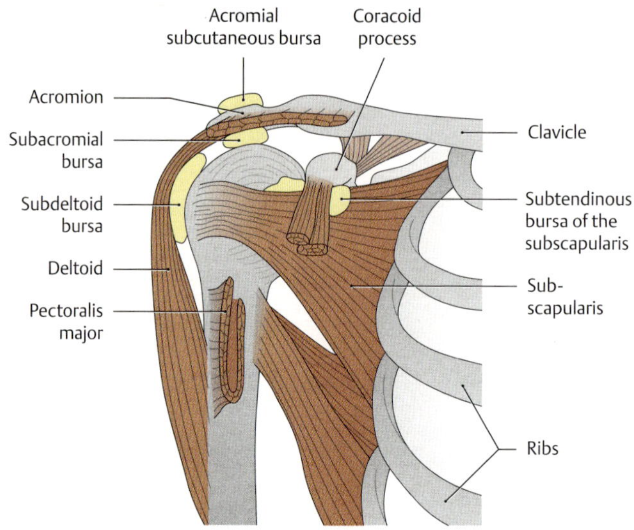

Fig. 10 Synovial bursae in the shoulder region.

5. Irregular bones (e.g., vertebrae)
6. Pneumatic bones (e.g., ethmoid and maxilla)
7. Sesamoid bones (e.g., patella and fabella)

Long bones: They are found in limbs (**Fig. 11**). Each has shaft, diaphysis, and two ends, epiphyses.

The shaft usually develops from a primary centre of ossification. The ends develop from the secondary centres (one or more) of ossification. Ossification is the process of laying down of bone. The primary centres appear before birth, that is in prenatal life, and the secondary centres of ossification appear after birth (post-natally). The ossification of the bone can be in either cartilage or a membrane, and accordingly it is called:

1. Endochondral ossification
2. Intramembranous ossification

In endochondral ossification, cartilaginous model is formed and then cartilage is replaced by bone formation. Bone formation is done by osteoblasts. The remodelling by resorption is done by osteoclasts. The growth in length of bone occurs at cartilaginous ends which then calcifies and then replaced by bone. The epiphyseal end of the diaphysis is called metaphysis, the zone of active growth. The growth in diameter of the shaft is done by inner osteogenic layer of the periosteum (outer covering of bone) by proliferation of the cells in this layer. This adds to the outer side, while inner (marrow side) layers of cancellous bone disappear, that is resorption on inner side and deposition on the outer side adds to the girth of the bone.

The bone occurs in two forms:

1. *Compact bone*: It consists of longitudinal laminated tubules with passage of a capillary in the centre. This is Haversian system with the Haversian canal transmitting the capillary. The laminae are concentrically arranged around it. They contain spaces called lacunae. The lacunae contain bone cells osteoblasts/osteocytes. In between the Haversian system, there are interstitial lamellae.
2. *Cancellous bone*: It consists of a lattice of bony spicules. It occurs in flat bones, irregular bone and at the ends of long bones. The spaces in between the bony spicules contain bone marrow which forms blood cells.

Joint

Joint is formed where two bones come together. The joints are classified according to the structure as follows.

1. *Fibrous joints* (**Figs. 12** and **13**): For example, gomphosis, that is the joint between the tooth and socket (alveolar margin of jaw bone). Sutures in between the skull bones also belong to this type. Fibrous joints do not permit movement.

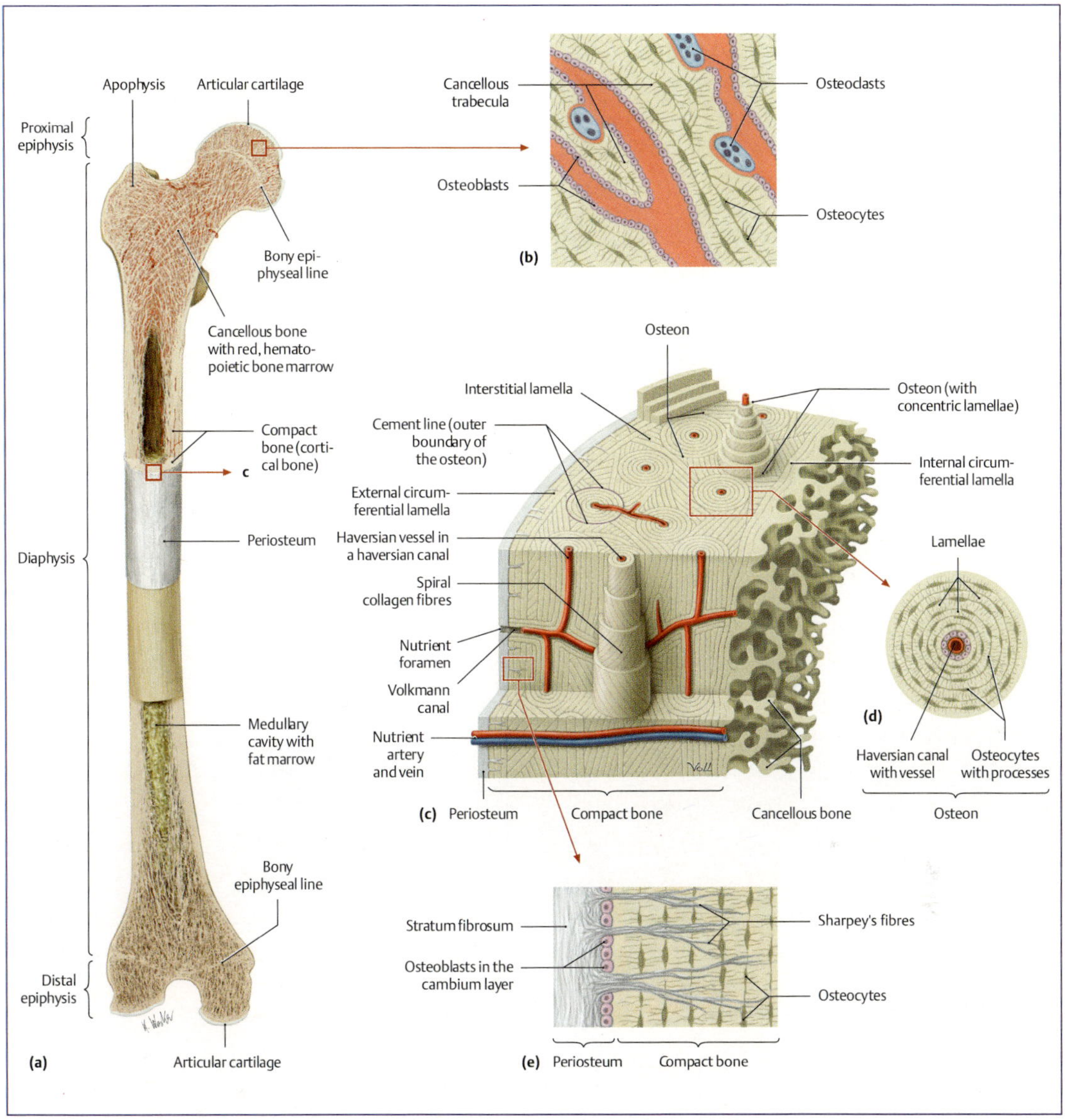

Fig. 11 Structure of a typical tubular bone, illustrated for the femur. **(a)** Coronal saw cuts have been made through the proximal and distal parts of an adult femur (without sectioning the midshaft region). **(b)** Detail from '**a**': The sectioned areas display the lamellar architecture ("lamellar bone") of the cancellous trabeculae. The lamellae are arranged in contiguous plates, similar to plywood. Since the cancellous trabeculae do not have an actual vascular supply and are nourished by diffusion from the adjacent medullary cavity, the trabeculae attain a thickness of only about 200 to 300 µm. **(c)** Detail from '**a**': Three-dimensional representation of compact bone, whose structural units consist of vascularized osteons approximately 1 cm long and 250 to 350 µm in diameter. The Haversian canals, which tend to run longitudinally in the bone, are connected to one another by short transverse and oblique Volkmann canals and also to the vessels of the periosteum and medullary cavity. **(d)** Detail from '**c**', demonstrating the microstructure of an osteon. The Haversian canal at the centre is surrounded by approximately 5–20 concentric lamellar systems composed of osteocytes and extracellular matrix. The osteocytes are interconnected by numerous fine cytoplasmic processes. **(e)** Detail from '**c**', showing the structure of the periosteum.

2. *Cartilaginous joints*: These are further split into the following:
   - *Primary cartilaginous joints* (**Fig. 14**): For example, joint between an epiphysis and the diaphysis of a long bone. In this, the cartilage is transient, that is, it is replaced by bone.
   - *Secondary cartilaginous joints* (**Fig. 15**): For example, pubic symphysis, intervertebral discs, manubriosternal joint, etc. In this, there is fibrocartilage between two bones covered by thin plates of hyaline cartilage. The cartilage remains permanently. These joints are placed in midline.

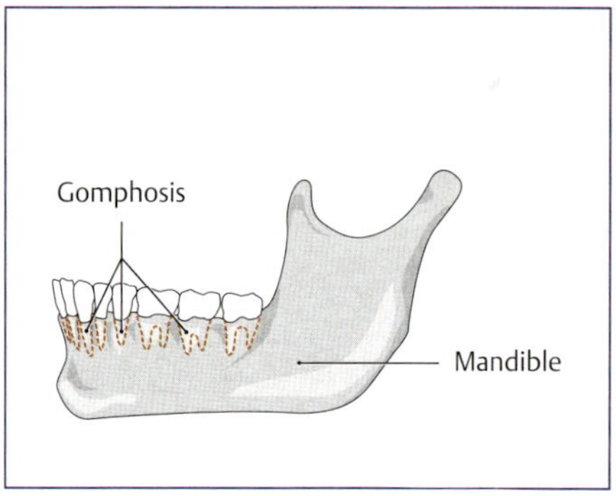

Fig. 12 Gomphosis.

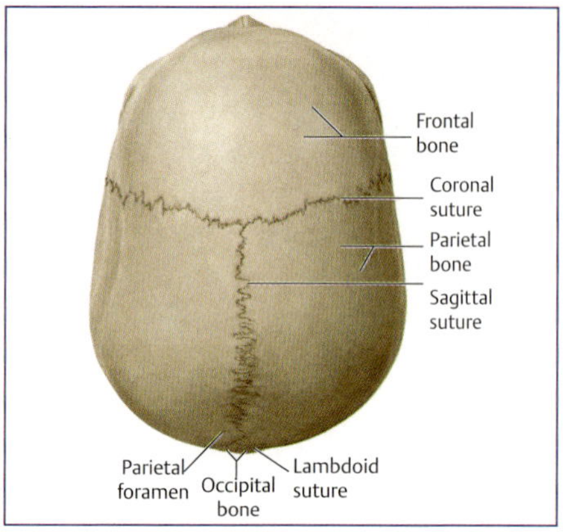

Fig. 13 Sutures.

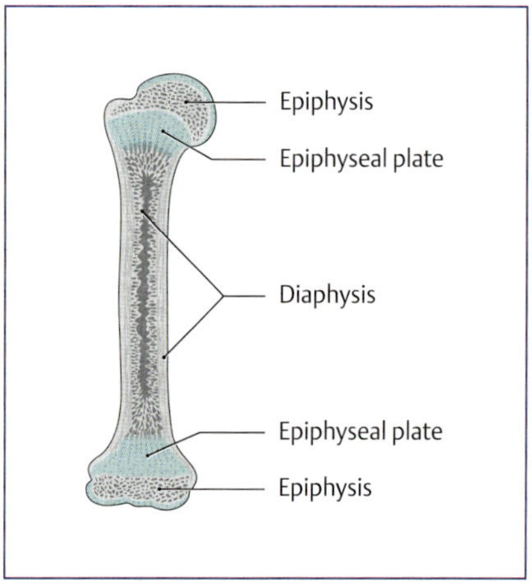

Fig. 14 Epiphyseal plates prior to closure.

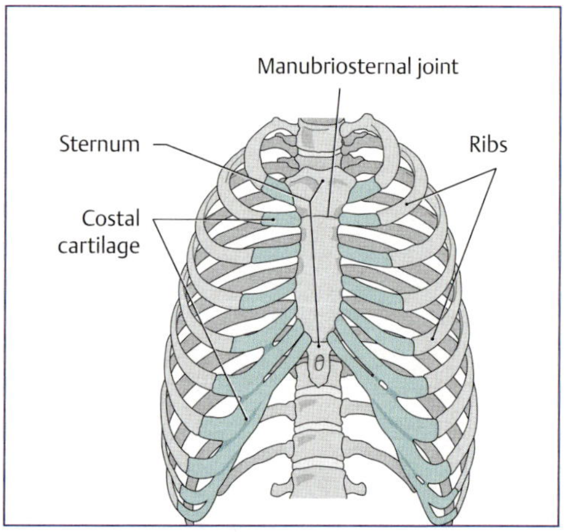

Fig. 15 Costal cartilages and manubriosternal joint.

- *Synovial joints* (**Fig. 16**): These joints permit wide range of movement. In this, the bones participating are covered by articular cartilage and slide on each other. There is a cavity with synovial fluid, and a fibrous capsule covers and holds the ends of the bones meeting at the joint. The capsule is strengthened by these fibrous bands called ligaments.

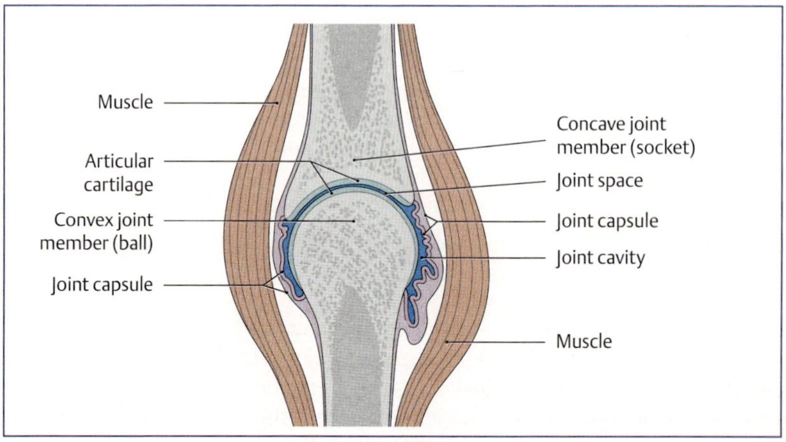

Fig. 16 Structure of a true synovial joint.

The synovial joints are further subclassified into various types:

1. Ball and socket type (**Fig. 17**), for example shoulder joint, hip joint
2. Hinge type (**Fig. 18**), for example elbow joint
3. Condylar type, for example temporomandibular joint
4. Saddle type (**Fig. 19**), for example the first carpometacarpal joint, calcaneocuboid joint
5. Plane type (**Fig. 20**), for example acromioclavicular joint
6. Condyloid type, for example metacarpophalangeal joint
7. Ellipsoid type, for example wrist joint
8. Pivot type (**Fig. 21**), for example superior and inferior radioulnar joints, median atlantoaxial joint

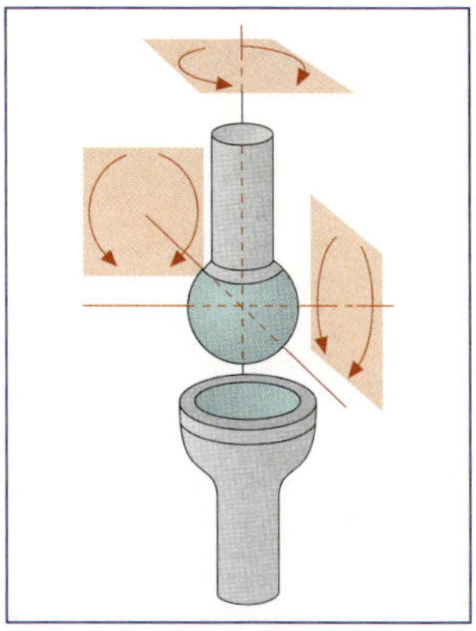

Fig. 17 Spheroidal joint.

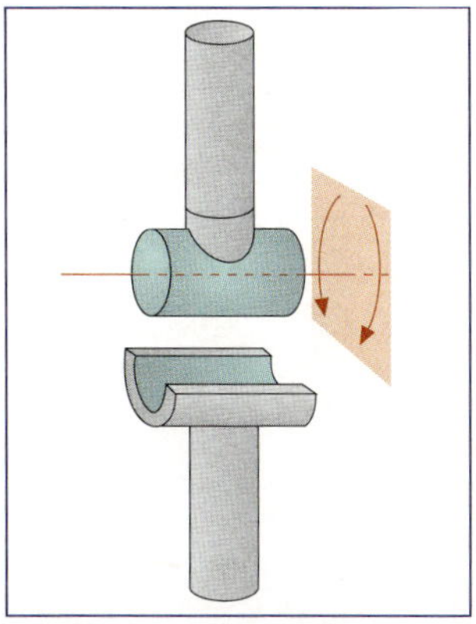

Fig. 18 Hinge joint.

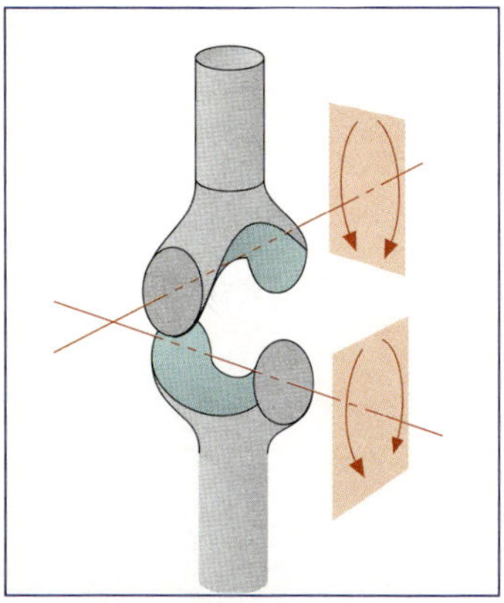

Fig. 19 Saddle joint.

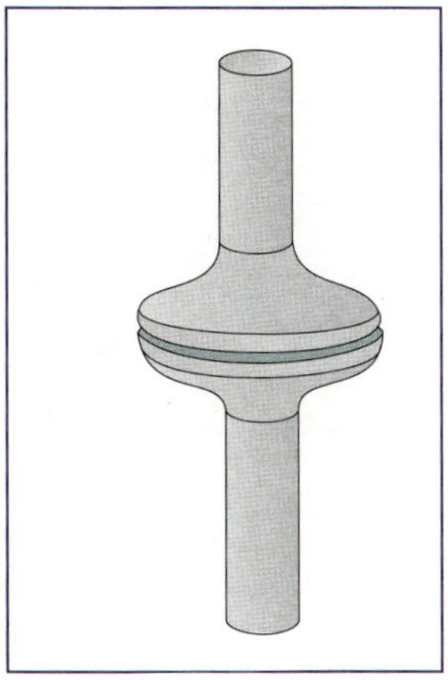

Fig. 20 Plane joint.

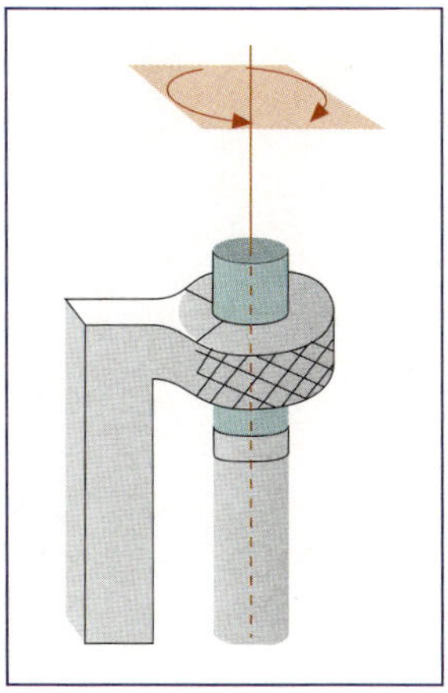

Fig. 21 Pivot joint.

General Instructions for Dissection

1. Daily dissection schedule should be prepared so that the entire exercise is complete in stipulated time.
2. Prepare yourself by reading about the part you are going to dissect. This will help you in identifying the structure that you meet in dissection.
3. Illustrations in a good atlas are a great help in getting visual impression of the structures that you have dissected.

Instruments Required

Among these, the large instruments provided in the dissection room include saws, chisels, hammers, etc. However, the dissector should have the following set of instruments (**Fig. 22**):

1. *Forceps*: Two pairs of forceps are necessary. One pair of serrated-tip forceps is needed for lifting vessels, nerves or other structures while doing blunt dissection. Another pair of toothed forceps essential for firm grip on the structure that one needs while doing dissection.
2. *Probe*: It is helpful in blunt dissection while cleaning various structures, for example, the vessels and nerves.
3. *Scalpel*: It is used for incisions. It should have a detachable blade of about 3 to 4 cm. To do better dissection, a sharp blade is necessary, because dull scalpel will not yield good results. Scalpel handle should be metallic (not plastic).
4. *Scissors*: They are useful in cutting and even in blunt dissection (for opening the bladder). Two pairs of scissors are recommended, one large about 15 cm and another smaller one with sharp points.

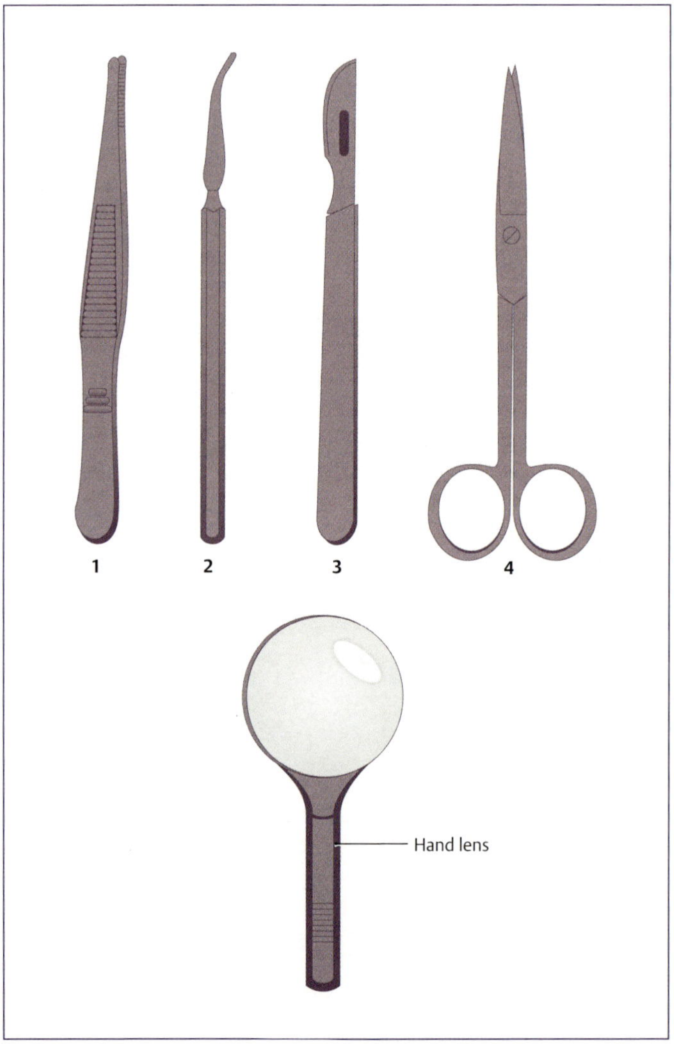

Fig. 22 Instruments required for dissection.

Dissection Technique

This forms the first step in dissection. During the removal of skin, it needs to be separated from the underlying superficial fascia. To separate these, the incisions are made in a series to get skin flaps which can be reposed back to avoid drying of the part. Please remember that the thickness of the skin differs from region to region; for example, on anterior side of the forearm it is thin but relatively thick on the posterior side. Skin removal in the region of the palm and sole poses problem because in these regions it is firmly anchored to the underlying structures. The process of skin removal starts with skin incision. Then using the toothed forceps, it is firmly grasped and separated, starting from the underlying tissues using scalpel (**Fig. 23**).

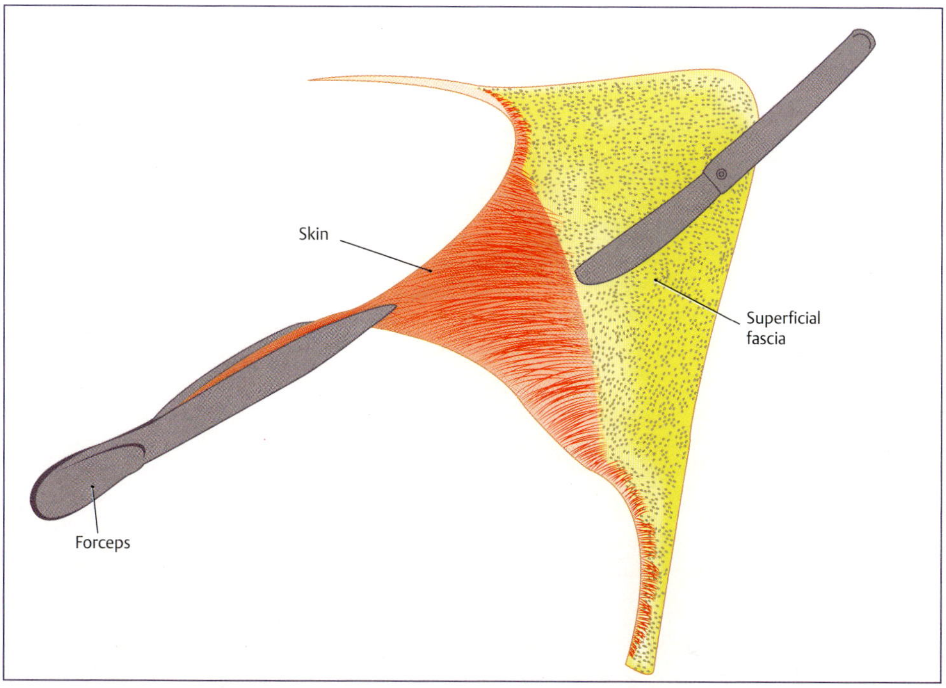

Fig. 23 Process of reflection of skin from the superficial fascia.

Embedded in the superficial fascia, beneath the skin, are the cutaneous nerves and vessels. Note that the distribution of cutaneous nerves is clinically important (to localize segment involved in lesion) and can best be learnt from the illustrations. Among these cutaneous nerves, the larger ones can be identified and traced. The identification of these nerves shall be easy if you remember that they are often accompanied by a small artery and vein. Larger vein in the superficial fascia can be identified easily. They terminate in deeper veins, the junction being provided with valves to ensure flow from superficial to deep vein. If these valves fail to work, it results in varicose veins.

As we approach deep fascia, proceed with its removal. This may be little difficult where the deep fascia sends in septa between the muscles and at the places where the muscle(s) is attached to it. Removal of deep fascia exposes the muscles. Identify each one of the muscles. Note the relation of the muscle to the joint that it crosses. This will help you to understand its action on the joint. Follow the major nerve and the accompanying vessels. Trace their branches to know their area of distribution.

During the dissection, a keen observer can note the variations in size, shape, extent, course, branching pattern of nerves and vessels. Note them carefully. These variations are little different from the congenital anomalies, commonly called birth defects. They refer to the developmental error and are present at birth. The anomaly may be severe, leading to death, or it may be minor and compatible with life. This can be observed in the dissecting room.

Before you start dissecting, remember that dissection is only a means to have further understanding of the function. This will form the basis to understand the disease process and subsequently help in management and treatment of the disease in an effective manner.

CHAPTER 1

Osteology of the Upper Limb

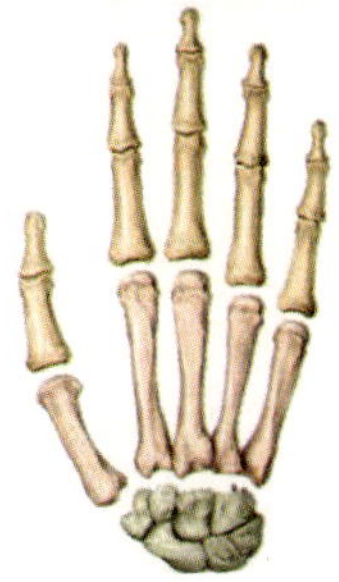

Learning Objectives

After reading this chapter, students should be able to identify the following:

- Bones in anatomical position.
- Muscular and ligamentous attachments.
- Important relations like nerves (e.g., ulnar nerve, axillary nerve, radial nerve) related to humerus.
- Anatomical aspect of applied anatomy (e.g., fractures involving bones like surgical neck of humerus).

Introduction

The bones of the pectoral girdle and upper limb form the superior appendicular skeleton. It articulates with the axial skeleton only at a small sternoclavicular joint, thus permitting greater range of mobility.

Bones of the Pectoral Girdle

Bones of the pectoral girdle are clavicle and scapula.

Clavicle (Collar Bone)

The clavicle is sinuously curved in the horizontal plane (**Fig. 1.1**). Its medial two-thirds is convex anteriorly while the lateral one-third is concave anteriorly. It has an enlarged triangular *sternal end* that articulates with the manubrium at the sternoclavicular joint. Its lateral flat *acromial end* articulates with the acromion of the scapula at the acromioclavicular joint. It serves as a strut (rigid support), suspending the free upper limb away from the trunk with freedom of motion.

Inferior Surface

The inferior surface is rough at the *sternal end* for the attachment of the costoclavicular ligament. In the middle third, it presents the *subclavian groove* that gives attachment to the subclavius muscle. The lips of the groove give attachment to the *clavipectoral fascia*. At the acromial end, it presents the *conoid tubercle*, extending obliquely forwards from it is the *trapezoid line*, which gives attachment to the conoid and trapezoid parts of the coracoclavicular ligament, respectively.

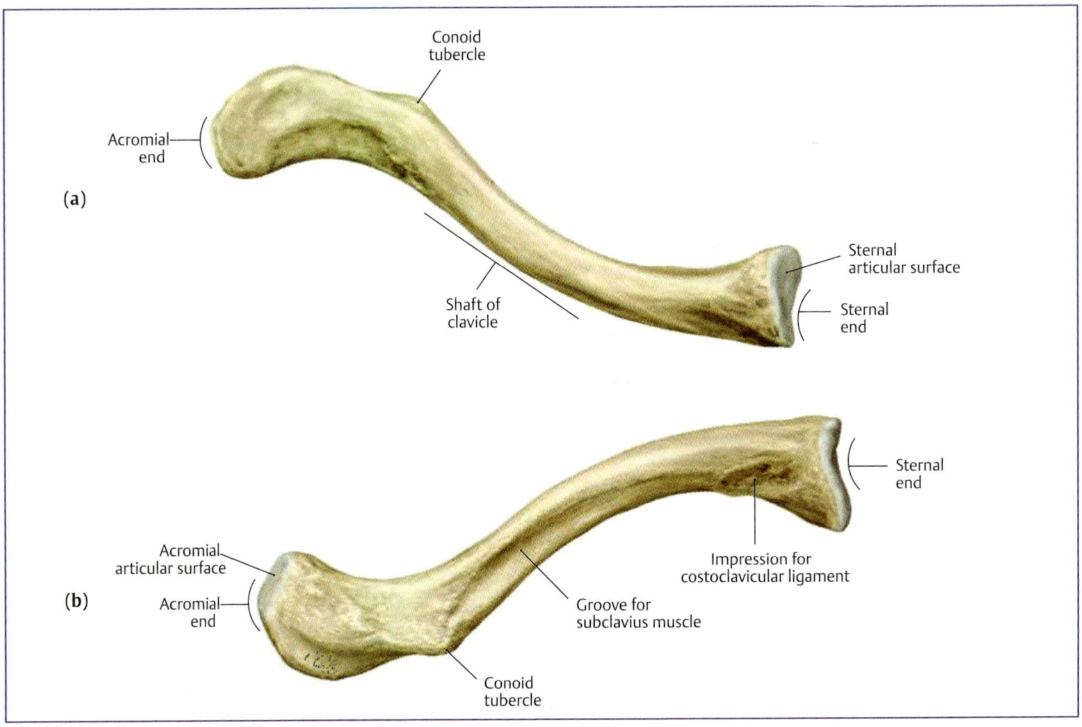

Fig. 1.1 Clavicle: **(a)** Superior view and **(b)** inferior view.

Superior Surface

The superior surface is smooth and featureless and lies just deep to the skin and platysma.

Scapula

The scapula is a flat triangular bone, lying along the posterolateral aspect of the thorax (**Fig. 1.2**). It rests on the second to the seventh rib. Its posterior surface is convex and presents the *spine of the scapula* with the *supraspinous fossa* above and *infraspinous fossa* below. Its anterior surface/costal surface is concave and forms the large *subscapular fossa*. The spine of the scapula is continuous and presents itself as a flat, expanded *acromion process*. The flat triangular body presents *three angles* and *three borders*. The three angles are superior, inferior and lateral. The *lateral angle* is truncated forming the shallow *glenoid cavity* that articulates with the head of the humerus forming the shoulder joint. The three borders of the scapula are *medial (vertebral)*, *lateral (axillary)* and *superior borders*. The superior border presents the *suprascapular notch*.

Coracoid process: It is a beak-like process projecting forward and provides attachment to an important coracoclavicular ligament. It forms an example of the *atavistic epiphysis*.

Bone of the Brachium or Arm

Humerus

Humerus is a bone of the *brachium* or *arm* (**Fig. 1.3**).

1. *Upper end*: At its upper end, the humerus presents the *head* that articulates with the glenoid cavity of the scapula at the shoulder joint. The articular surface is less than a hemisphere; close to it is the groove that marks the *anatomical neck*. The upper end has a *greater tubercle* and a *lesser tubercle* with *intertubercular sulcus (bicipital groove)* between them.
2. *Surgical neck*: It is narrowing at the upper end, about 1 cm zone running circumferentially around the bone between the muscular attachments of the subscapularis and teres major muscles. The surgical neck is related to the *axillary nerve* and *posterior circumflex humeral artery*.

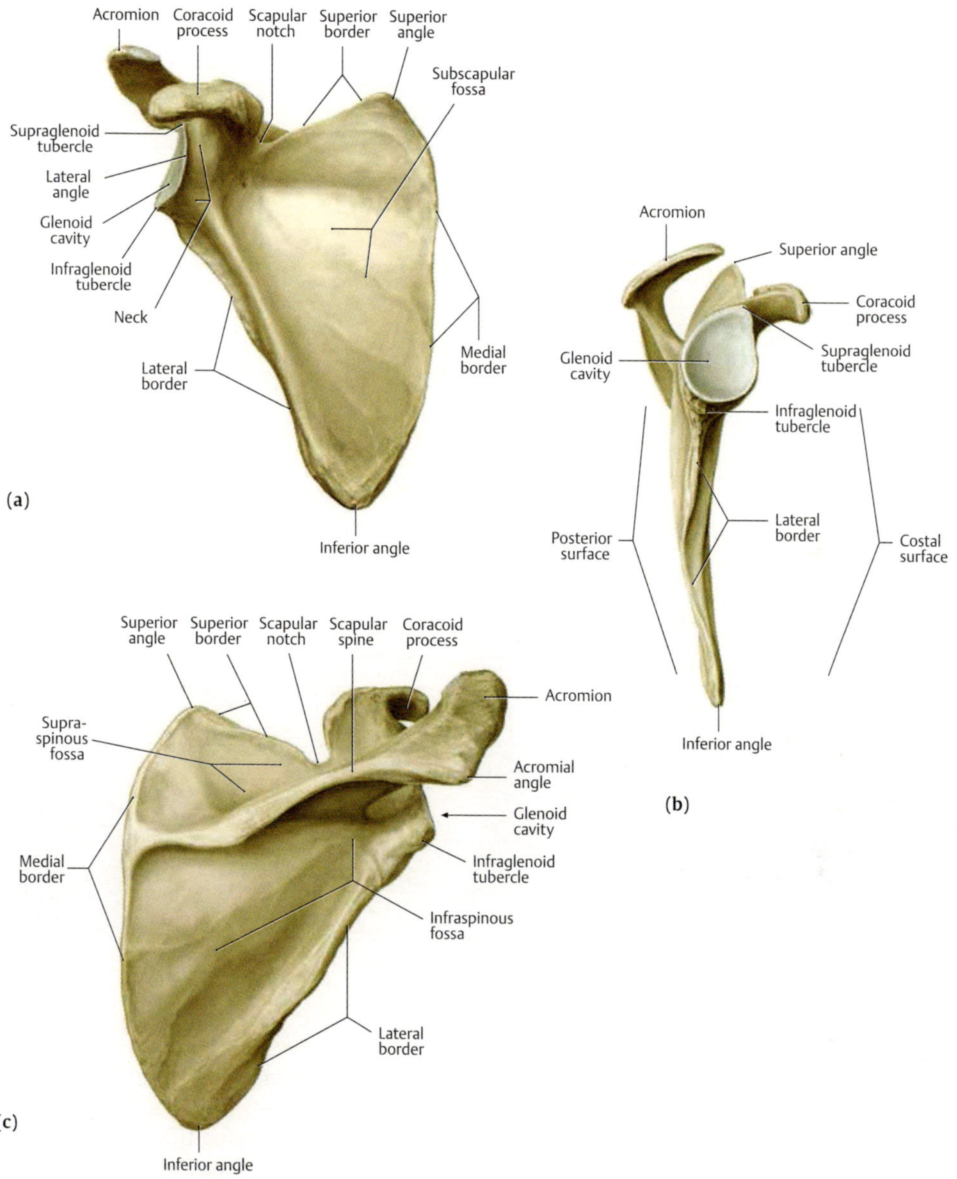

Fig. 1.2 Scapula (right): **(a)** Anterior view, **(b)** right lateral view and **(c)** posterior view.

3. *Spiral/radial groove* runs spirally across the back of the bone and is related to the *radial nerve* and *profunda brachii artery*.
4. *Lower end* of the bone presents the *lateral* and more prominent *medial epicondyles* with *lateral* and *medial supracondylar ridges* running upwards, respectively. In addition, at the lower end there is *capitulum*, rounded structure with articular surface engaged by the radial head. Medial to it is the *trochlea* (pulley shaped) with medial flange projecting lower down. Trochlea articulates with the trochlear notch of the ulna. On the anterior surface above the trochlea is the *coronoid fossa* and above the capitulum is the *radial fossa*. On the posterior surface at the lower end is the deep *olecranon fossa*, occupied by the olecranon. In the extended elbow, behind the *medial epicondyle*, ulnar nerve is palpated.

Bones of the Forearm or Antebrachium

Bones of the forearm are the radius and ulna. They are parallel to each other in the supinated forearm. The radius lies laterally and the ulna medially.

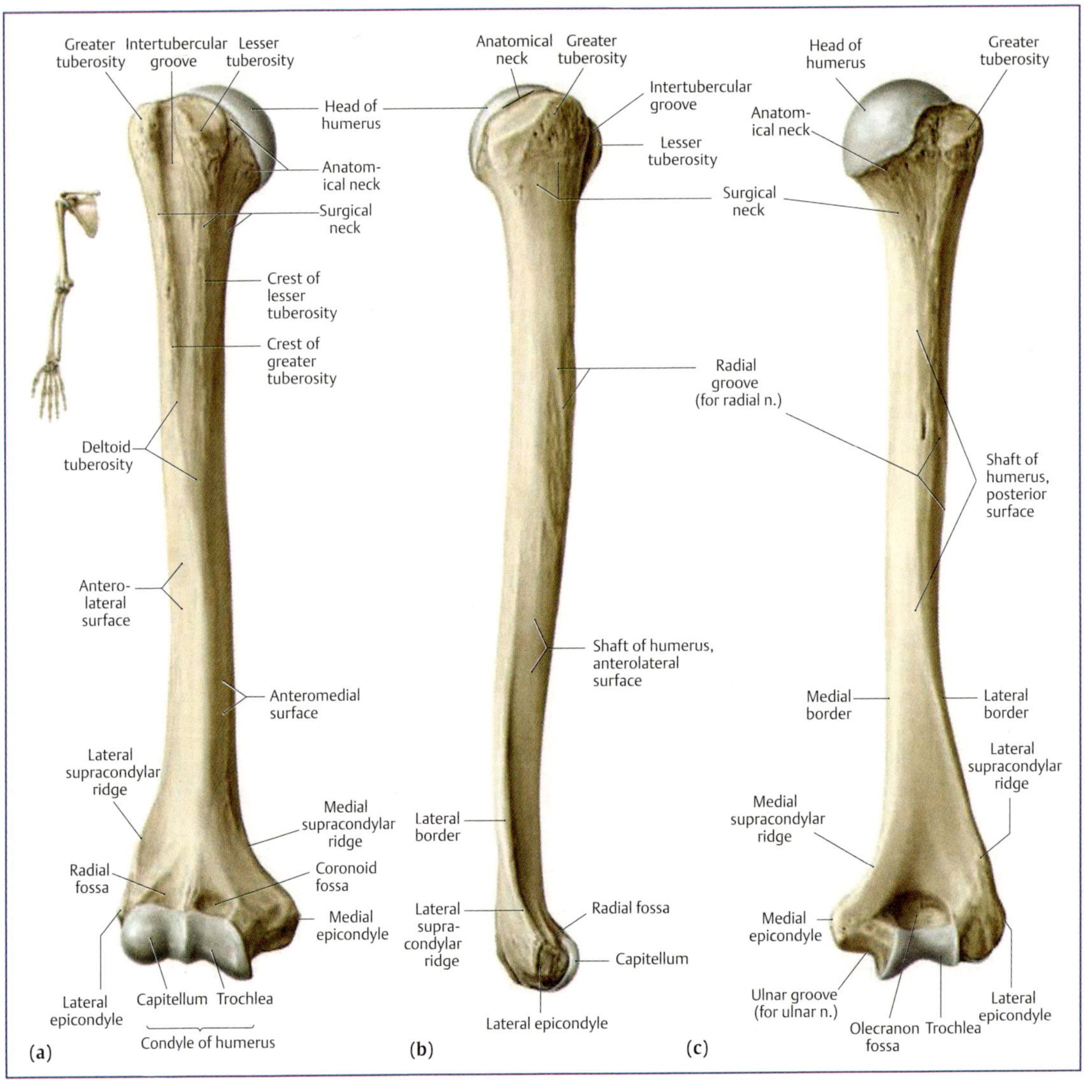

Fig. 1.3 Humerus (right): **(a)** Anterior view, **(b)** lateral view and **(c)** posterior view.

Radius (Fig. 1.4)

Upper end: It has a *discoid head* at the *upper end*. Its upper concave surface articulates with the capitulum of the humerus at the elbow joint. The rim of the discoid head articulates with the radial notch of the ulna at the superior radioulnar joint, a pivot type. *Radial tuberosity* projects from the medial side and offers attachment to the biceps brachii tendon.

The shaft of the radius is convex laterally, presenting a rough impression for attachment of the pronator teres.

Lower end: It is broad and presents a projection called the *styloid process* that projects lower down. The lower articular surface articulates with the scaphoid and lunate, the carpal bones, *forming the radiocarpal joint (wrist joint). The lower end has an additional triangular surface.* It also has an articular strip for the head of the ulna where it forms the inferior radioulnar joint. The dorsal aspect of the lower end has a *dorsal tubercle (Lister's tubercle)* with grooves for extensor tendons.

Ulna (Fig. 1.4)

Upper end: The ulna has an expanded upper end with beak-like *olecranon process*, shelf-like *coronoid process* projecting forward. Together they form the *trochlear notch* that articulates with the trochlea of the humerus at the *elbow joint*. Lateral aspect of the coronoid presents the *radial notch* forming the *superior radioulnar joint* with the head of the radius.

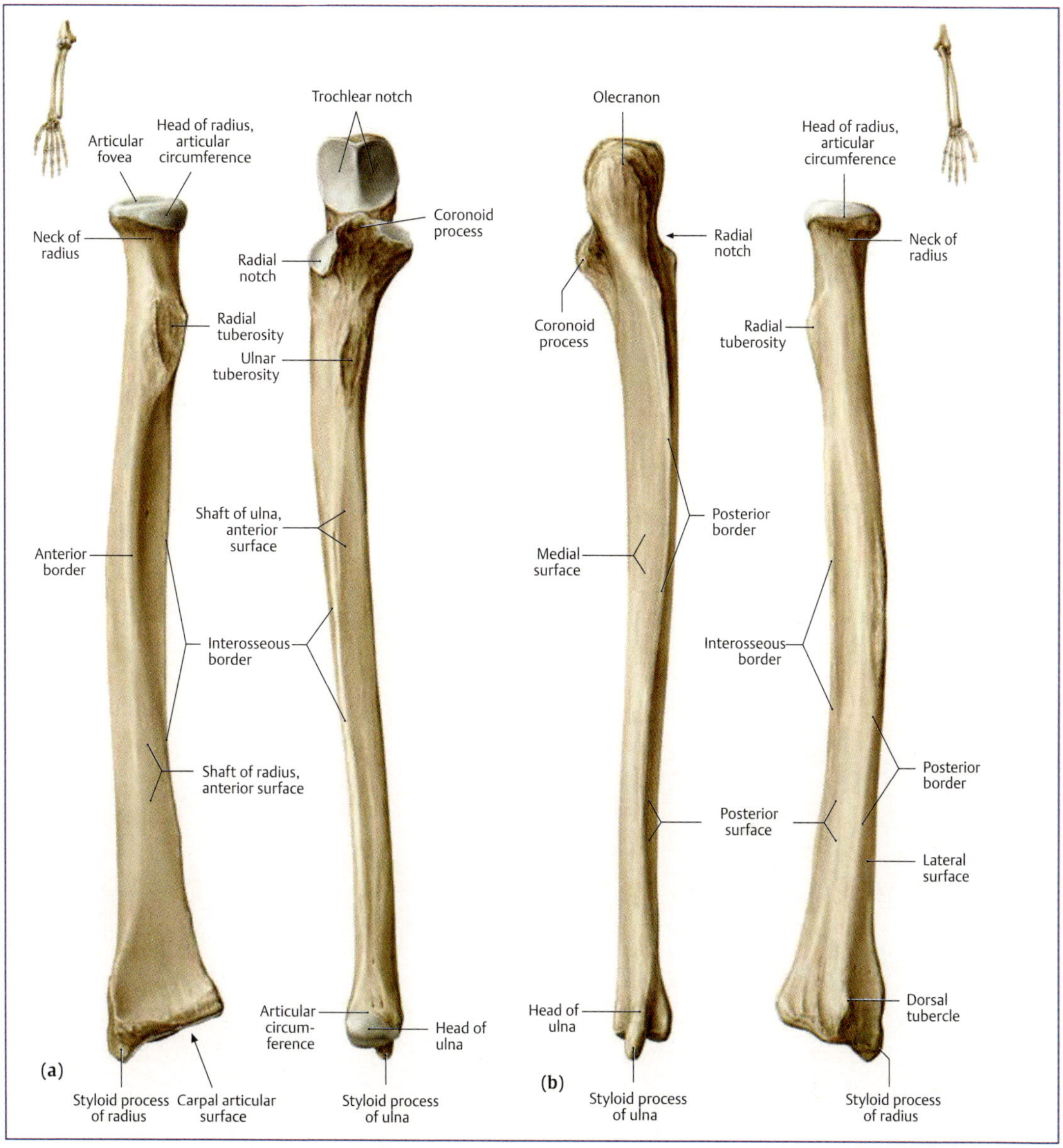

Fig. 1.4 Radius and ulna: **(a)** Anterior view and **(b)** posterior view.

The shaft presents a sharp *interosseous border* laterally giving attachment to the interosseous membrane. Inferior to the coronoid process is a roughened area called the *tuberosity of the ulna* with attachment of the brachialis muscle. *Supinator crest* is a prominent ridge below the radial notch on the lateral surface of the shaft of the ulna, meant for attachment of the supinator muscle.

Lower end: *The lower end* of the ulna has a small disc-like head with a small conical projection called the *styloid process of the ulna.*

Bones of the Wrist and Hand

The bones of the wrist and hand comprise carpal bones, metacarpals and phalanges (**Fig. 1.5**).

Carpal Bones

The carpal bones are eight in number and are arranged in two rows, proximal and distal (**Figs. 1.5** and **1.6**). They articulate with each other in such a way that the carpus is convex posteriorly from side to side and concave anteriorly. The anterior concavity provides room for nerves and vessels entering through the carpal tunnel.

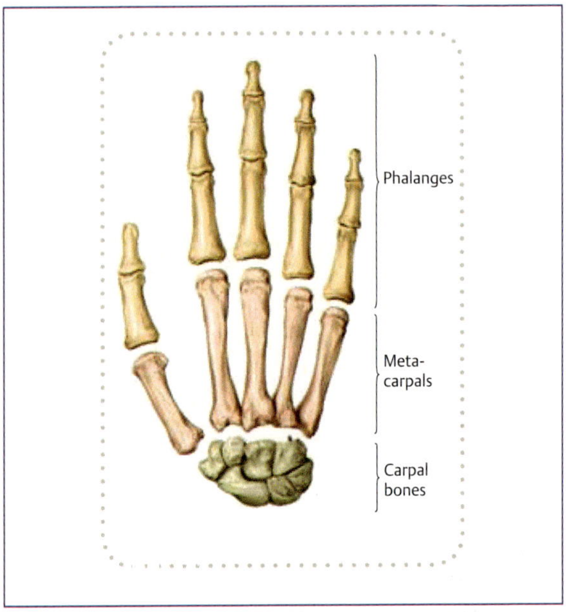

Fig. 1.5 Overview of the bones of the wrist and hand.

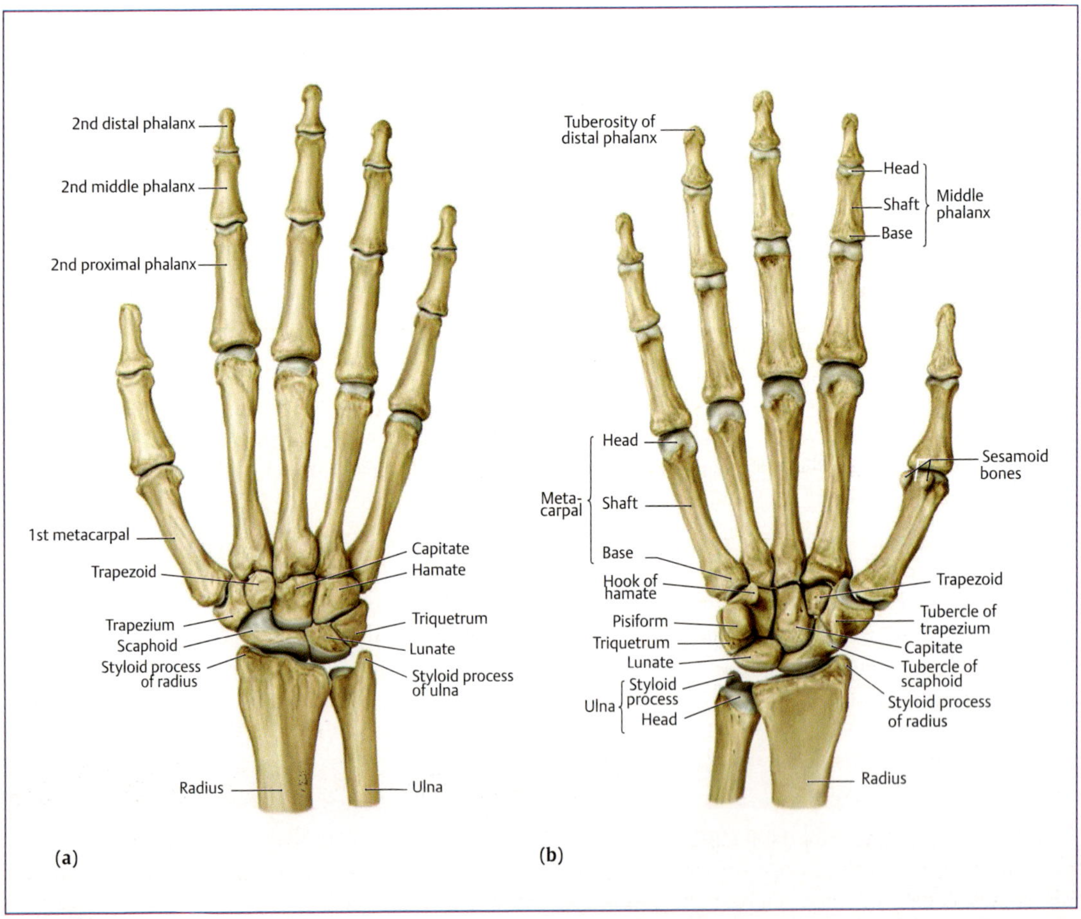

Fig. 1.6 Bones of the wrist and hand. **(a)** Dorsal view and **(b)** palmar view.

Bones of the Proximal Row from the Lateral to the Medial Side

Scaphoid (Boat Shaped)

The scaphoid has a prominent tubercle and a narrow waist making it vulnerable to fractures. It articulates with the radius proximally.

Lunate (Moon Shaped)

The lunate lies between the scaphoid and triquetrum. It articulates proximally with the radius. It has a broader anterior surface than the posterior, making it vulnerable to dislocation.

Triquetrum (Three-Cornered Bone)

The triquetrum is pyramidal in shape. Proximally, it articulates with the triangular articular disc.

Pisiform

The pisiform is a pea-like, small bone on the palmar surface of the triquetrum. It is regarded as the sesamoid bone in the tendon of the flexor carpi ulnaris muscle by some researchers.

Bones of the Distal Row from the Lateral to the Medial Side

Trapezium (Trapeze Table)

The trapezium has a crest and a groove on the palmar aspect. It articulates with the first and second metacarpals and the two carpals, the scaphoid and trapezoid.

Trapezoid

The trapezoid is a wedge-shaped bone. It articulates with the base of the second metacarpal and the three carpals, that is, the trapezium, capitate and scaphoid.

Capitate (Caput Head)

The capitate is the largest among the carpal bones. Distally, it articulates with the bases of the second, third and fourth metacarpals; proximally with the scaphoid and lunate; laterally with the trapezoid and medially with the hamate.

Hamate

The hamate is a wedge-shaped bone with a hook. Distally, it articulates with the fourth and fifth metacarpals.

Metacarpals

The skeleton of the palm of the hand is formed by five bones, numbered from the lateral to the medial side as first to fifth metacarpal bones. Each metacarpal has a base, shaft and head. Their bases articulate with the carpal bones and the heads of the metacarpals articulate with the proximal phalanges forming the knuckles. The first metacarpal is the shortest among them (regarded as the modified phalanx with basal epiphysis). The second metacarpal has a grooved base. The third metacarpal has a remarkable feature of styloid process on lateral side of its base.

Phalanges

Each digit has three phalanges: proximal, middle and distal, except the first (thumb) which has only two phalanges. Each phalanx has a base proximally, a shaft and a distal head.

CHAPTER 2

Pectoral Region and Axilla

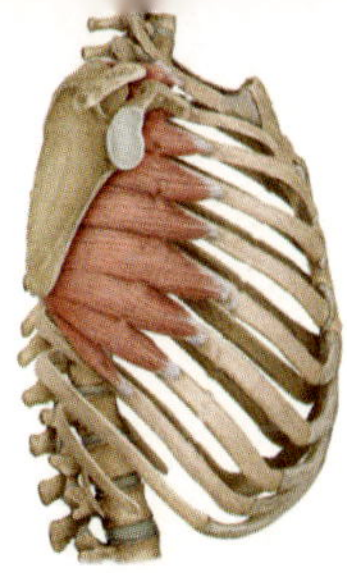

Learning Objectives

At the end of the dissection of the pectoral region and axilla, students should be able to identify the following:

- *Nerves*: Supraclavicular nerves, medial and lateral pectoral nerves, long thoracic nerve and branches of the intercostal nerves.
- *Vessels*: Branches of the internal thoracic artery, *thoracoacromial artery and its branches, superior thoracic artery* and *cephalic vein.*
- *Muscles*: Pectoralis major, pectoralis minor, subclavius and serratus anterior.
- The anatomical basis of the clinical signs and conditions (e.g., Peau d'orange skin in carcinoma of the breast and policeman's tip position of the upper limb in Erb's palsy).

Introduction

The upper limb is adapted to great freedom of movement in order to perform skillful/prehensile acts. Its importance is duly reflected by the sizeable area of representation it occupies in the cerebral cortex. The upper limb for the purpose of dissection is divisible into the following:

Shoulder region: It includes the axilla or armpit, scapular region and pectoral region.

Arm (brachium): The part between the shoulder and elbow, with humerus as its bone.

Forearm (antebrachium): It extends from the elbow to the wrist. It has two bones, the radius and ulna. Distally, they articulate with the carpal bones to form the wrist joint. The forearm bones articulate at the superior, middle and inferior radioulnar joints. The movements of pronation and supination occur at these joints.

Hand (manus): It consists of the wrist/carpus, metacarpus and digits (fingers and thumbs). The forearm bones, radius and ulna, articulate with the carpal bones. The carpals distally articulate with the metacarpals and the metacarpals articulate with the phalanges. The hand presents ball of the thumb, thenar eminence and ball of the little finger, that is, the hypothenar eminence.

The upper limb is attached to the thorax by muscles which form the *anterior* and *posterior axillary folds*. When the upper limb is moved away, the axilla (pyramidal shape) or armpit becomes evident.

The pectoral region covers the anterior thoracic wall presenting mammary glands. In females, breasts or mammary glands are well developed, while in males, they are rudimentary.

Surface Landmarks

1. *Clavicle*: It is the collar bone. It is subcutaneous and palpable throughout its length. It is concave along the lateral one-third and convex along the medial two-thirds for vessels and nerves to pass between the axilla and root of neck. It articulates with the manubrium at the sternoclavicular joint and laterally with the acromion of the scapula at the acromioclavicular joint (**Fig. 2.1**).
2. *Acromion* (Acron: summit; omos: shoulder): It can be felt as a flat subcutaneous bone on the top of the shoulder.
3. *Acromioclavicular joint*: A plane synovial joint is felt as a slight depression between the lateral end of the clavicle and acromion.
4. *Jugular notch*: It lies between the medial ends of the clavicle along the superior margin of the manubrium.
5. *Sternal angle*: It can be felt as a transverse ridge at the junction of the manubrium with the body of the sternum. It lies at the level of the second costal cartilage. Other ribs are counted downwards from the second.

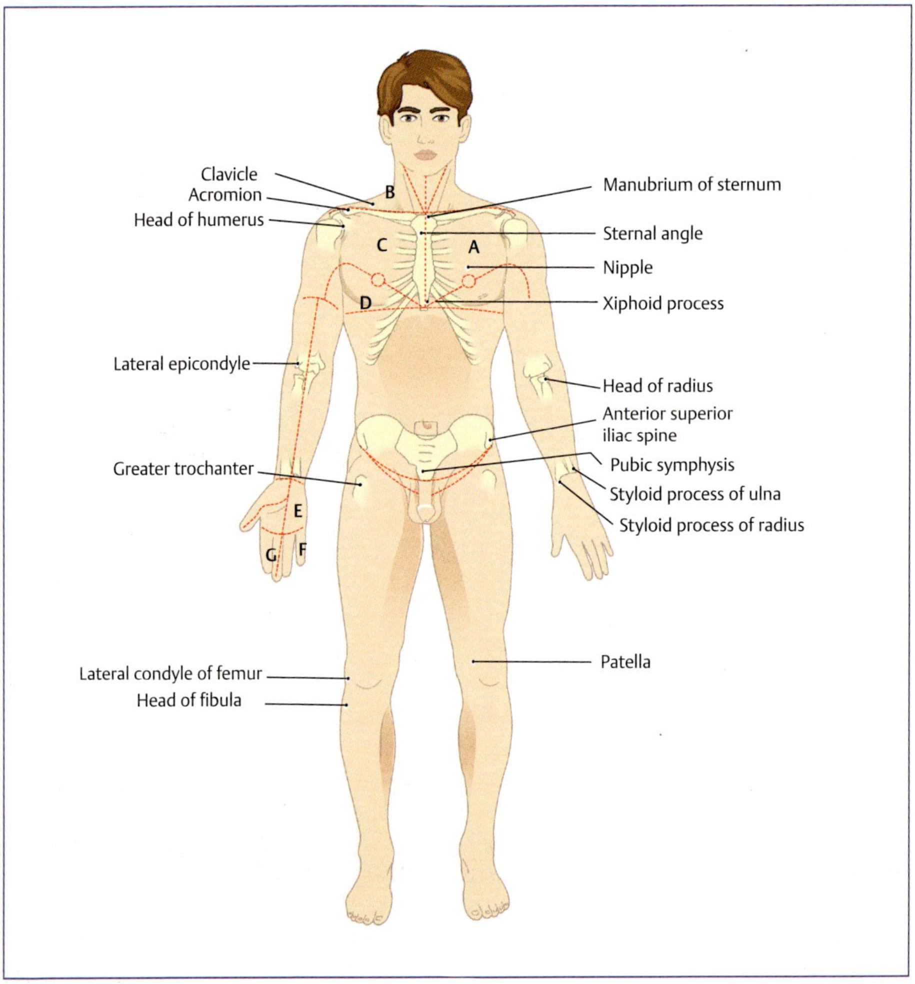

Fig. 2.1 Surface landmarks and incisions.

6. *Xiphoid process*: It is the lower part of the sternum lying in the epigastric fossa between the cartilages of the seventh ribs.
7. *Nipple*: It is variable in position, usually at the fourth intercostal space slightly medial to the midclavicular line.
8. *Infraclavicular fossa*: It is a depression inferior to the junction of the middle with lateral one-third of the clavicle.
9. *Coracoid process of the scapula*: It can be felt 2 cm below the clavicle just lateral to the infraclavicular fossa, under the muscle fibres of the deltoid.
10. *Axilla* (armpit): It is a hollow pyramidal space between the abducted upper limb and side of the thorax.
11. *Anterior axillary fold*: It is formed by the pectoralis major muscle.
12. *Posterior axillary fold*: It is formed by the latissimus dorsi and teres major muscles.

Dissection and Identification

In the supine position of the cadaver, as shown in **Fig. 2.1**, give the following *skin incisions*:

https://www.winkingskull.com/dissector/V1/video.aspx?vid=73

1. *Incision A*: Along the midline from the jugular notch to the xiphisternum.
2. *Incision B*: From the jugular notch along the clavicle to the acromion; in this, avoid (refrain) cutting through the platysma muscle and supraclavicular nerves.
3. *The platysma* is a thin sheet of muscle present in the superficial fascia of the neck region and helps in facial expressions. The muscle may extend below the clavicle into the superficial fascia of the upper part of the thorax and will be studied in detail with the head and neck regions.
4. *Incision C*: From the xiphisternal junction encircling the nipple and then along the anterior axillary fold to the arm.
5. *Incision D*: Horizontal incision from the xiphisternal junction to the posterior axillary fold.
6. Reflect the skin flaps and the superficial fascia laterally by blunt dissection.
7. While separating the skin flap along the clavicle (incision B), identify the *supraclavicular nerves* by doing blunt dissection through the superficial fascia.
8. While reflecting the skin flap at incision C, close to the anterior axillary fold, identify the *lateral cutaneous branches of the intercostal nerves* emerging serially in a vertical line. Trace their branches anteriorly and posteriorly.
9. The *nipple* and surrounding skin should be left as a landmark.
10. In female cadavers, an attempt can be made to dissect the mammary gland.

Mammary Gland

The mammary gland is a *modified sweat gland* extending vertically between the second and the sixth rib in the midclavicular line and sideways from the lateral border of the sternum to the midaxillary line. It lies within the superficial fascia anterior to the pectoralis major muscle. The pectoral fascia covers the anterior surface of the pectoralis major and is connected to the overlying skin by the *suspensory ligaments of the breast* (*ligaments of Cooper*), which pass between the lobes of the mammary gland (**Fig. 2.2**).

The mammary gland consists of 15 to 20 lobes; each lobe has a *lactiferous duct* which is dilated to form the *lactiferous sinus* at the base of the nipple and opens separately at the apex. *Axillary tail (tail of Spence)* of the gland passes superolaterally into the axilla to the level of the third rib. The gland is surmounted by the *nipple* lying at the level of the fourth intercostal space. It is surrounded by the *areola*, which is pink in colour at young age. In the early stages of pregnancy and shortly thereafter owing to pigmentation, both nipple and areola become dark permanently (**Fig. 2.3**).

Blood Supply

Blood supply to this region occurs by the perforating branches of the *intercostal* and *internal thoracic arteries* medially and the *lateral thoracic artery* laterally (**Fig. 2.4**).

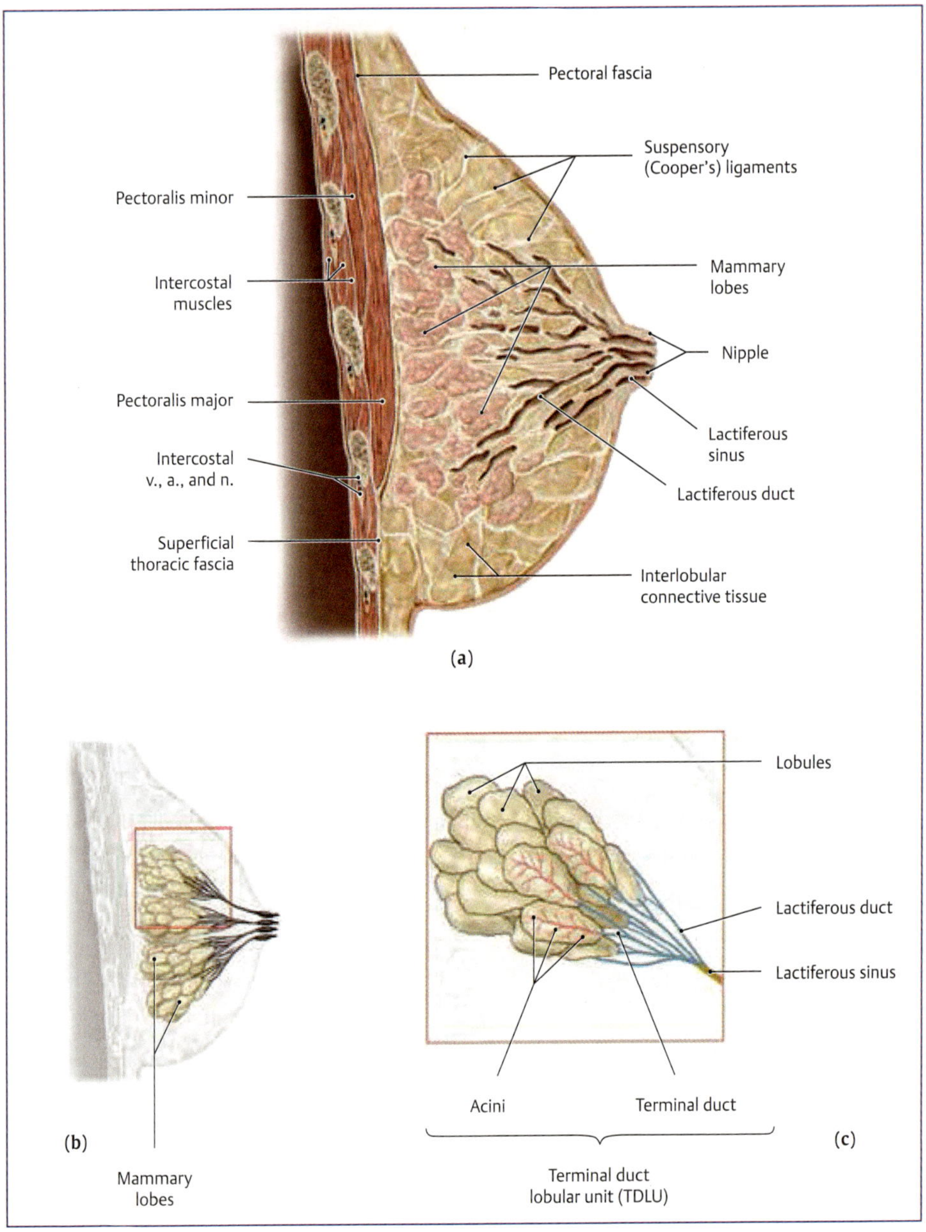

Fig. 2.2 **(a, b, c)** Structures of the mammary gland (breast).

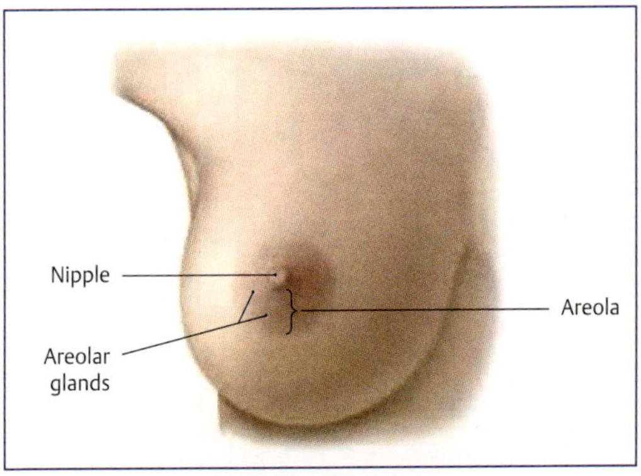

Fig. 2.3 External features of the right breast.

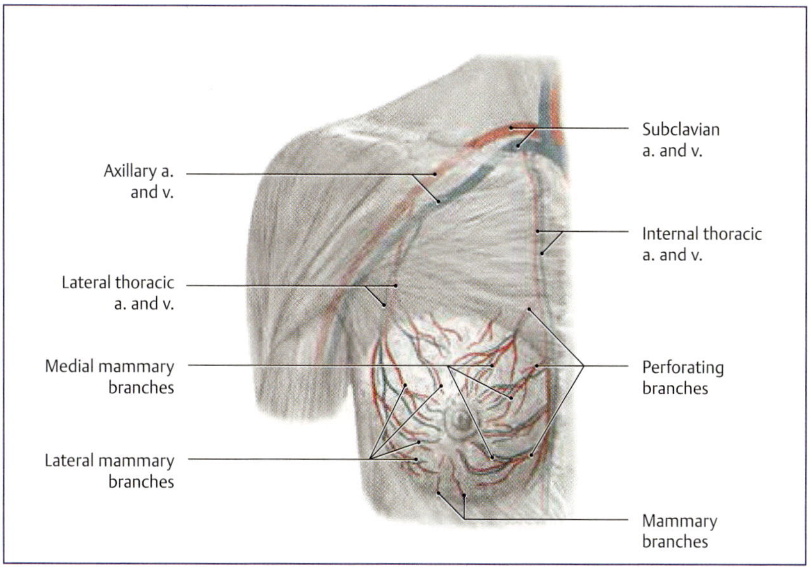

Fig. 2.4 Blood supply of the breast.

Lymphatic Drainage of the Breast

Considering the frequency of occurrence of the carcinoma of the breast in females and its spread through the lymphatics, it is necessary to study the lymphatic drainage of the breast (**Fig. 2.5**).

From the superficial part of the gland, the lymphatics drain into the *subareolar plexus of Sappy*. From the deep part of carcinoma involving the *inferomedial quadrant of the breast*, the malignant cells may pass through the rectus sheath to the umbilicus, then along the ligamentum teres hepatis to the liver and from there the cells fall on the ovary, forming a secondary tumour called the *Krukenberg's tumour*. Lymphatics from the mammary gland pass to the *pectoral lymph nodes* along the axillary tail through the pectoralis major to the apical axillary nodes via *infraclavicular nodes* and to the *parasternal nodes* along the internal thoracic artery of the same as well as the opposite side.

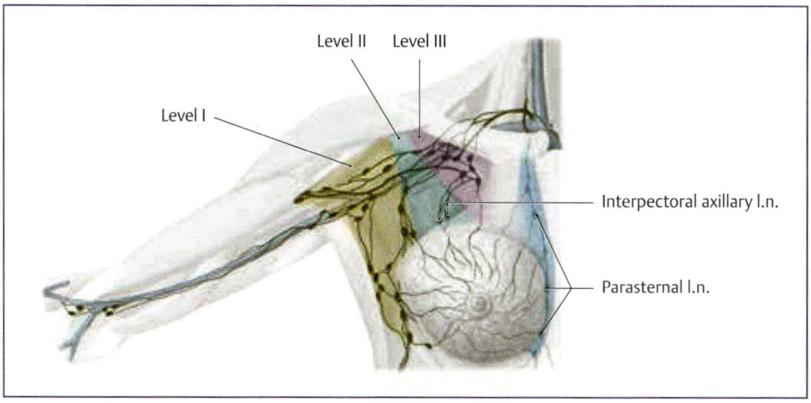

Fig. 2.5 Lymphatic drainage of the breast.

Dissection and Identification

1. Identify the *nipple and areola*.
2. Scoop the fat out by blunt dissection between the *suspensory ligaments of the breast*, where lobes of the functional glandular tissue existed earlier.

3. About *15 to 20 lactiferous ducts*, each arising from a lobe of the gland, converge on the nipple and expand into the *lactiferous sinus* deep to the nipple.
4. Attempt to pass a bristle through one of the ducts of the nipple and try to identify a lobe of the gland. The attempt may not be very successful in elderly females.
5. At the anterior ends of the intercostal spaces deep to the breast, small *neurovascular bundles* exist. Trace the branches of these nerves medially and laterally.

At this stage, it would be pertinent to have short descriptions of the cutaneous nerves, vessels and deep fascia in the region before we explore the deeper structures.

Cutaneous Nerves

Table 2.1 provides an account of the cutaneous nerves, their origin and distribution (**Fig. 2.6**).

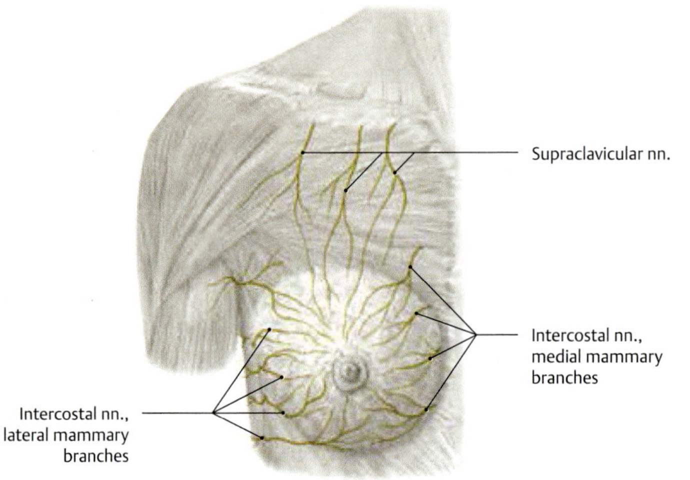

Fig. 2.6 Cutaneous innervation of the breast.

Table 2.1 Cutaneous nerves

Name of nerve	Origin/Source	Distribution
Supraclavicular	Branches from the third and fourth cervical nerves	Piercing the deep fascia in the neck, then crossing over the clavicle to supply the *skin in front of the chest* (up to the second costal cartilage) and *shoulder* They are grouped as *medial, intermediate* and *lateral* as per their placement
Anterior cutaneous branches of the intercostal nerves	Branches from the *intercostal nerves* emerge from the intercostal spaces (except T1 or at times T2)	Piercing the pectoralis major and deep fascia. They supply the *skin, from the anterior midline to the midclavicular line*
Lateral cutaneous branches of the intercostal nerves	Branches from the *intercostal nerves*	They pierce the deep fascia in a vertical line little behind the anterior axillary fold, supplying the overlying strip of the skin

Deep Fascia

The deep fascia covering the pectoralis major (pectoral fascia) blends with the periosteum of the clavicle and sternum, and then passes over the deltopectoral groove to be continuous with the fascia over the deltoid. At the lower border of the pectoralis major, it is continuous along the axillary floor as *axillary fascia*.

Clavipectoral Fascia

It is a strong sheet of fascia, lying deep to the pectoralis major muscle (**Fig. 2.7**). It is attached to the clavicle above and splits to enclose the subclavius and pectoralis minor muscles. Lower down, it continues as a suspensory ligament of the axilla which blends with the *axillary fascia*. Between the subclavius and pectoralis minor, it is pierced by the following structures:

1. Lateral pectoral nerve
2. Thoracoacromial trunk/artery
3. Cephalic vein
4. Lymphatics from the deep part of the breast

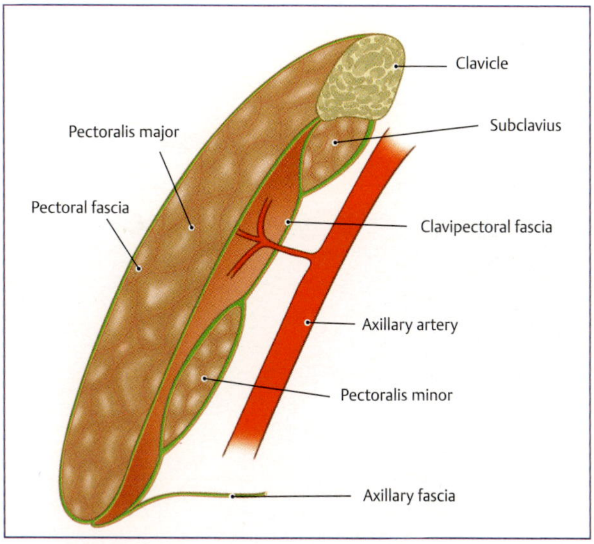

Fig. 2.7 Clavipectoral fascia as seen in oblique section parallel to the axillary artery.

Muscles of the Pectoral Region

Muscles of the pectoral region (**Fig. 2.8**) are described in **Table 2.2**.

Table 2.2 Muscles of the pectoral region

Name of muscle	Origin	Insertion	Nerve supply	Action/Function
Pectoralis major (**Fig. 2.8**)	*Clavicular head*: Anterior surface of the medial half of the clavicle *Sternocostal head:* Anterior surface of the sternum, upper six costal cartilages, aponeurosis of the external oblique muscle	Lateral lip of the intertubercular sulcus of the humerus	Lateral and medial pectoral nerves, clavicular head (C5, C6), sternocostal head (C7, C8 and T1)	1. *Adducts and medially rotates* the humerus; draws the scapula anteriorly and inferiorly 2. Acting alone, the clavicular head *flexes the humerus* and the sternocostal head *extends it* from the flexed position

(continued)

Table 2.2 (*continued*) Muscles of the pectoral region

Name of muscle	Origin	Insertion	Nerve supply	Action/Function
Pectoralis minor (**Fig. 2.9**)	Third to fifth ribs near their costal cartilages	Medial border and superior surface of the coracoid process of the scapula	Medial pectoral nerve (C8, T1)	*Stabilizes the scapula* by drawing it inferiorly and anteriorly against the thoracic wall
Subclavius (**Fig. 2.9**)	Junction of the first rib and its costal cartilage	Inferior surface of the middle third of the clavicle	Nerve to the subclavius (C5, C6)	*Anchors* and *depresses* the clavicle
Serratus anterior (**Fig. 2.10**)	External surface of the upper eight ribs	Anterior surface of the medial border of the scapula	Long thoracic nerve (C5, C6, C7)	*Protracts* the scapula and holds it against the thoracic wall; rotates the scapula

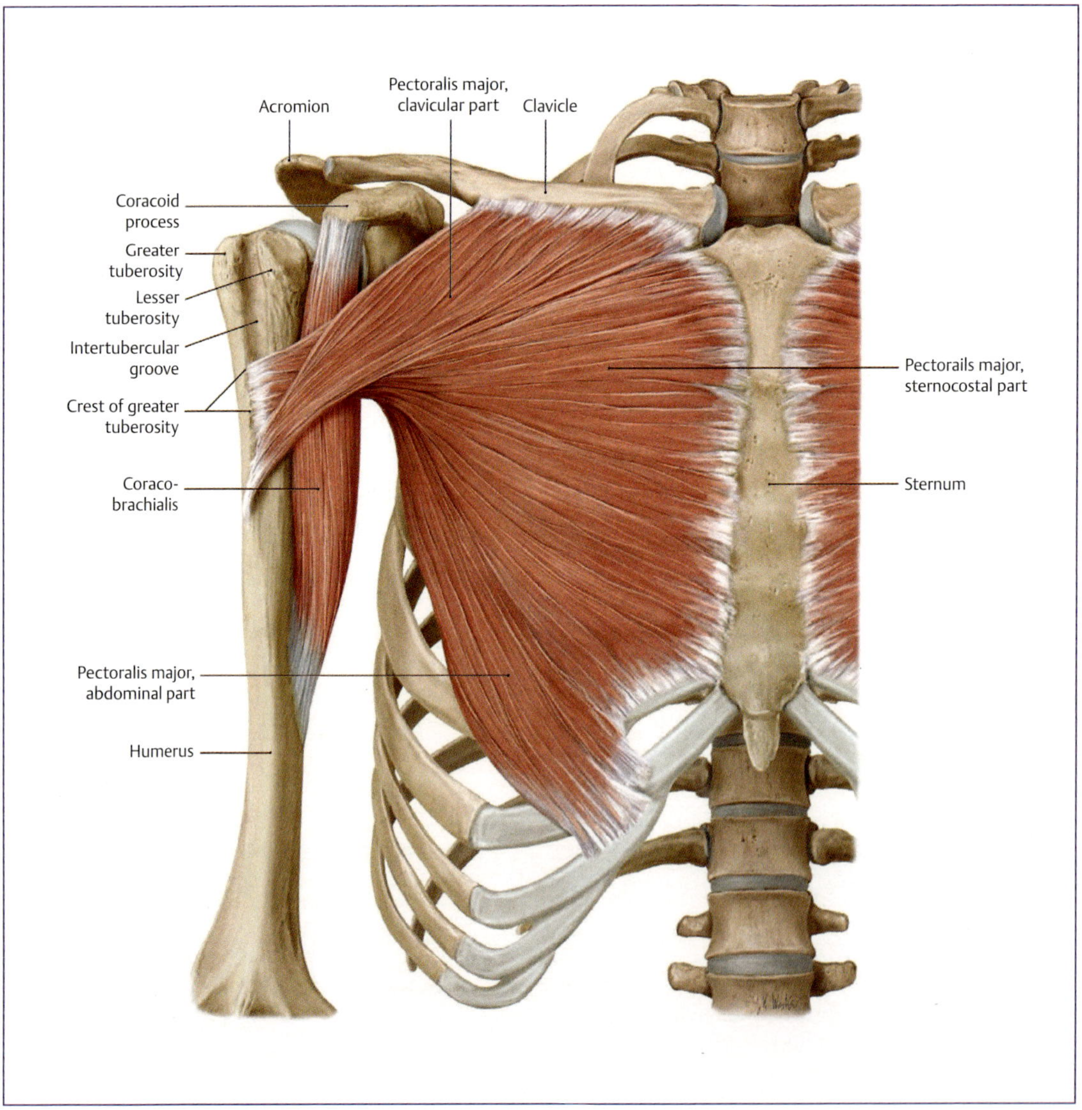

Fig. 2.8 Pectoralis major.

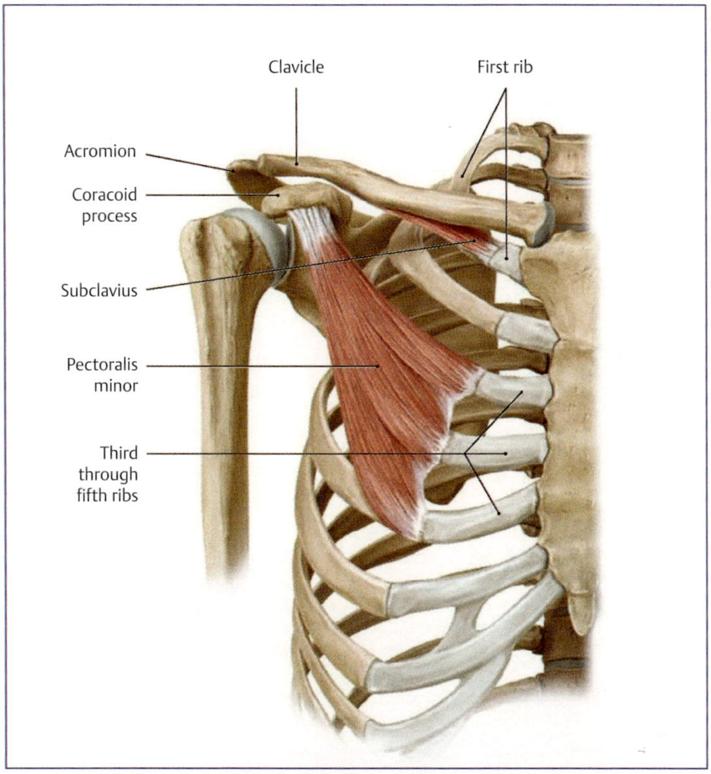

Fig. 2.9 Pectoralis minor and subclavius.

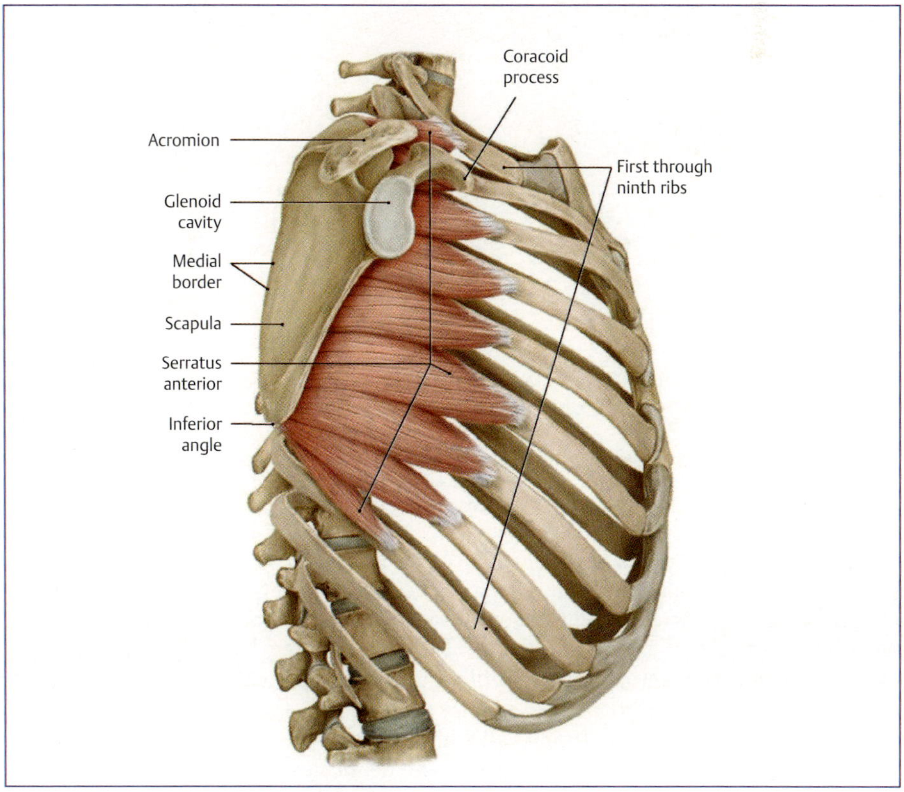

Fig. 2.10 Serratus anterior muscle.

Dissection and Identification

1. Remove the fascia from the anterior surfaces of the pectoralis major and deltoid to define their attachments.
2. Identify the clavicular and sternocostal head of the pectoralis major and trace the muscle up to its insertion on the humerus.
3. Divide the deep fascia by blunt dissection along the *deltopectoral groove* to reveal the *cephalic vein* (**Fig. 2.11**).
4. Identify the *deltopectoral triangle* (**Fig. 2.11**) bounded by the deltoid, pectoralis major and clavicle.

https://www.winkingskull.com/dissector/V1/video.aspx?vid=242

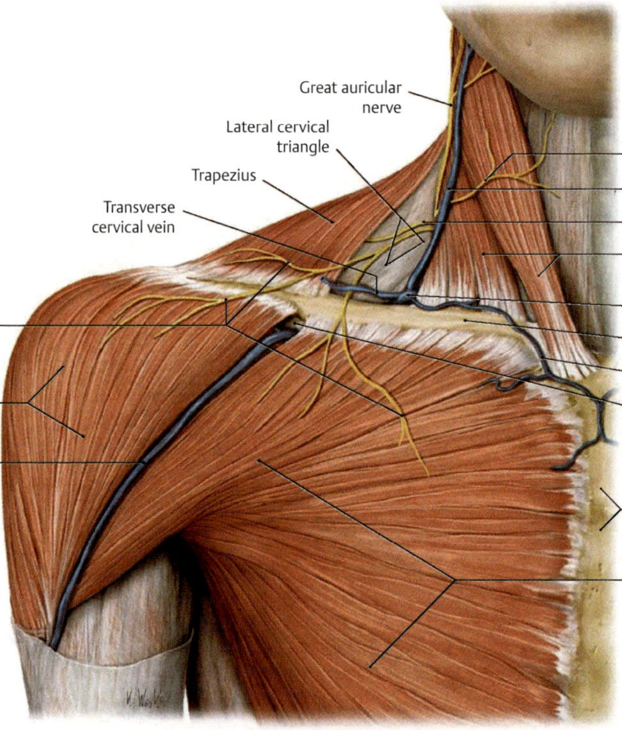

Fig. 2.11 Superficial veins and nerves of the right shoulder region.

5. Cut through the clavicular head of the pectoralis major (**Fig. 2.12**) just below the clavicle and lift it laterally. This exposes the *lateral pectoral nerve* and *thoracoacromial artery* piercing the clavipectoral fascia.

https://www.winkingskull.com/dissector/V1/video.aspx?vid=81

6. Cut through the sternocostal head of the pectoralis major (**Fig. 2.12**) and lift it carefully so that the underlying structures are not damaged. Reflect the cut parts to expose the medial pectoral nerve that pierces the pectoralis minor and then the pectoralis major thus innervating both muscles.
7. Find under the reflected pectoralis major muscle the *clavipectoral fascia, pectoralis minor muscle* and *subclavius muscle.*
8. Trace the *cephalic vein* and *lateral pectoral nerve* through the clavipectoral fascia. Trace the cephalic vein to its termination into the *axillary vein.*
9. Trace the *pectoralis minor muscle* to its attachments.
10. Before you reflect the pectoralis minor, note that it delineates the *three parts of the axillary artery.*
11. Trace the branches of the *thoracoacromial artery.*
12. First, trace the *pectoral branch* which passes downwards and medially between the pectoralis major and minor and supplies them, then trace it proximally and identify the *acromial branch*

which passes upwards and laterally deep to the deltoid, crossing the tip of coracoid process to the acromion.

13. Find out the *clavicular branch* ascending medially to supply the sternoclavicular joint and *deltoid branch* in the deltopectoral groove accompanying the cephalic vein.
14. Trace the lateral thoracic artery, a branch of the second part of the axillary artery, along the lateral border of the pectoralis minor muscle.

https://www.winkingskull.com/dissector/V1/video.aspx?vid=243

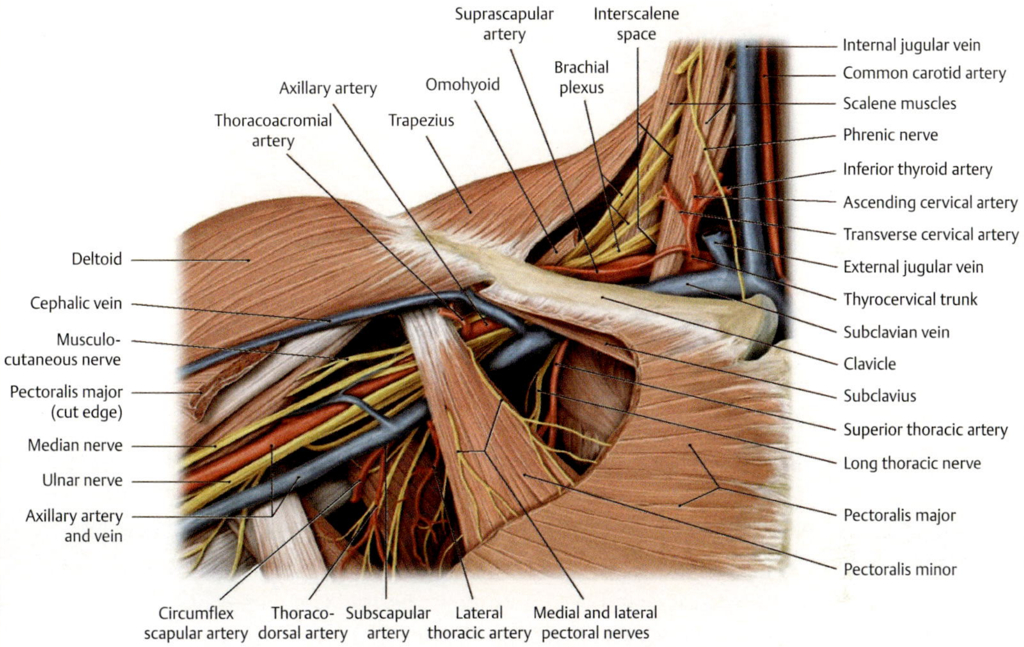

Fig. 2.12 Clavicular and sternocostal heads of pectoralis major muscle are cut to explore the underlying structures.

Axilla

The axilla (armpit) is a pyramidal-shaped space between the upper part of the arm and the lateral thoracic wall.

Boundaries and Contents

Anterior wall: Pectoralis major, pectoralis minor and subclavius with enclosing investing fascia.

Posterior wall: Subscapularis, teres major and latissimus dorsi (below).

Medial wall: Serratus anterior.

Lateral wall: Anterior and posterior walls approximate at the bicipital groove of the humerus.

Apex of the axilla: It is bounded by the clavicle, first rib and superior border of the scapula and is continuous with the root of the neck through which pass the axillary vessels and nerves of the brachial plexus. The contents of axilla include axillary vessels, axillary lymph nodes, nerves of brachial plexus and loose connective tissue (**Fig. 2.13**).

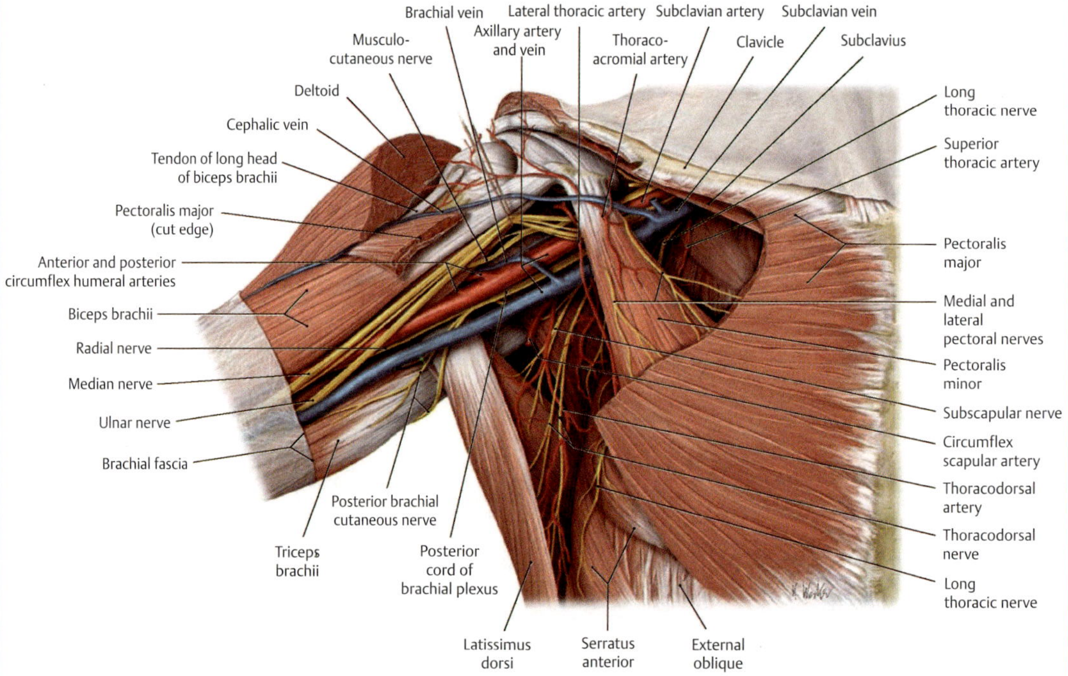

Fig. 2.13 Boundaries and contents of the axilla.

Dissection and Identification

1. Re-identify the previously dissected *pectoralis major, pectoralis minor, clavipectoral fascia*, the *medial and lateral pectoral nerves* and *thoracoacromial artery*.

   https://www.winkingskull.com/dissector/V1/video.aspx?vid=247

2. With the help of fingers, separate the *pectoralis minor* from the underlying thoracic wall.
3. Cut its medial attachments to the thoracic wall; reflect the muscle laterally retaining its attachment to the coracoid process and this exposes the contents of the axilla.
4. *Abduct the arm* to gain better access to the axilla and to appreciate the linear pathway of the brachial plexus into the upper limb.
5. Remove the fat from the axilla to expose *the axillary sheath*.
6. Subsequently, expose the vessels and nerves in the axilla, superior to the pectoralis minor (**Fig. 2.14**).
7. Cut through the anterior layer of the clavipectoral fascia just inferior to the clavicle to expose the *subclavius muscle*.
8. Expose the contents of the axilla by removing the loose connective tissue, fat and lymph nodes.
9. The lymph nodes cannot be seen unless enlarged by disease.
10. Identify the extensive *axillary venous plexus*.
11. Remove the smaller tributaries of the vein in order to get better visualization of the brachial plexus and the axillary artery with its branches.

    https://www.winkingskull.com/dissector/V1/video.aspx?vid=131

12. Trace the branches of all three parts of the axillary artery.

    https://www.winkingskull.com/dissector/V1/video.aspx?vid=246

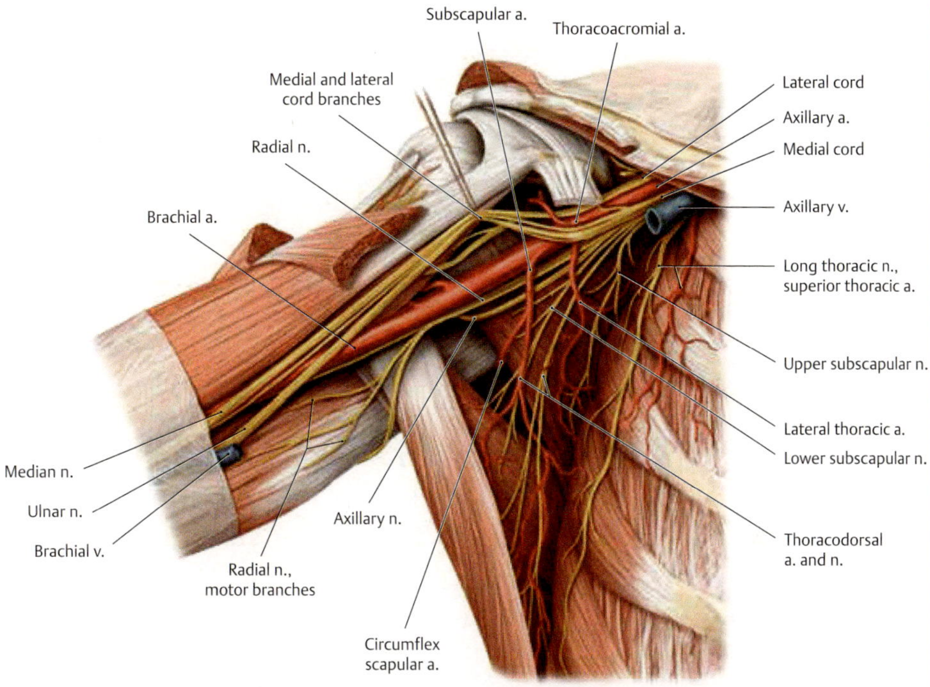

Fig. 2.14 *Removed*: Anterior wall (pectoral major and minor, and clavipectoral fascia). *Retracted*: Medial and lateral cords of the brachial plexus.

Axillary Artery

The *axillary artery* begins as a continuation of the third part of the *subclavian artery* at the outer border of the first rib and ends at the lower border of the teres major to continue as the *brachial artery* (**Fig 2.15**).

The proximal part of the axillary artery, axillary vein and brachial plexus and their branches are enclosed in the axillary sheath, derived from the prevertebral layer of the deep cervical fascia.

The axillary artery is surrounded by the brachial plexus and inferomedially it is related with the axillary vein throughout its course.

The axillary artery is divided into three parts by the pectoralis minor muscle.

First part of the axillary artery: It lies proximal to the pectoralis minor muscle and extends from the outer border of the first rib to the medial border of the pectoralis minor muscle.

Branches from the first part: The superior thoracic artery is the only branch given by the first part of the axillary artery. It arises near the apex of the axilla and supplies blood to the first and second intercostal spaces.

Second part of the axillary artery: It lies behind the pectoralis minor muscle. It gives two branches, the thoracoacromial artery and lateral thoracic artery. The thoracoacromial artery is divided into four branches:

1. Pectoral branch
2. Acromial branch
3. Deltoid branch
4. Clavicular branch

The lateral thoracic artery arises at the lateral border of the pectoralis minor muscle and descends along the lateral border of the pectoralis minor, and provides, in females, large lateral mammary branches to supply the breast.

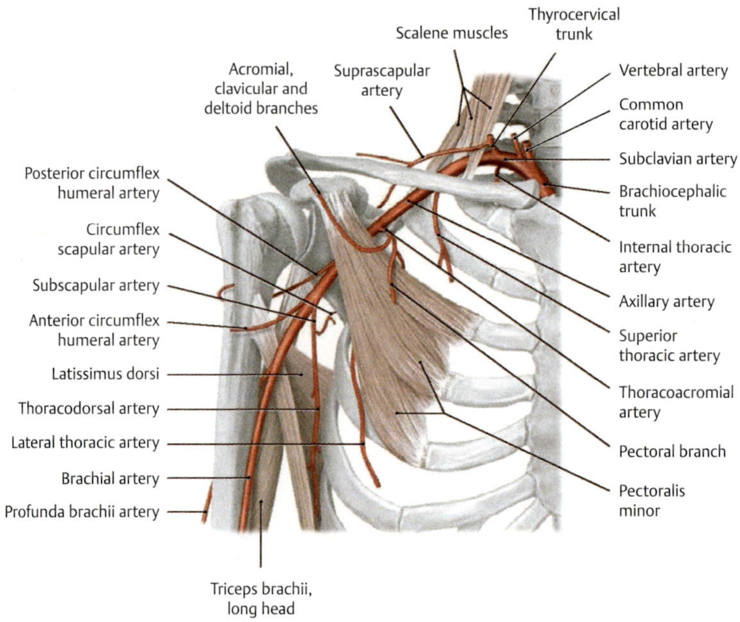

Fig. 2.15 Origin and branches of the axillary artery.

Third part of the axillary artery: It extends from the lateral border of the pectoralis minor to the lower border of the teres major muscle. The third part of the axillary artery gives three branches:

Subscapular artery: It is the largest of all branches. It runs along the lower border of the subscapularis to the inferior angle of the scapula.

Anterior circumflex humeral artery: It passes laterally and deep to the coracobrachialis, short and long head of the biceps, around the surgical neck of the humerus and anastomoses with the posterior circumflex humeral artery.

Posterior circumflex humeral artery: It passes posteriorly to the surgical neck of the humerus with the axillary nerve and leaves the posterior wall of the axilla through the quadrangular space.

Having seen and traced the axillary artery with its branches, let us now follow the nerves (derived from the brachial plexus) in the region of the axilla further destined to the upper limb.

Brachial Plexus

Brachial plexus is derived from the ventral rami of C5 to C8 and T1. The rami subsequently unite to form three trunks, namely upper, middle and lower. Each trunk divides into two divisions, anterior and posterior. The divisions then form cords which give branches that are distributed to the upper limb (**Fig. 2.16**). The branches of brachial plexus are given in **Table 2.3**.

Table 2.3 Brachial plexus

Name of nerve	Source with root value	Course	Distribution
Lateral pectoral	*Lateral cord*, C5, C6 and C7	Pierces the clavipectoral fascia to reach the deep surface of the pectoralis major	Pectoralis major
Musculocutaneous	Terminal branch of the *lateral cord* (C5–C7)	Exits the axilla by piercing the coracobrachialis; descending between the biceps and brachialis, it continues as the lateral cutaneous nerve of the forearm	Coracobrachialis, biceps brachii and brachialis muscle and lateral forearm skin
Median	Lateral root of the median nerve from the *lateral cord* (C5–C7) and medial root from *medial cord* (C8, T1)	Lateral and medial roots unite to form the median nerve lateral to the axillary artery, then descends through the arm adjacent to the brachial artery	Muscles of the flexor compartment of the forearm (except for the flexor carpi ulnaris, medial half of the flexor digitorum profundus), intrinsic muscles of the thenar part and palmar skin
Medial pectoral	*Medial cord* (C8, T1)	Passes between the axillary artery and vein, pierces the pectoralis minor and then pierces the deep surface of the pectoralis major muscle	Pectoralis major (sternocostal part) and pectoralis minor
Medial cutaneous nerve of the arm		Runs by the medial side of the axillary and brachial veins and communicates with the intercostobrachial nerve	Skin of the medial side of the arm up to the medial epicondyle of the humerus and olecranon process of the ulna
Medial cutaneous nerve of the forearm		In close relation with the ulnar nerve, pierces the deep fascia along with the basilic vein and then divides into anterior and posterior branches	Skin of the medial side of the forearm up to the wrist
Ulnar	*Medial cord* (C7, C8 and T1)	Terminal branch of the medial cord of the brachial plexus descends on the medial side of the arm; running behind the medial epicondyle of the humerus, it supplies the medial aspect of the forearm and hand	Flexor carpi ulnaris and medial half of the flexor digitorum profundus, intrinsic muscles of the hand, medial half of the skin of the hand
Upper subscapular	*Posterior cord* (C5)	Passes posteriorly and enters the subscapularis muscle directly	Upper part of the subscapularis muscle
Lower subscapular	*Posterior cord* (C6)	Runs inferolaterally, deep to the subscapular artery and vein	Lower part of the subscapularis and teres major muscles
Thoracodorsal	*Posterior cord* (C6, C7 and C8)	Arises between the upper and lower subscapular nerves, passes along the posterior axillary wall to the latissimus dorsi muscle	Latissimus dorsi muscle
Axillary	Terminal branch of the *posterior cord* (C5, C6)	Exits the axilla through the quadrangular space. Winds around the surgical neck of the humerus	Shoulder joint, deltoid, teres minor muscles and skin overlying the inferior part of the deltoid
Radial	Terminal branch of the *posterior cord* (C5–T1)	Exits the axilla lying posterior to the axillary artery, passes into the radial groove, perforates the lateral intermuscular septum and enters the cubital fossa	All the muscles of the *extensor compartment of the forearm*, skin of the posterior and inferolateral arm

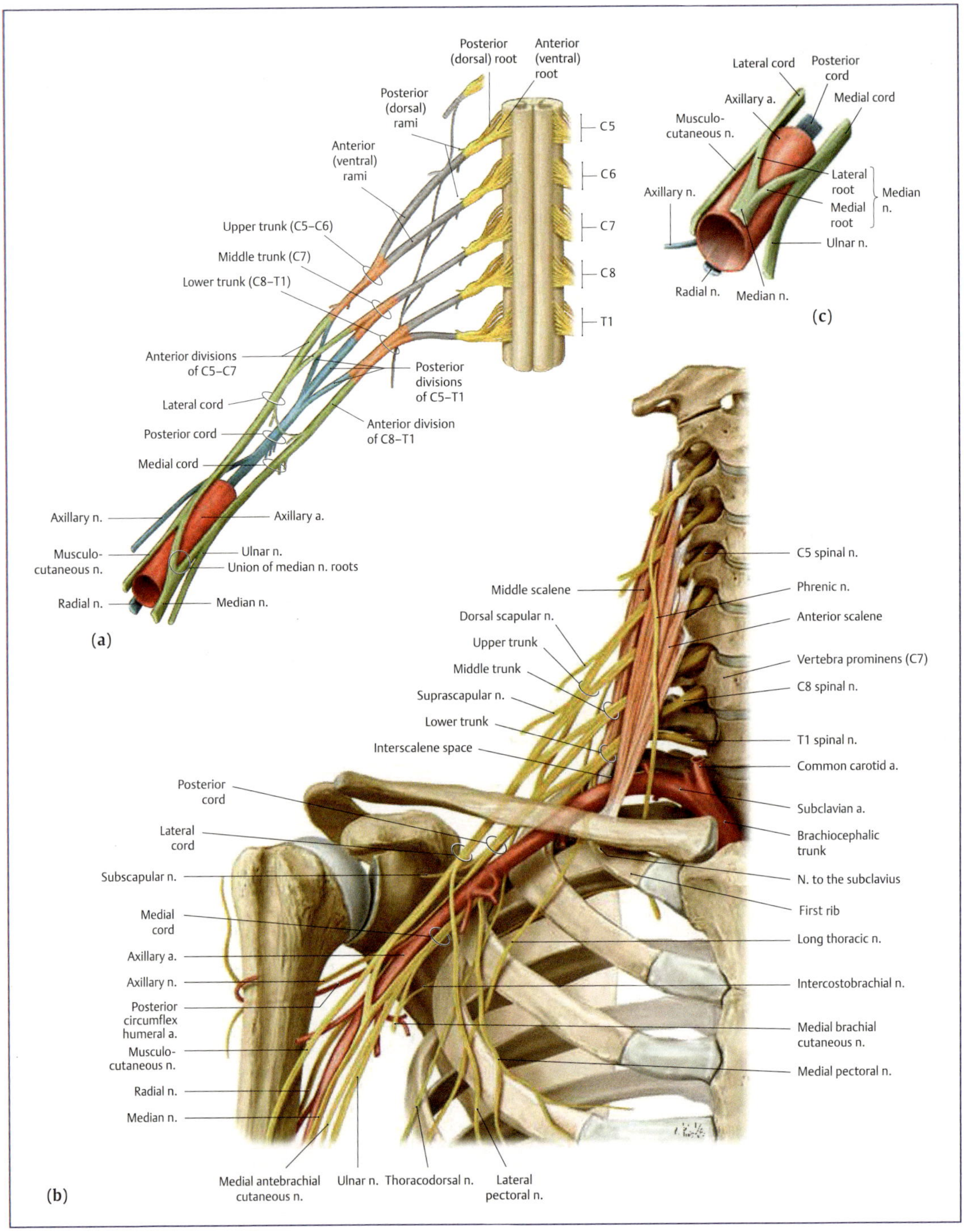

Fig. 2.16 Brachial plexus. **(a and b)** Formation and structure. **(c)** Course in relation to axillary artery stretched for clarity.

Dissection and Identification

Let us now trace the branches of the brachial plexus.

https://www.winkingskull.com/dissector/V1/video.aspx?vid=245

Lateral cord of the brachial plexus:

1. Trace the *coracobrachialis* and *short head of the biceps* springing from the tip of the coracoid process.

2. Find the *musculocutaneous nerve* entering the coracobrachialis, and trace this nerve upwards to find the lateral cord of the brachial plexus.
3. *Lateral root of the median nerve* also arises from the lateral cord of the brachial plexus. To find out the median nerve, trace the lateral root distally.
4. Find the *axillary artery* and *median nerve* medial to the coracobrachialis muscle.

Medial cord of the brachial plexus:

1. Trace the *medial root of the median nerve* proximally to find out the medial cord of the brachial plexus.
2. Identify the *ulnar nerve* from the medial cord of the brachial plexus.
3. Trace the previously identified medial and lateral pectoral nerves to the medial and lateral cords of the brachial plexus, respectively.
4. Identify the *medial cutaneous nerve of the forearm, medial cutaneous nerve of the arm* and branches from the medial cord of the brachial plexus by tracing them to a short distance into the arm.

Posterior cord of the brachial plexus:

1. To get a better view of the posterior cord of the brachial plexus, retract the axillary artery, the medial and lateral cords of the brachial plexus superiorly.
2. With the help of blunt dissection, clean the *axillary nerve* passing posterior to the humerus accompanied by the posterior circumflex humeral artery.
3. Identify the *radial nerve*, which passes behind the humerus but anterior to the latissimus dorsi and teres major muscles.
4. Identify the *subscapular nerves* arising from the posterior cord of the brachial plexus and supplying the subscapularis muscle.
5. At this stage, one can also see the teres major and latissimus dorsi along with the subscapularis, forming the post axillary wall.
6. Please note that the medial, lateral and posterior cords of the brachial plexus are disposed around the second part of the axillary artery in their respective positions behind the pectoralis minor.

Clinical Notes

1. *Carcinoma of the breast* is a common cancer in females. It can cause *dimpling of the skin* from the malignant infiltration and contraction of the suspensory ligaments of the breast (ligaments of Cooper).
2. *Peau d'orange sign*: An orange peel appearance of the skin because of cancer cells interfering with the lymph drainage leading to lymph edema with puffy skin between the dimpled pores.
3. *Radical mastectomy*: In radical mastectomy, excision of the breast tumour is done with pectoralis major and axillary node clearance. The clavicular head of the pectoralis major is usually spared for cosmetic reasons.
4. *Breast abscess* is drained by radial incisions to avoid cutting through a number of lactiferous ducts.
5. *Krukenberg's tumour* is a secondary ovarian tumour and may occur in case of carcinoma of the breast, involving the inferomedial quadrant of the breast.
6. *Erb–Duchenne palsy*: Injury to the upper part of the brachial plexus (C5, C6) results in the paralysis of the shoulder and arm muscles. The upper limb is adducted in the shoulder, arm is medially rotated and the elbow extended (Porter's tip hand/Policeman's tip hand).
7. *Klumpke's paralysis*: Injury to the lower part of the brachial plexus, damaging the lower trunk (C8, T1), results in claw hand due to paralysis of the short muscles of the hand.

CHAPTER 3

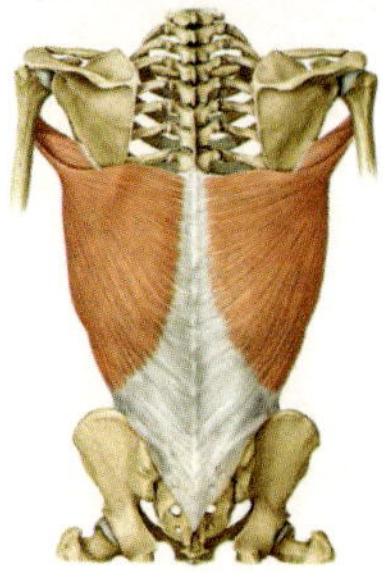

Dissection of the Back

Learning Objectives

At the end of the dissection, students should be able to identify the following:

- *Muscles*: Trapezius, latissimus dorsi, levator scapulae, rhomboideus major, rhomboideus minor, longissimus capitis, erector spinae and iliocostalis.
- *Vessels and nerves*: Dorsal scapular nerve, posterior cutaneous branches of the dorsal rami and deep branch of the transverse cervical artery.

Introduction

The back region of the body presents the posterior axioappendicular muscles in two groups: the *superficial* and *intermediate*. These are extrinsic muscles and extend from the axial to the appendicular skeleton.

The deep group of muscles of the back are intrinsic muscles that maintain the posture and control the movements of the vertebral column.

Surface Landmarks (Fig. 3.1)

1. *External occipital protuberance*: It is a bony prominence on the lower part of the back of the head where the nuchal groove meets the skull.
2. *Superior nuchal line*: It is a curved bony ridge extending laterally from the external occipital protuberance.
3. *Ligamentum nuchae*: It is a median fibrous structure extending from the external occipital protuberance to the spine of C7.
4. Spinous process of C7 vertebra (vertebra prominence).
5. *Spine of the scapula*: It corresponds to the spine of T3 vertebra.
6. Medial border of the scapula.
7. Inferior angle of the scapula: It corresponds to the spine of T7 vertebra.
8. Spines of the thoracic vertebrae: They can be palpated in the median furrow of the back.

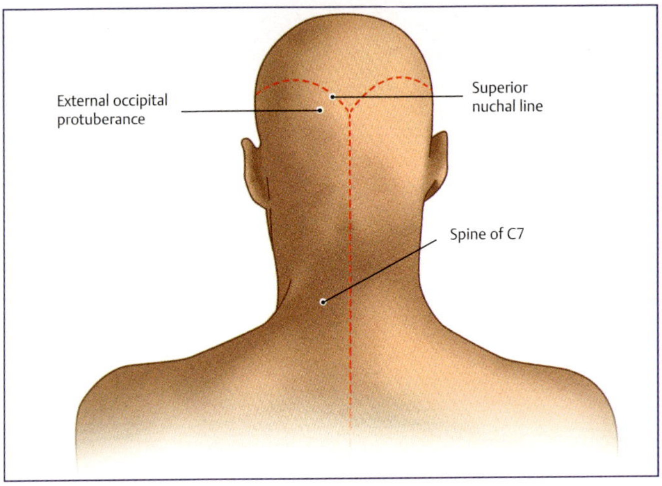

Fig. 3.1 Surface landmarks of the back.

9. *Twelfth rib*: Its tip can be felt 3 cm above the iliac crest.
10. *Iliac crest*: The curved bony ridge felt below the waist can be traced from the posterior to the anterior superior iliac spine.
11. *Posterior superior iliac spine*: It is felt in the dimple about 5 cm from the median plane at the level of S2 vertebra.
12. *Sacrum*: Usually three palpable spines can be felt in the median plane.
13. *Coccyx*: It is felt deeply between the buttocks in the median plane.

Dissection and Identification

Give the following incisions (**Fig. 3.2**):

1. *Incision A*: Along the midline from the spine of C7 to the tip of the coccyx (**Fig. 3.2**).
2. *Incision B*: Make a transverse incision from the spine of C7 to the acromion process of the scapula.
3. *Incision C*: An oblique skin incision starting from the spine of T12 obliquely upwards to the midaxillary line at the intersection of the seventh rib.
4. *Incision D*: From the tip of the coccyx, a curved skin incision is taken along the iliac crest extending up to the anterior superior iliac spine.
5. *Incision E*: Extending from the external occipital protuberance to the mastoid processes of either side.
6. Reflect the skin flaps along with the superficial fascia from the deep fascia by blunt dissection. The flaps are reflected from the medial to the lateral side (**Fig. 3.2**).
7. The dense connection between the two fascia on the back poses difficulty in separation.
8. Observe the posterior cutaneous branches of the dorsal rami as they pierce the deep fascia.
9. Remove the deep fascia over the surface of the trapezius below the spine of C7.
10. Trace the trapezius to its medial attachment.
11. Observe the lateral attachment of the trapezius to the clavicle and scapula.
12. Reflect the trapezius by dividing the muscle horizontally between the clavicle and the spine of scapula, and vertically detaching the muscle from its medial attachment by using a pair of scissors.
13. While cutting, care should be taken to avoid injury to the underlying structures.
14. Now reflect the trapezius laterally and note the following:
    - Superior branch of the transverse cervical vessels
    - Accessory nerve (**Fig. 3.3**)
    - Cervical rami (C3 and C4) entering the deep surface of the trapezius
15. Remove the fascia over the *latissimus dorsi*. It is a bit difficult because the upper part of the muscle has an ill-defined margin and varying directions of its fibres (**Fig. 3.4**).
16. Trace the attachment of the muscle to the thoracolumbar fascia and to the iliac crest.
17. Trace the muscle to its lateral border and find its slips arising from the lower three to four ribs that interdigitate with the external oblique muscle of the abdomen.
18. To reflect the latissimus dorsi, insert your fingers deep to its superior border, medial to the inferior angle of the scapula, to break the loose connective tissue under it. Raise the muscle enough

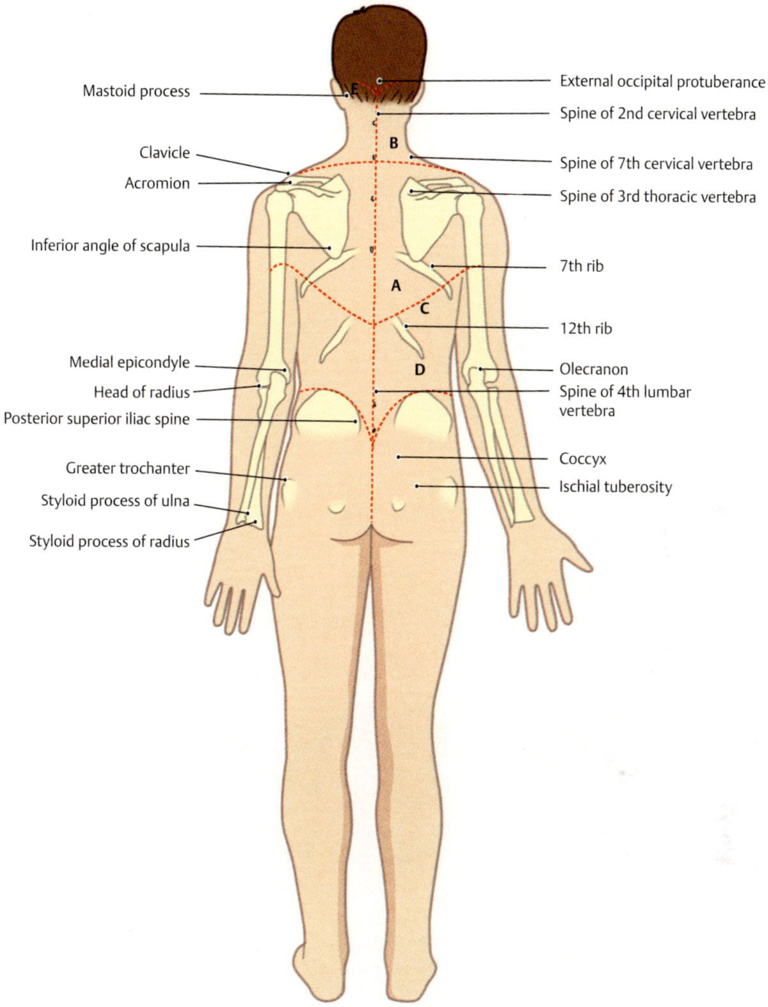

Fig. 3.2 Bony landmarks and skin incisions for dissection of the back.

to insert a pair of scissors and cut along the medial attachment of the muscle to the thoracolumbar fascia.

19. Reflect the latissimus dorsi laterally without severing its attachment to the lower ribs and inferior angle of the scapula. The distal attachment/insertion of the latissimus dorsi is along the floor of the intertubercular sulcus on the anterior side of the upper part of the humerus. The muscle receives its innervation from the thoracodorsal nerve and thoracodorsal artery supplying it. The insertion of the muscle and its nerve and blood supply shall be observed during the dissection of the upper limb.
20. Clear the surface and borders of the rhomboideus minor and major.
21. The rhomboideus minor is medially attached to the spinous processes of C7 and T1, and laterally to the medial border of the scapula on the dorsal aspect against the root of the spine.
22. The medial attachment of the rhomboideus major is to the spines of T2 to T5.
23. Lateral attachment of the rhomboideus major is to the medial border of the scapula on the dorsal aspect below the spine of the scapula.
24. To reflect the rhomboideus, insert your fingers deep to the inferior border of the rhomboideus major and clear it from deeper muscles using a pair of scissors. Detach the rhomboideus major from its medial attachment starting from its inferior border.

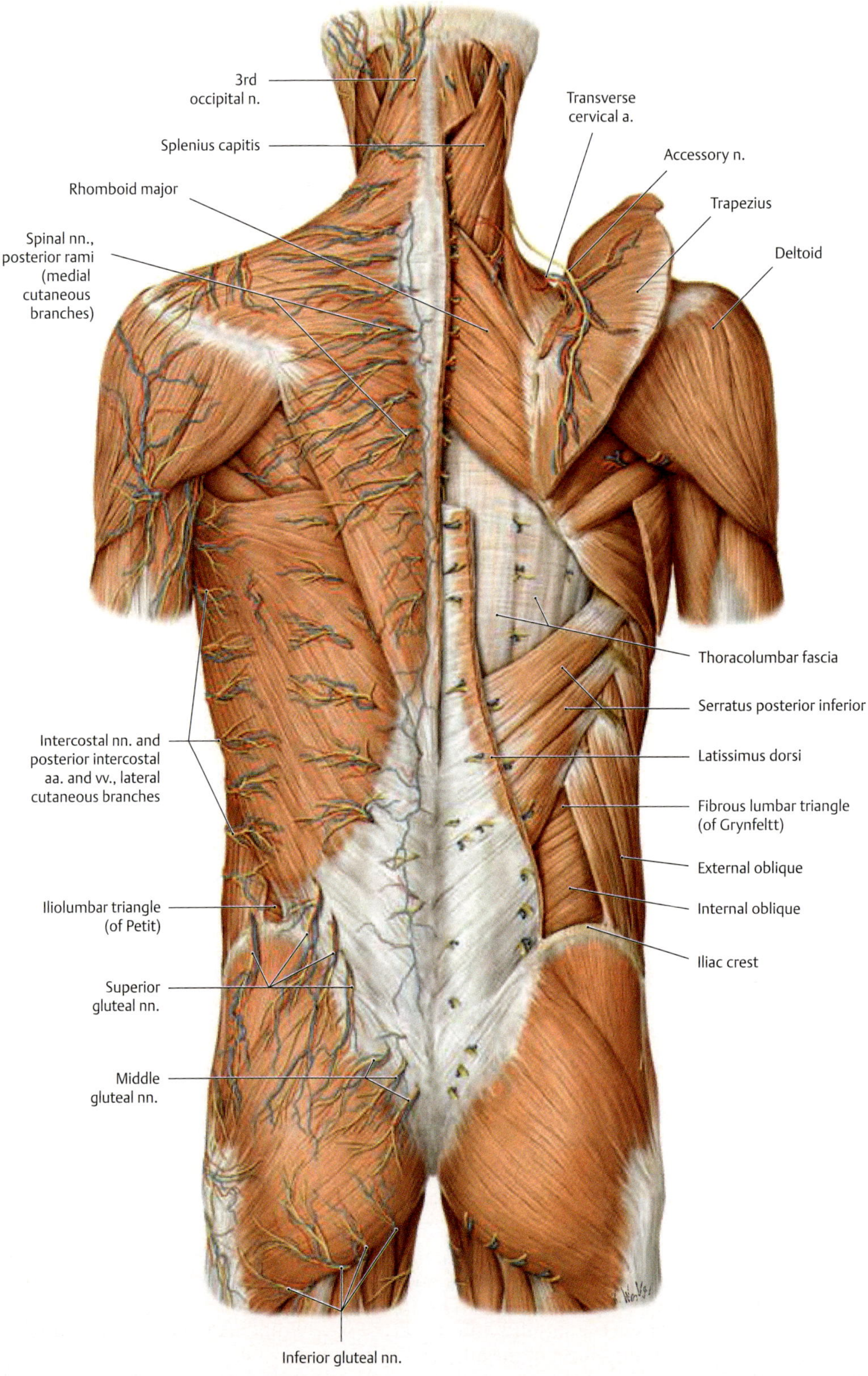

Fig. 3.3 Neurovasculature of the back.

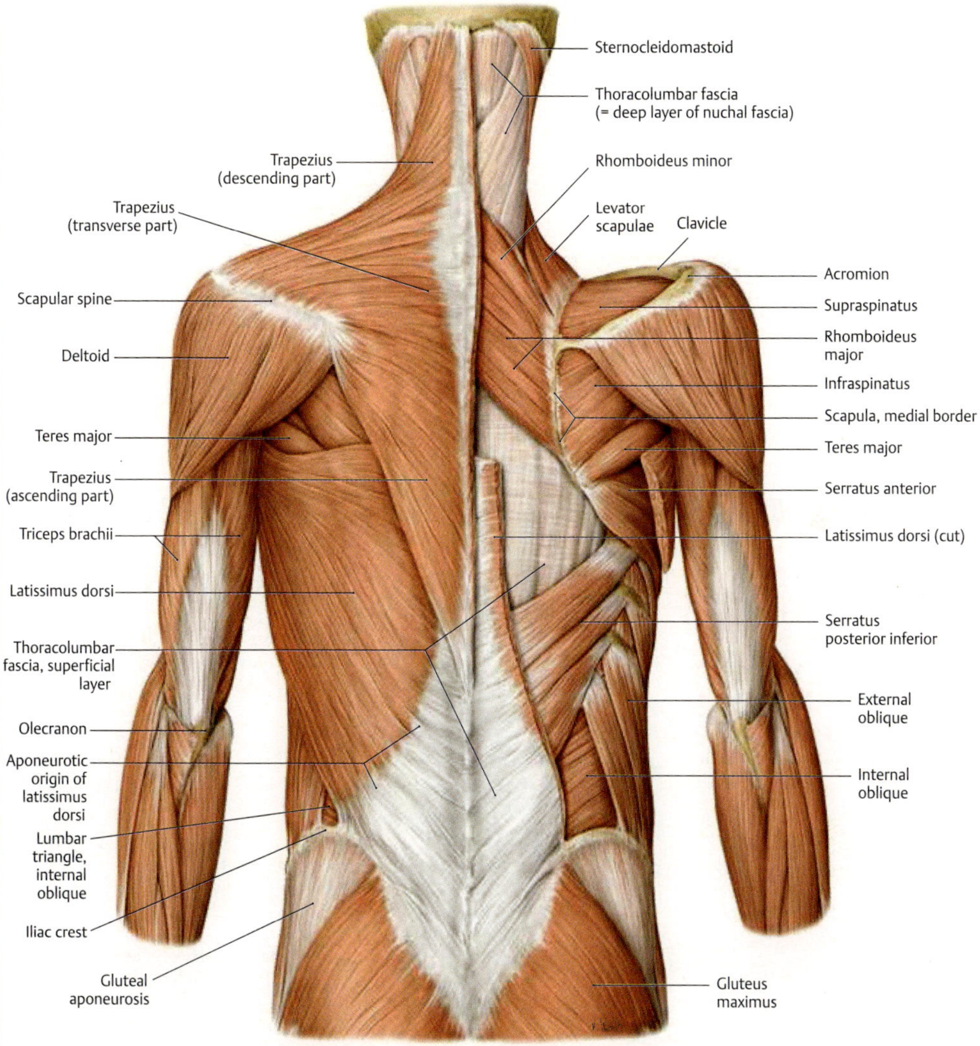

Fig. 3.4 Muscles of the back: an overview.

25. Continue to cut superiorly to detach the rhomboideus minor from its medial attachment to the spinous processes.

26. Reflect the two muscles laterally using blunt dissection; find the *dorsal scapular nerve* and deep branch of the transverse cervical artery on the deep surface of the rhomboideus near their lateral attachments. The nerve and vessels course parallel to the vertebral border of the scapula.

27. The *levator scapulae* muscle is attached to the dorsal aspect of the medial border of the scapula from the superior angle to the root of the spine. The superior attachment of this muscle is along the transverse processes of the upper four cervical vertebrae. The dorsal scapular nerve and artery supply it.

28. Raise the medial border of the scapula from the thoracic wall; it raises the serratus anterior muscle along.

29. Define the attachment of the serratus anterior to the scapula and note the lower digitations that converge on the anterior aspect of the inferior angle of the scapula.

30. Remove the fat and connective tissue from the suprascapular region under the cut edges of the trapezius to find the inferior belly of the omohyoid, the suprascapular nerve and vessels passing towards the suprascapular notch.

31. Observe the triangle of auscultation bounded by the latissimus dorsi, trapezius and rhomboideus major muscles. It overlies the sixth intercostal space.
32. Note the lumbar triangle bounded by the latissimus dorsi, external oblique muscles and iliac crest. It may form a site for lumbar herniation.

Muscles of the Back

Fig. 3.4 provides an overview of the muscles of the back.

Superficial Muscles of the Back

Superficial muscles of the back are trapezius, latissimus dorsi, levator scapulae, rhomboideus minor and rhomboideus major.

Table 3.1 provides an overview of superficial muscles of the back.

Table 3.1 Muscles of the back

Name of muscle	Origin	Insertion	Nerve supply	Action/Function
Trapezius (**Fig. 3.5**)	Medial third of the superior nuchal line, external occipital protuberance, nuchal ligament, spinous processes of the C7–T12 vertebrae	Lateral third of the clavicle, acromion and spine of the scapula	Spinal accessory nerve (cranial nerve XI) (motor fibres) and C3, C4 spinal nerves (pain and proprioceptive fibres)	Descending part *elevates*, ascending part *depresses* and middle part *retracts* the scapula Descending and ascending parts act together to *rotate the glenoid cavity superiorly*
Latissimus dorsi (**Fig. 3.6**)	Spinous processes of the inferior six thoracic vertebrae, thoracolumbar fascia, iliac crest and lower three to four ribs and inferior angle of scapula	Floor of the intertubercular sulcus of the humerus	Thoracodorsal nerve (C6, C7 and C8)	*Extends, adducts* and *medially rotates the humerus*. Raises the body towards the arms during climbing
Levator scapulae (**Fig. 3.7**)	Posterior tubercle of the transverse processes of the C1–C4 vertebrae	Medial border of the scapula superior to the root of the scapular spine	Dorsal scapular (C6) and cervical (C3, C4) nerves	*Elevates* the scapula and rotates the glenoid cavity inferiorly
Rhomboid minor (**Fig. 3.7**)	Nuchal ligament, spinous processes of C7 and T1 vertebrae	Smooth triangular area at the medial end of the scapular spine	Dorsal scapular nerve (C4, C5)	*Retracts* the scapula and rotates it to depress the glenoid cavity; fixes the scapula to the thoracic wall
Rhomboid major (**Fig. 3.7**)	Spinous processes of the T2–T5 vertebrae	Medial border of the scapula from the level of the spine to the inferior angle	Dorsal scapular nerve (C4, C5)	*Retracts* the scapula and rotates it to depress the glenoid cavity; fixes the scapula to the thoracic wall

Intermediate Muscles of the Back

1. *Serratus posterior superior* is medially attached to the nuchal ligament and the spinous processes of the C7 to T3 vertebrae. Lateral attachment/insertion is to the superior border of second to fifth ribs lateral to their angles.
2. *Serratus posterior inferior* is medially attached to the spines of T11 to L2. Lateral attachment of the muscle is to the inferior borders of the ninth to twelfth ribs lateral to their angles. They are innervated by the intercostal nerves and help in inspiration.

Deep Muscles of the Back

Deep muscles of the back act on the vertebral column. These include:

1. Splenius capitis
2. Splenius cervicis

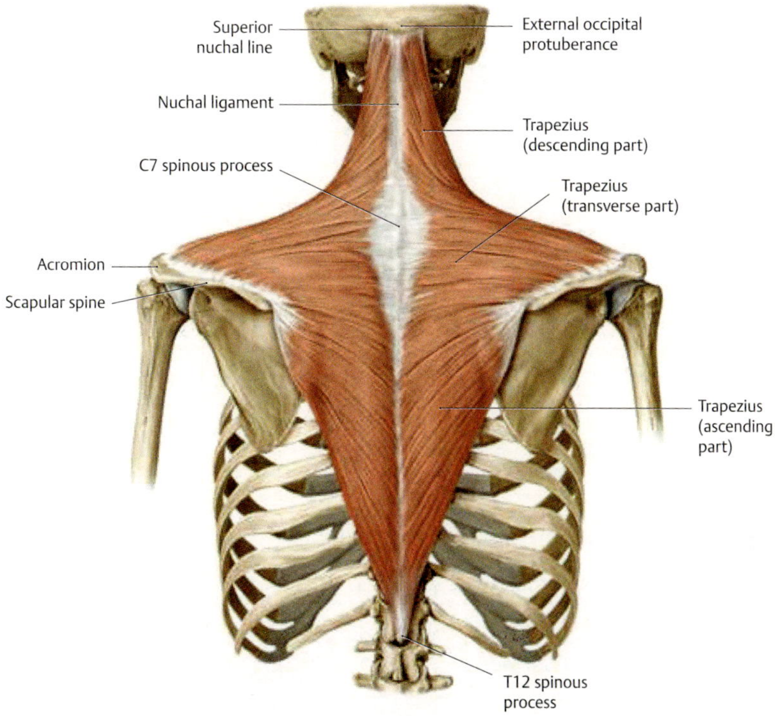

Fig. 3.5 Trapezius (posterior view).

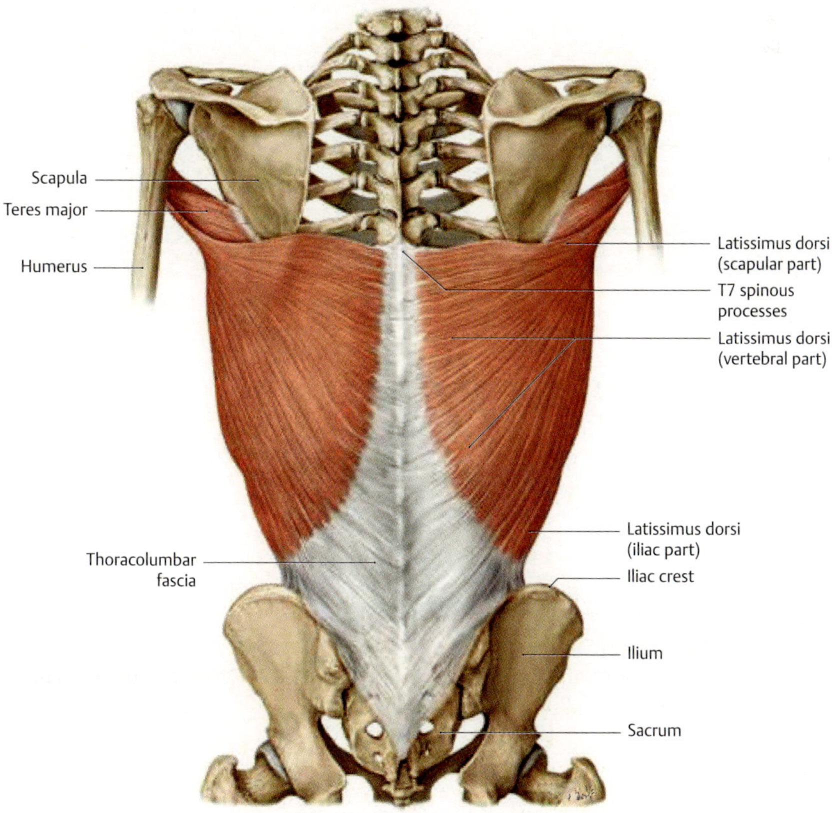

Fig. 3.6 Latissimus dorsi and teres major muscles.

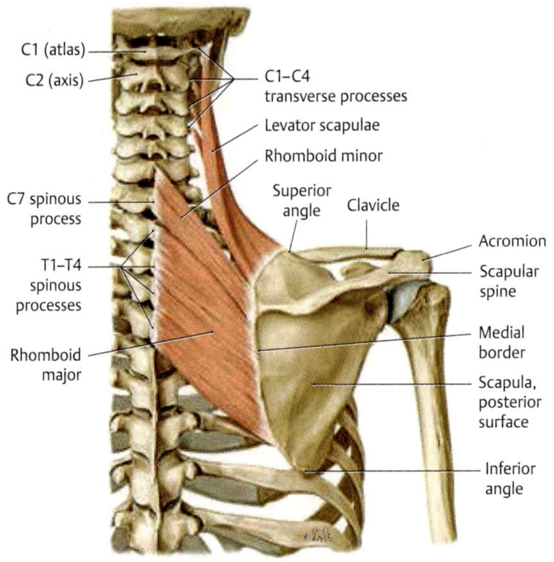

Fig. 3.7 Levator scapulae with rhomboids major and minor (right side, posterior view).

3. Semispinalis capitis
4. Erector spinae
5. Longissimus capitis
6. Iliocostalis

These will be dissected during the dissection of the vertebral column and spinal cord.

Clinical Notes

Scoliosis (Gr. crookedness of curved back): It is an abnormal lateral curvature of the vertebral column.

Lordosis: It is an accentuated lumbar curvature.

Kyphosis (hump back): It is an abnormally increased thoracic curvature.

Lumbar triangle: It may be the site of lumbar hernia.

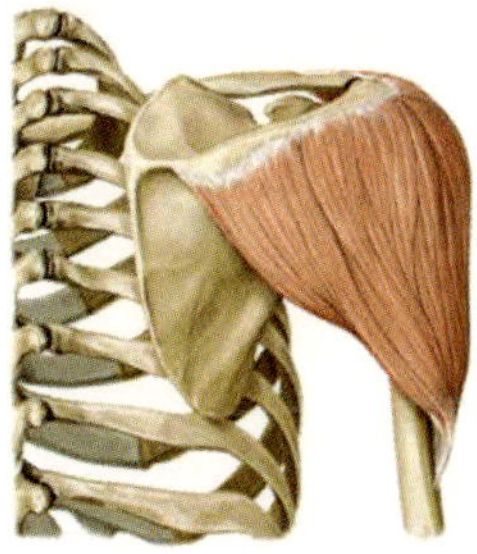

CHAPTER 4

Scapular Region and Shoulder

Learning Objectives

At the end of the dissection of this part, students should be able to identify the following:

- *Muscles:* Deltoid, subscapularis, supraspinatus, infraspinatus, teres minor, teres major, long head and short head of biceps, long head of triceps.
- *Nerves:* Axillary, radial, musculocutaneous, median and ulnar.
- *Arteries:* Subscapular, anterior and posterior circumflex humerals, profunda brachii.

Introduction

The scapular region comprises structures that are closely related to the area around the shoulder joint. It has six muscles: *deltoid, supraspinatus, infraspinatus, teres minor, teres major* and *subscapularis.*

Surface Landmarks

1. *Acromion*: *Crest* of the spine of the scapula, the *medial (vertebral), lateral (axillary) borders* of the scapula and its *inferior angle* can be felt through the skin.
2. *Deltoid*: The muscle covers nearly the upper half of the humerus and forms the rounded contour of the shoulder.
3. *Greater tubercle* of the humerus forms the most lateral bony landmark at the shoulder. It is advisable to identify the bony features associated with the scapula and humerus using the skeleton before dissection of the region (**Fig. 4.1**).

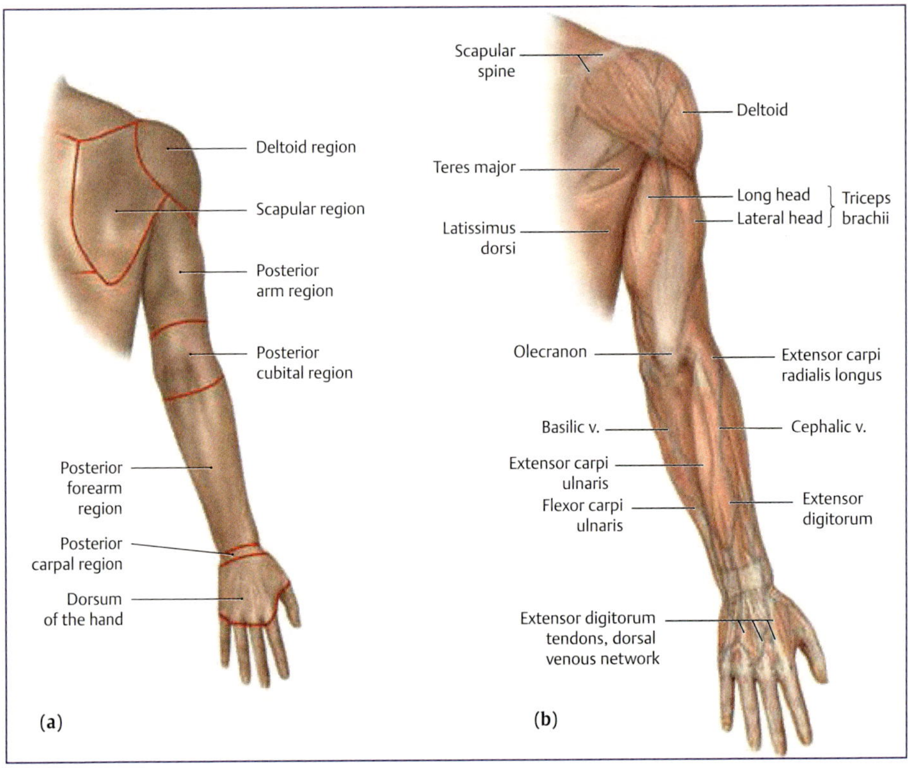

Fig. 4.1 **(a)** Region of the upper limb. **(b)** Palpable musculature.

Dissection and Identification

1. Place the cadaver in the prone position; abduct the upper limb to 45 degrees. Place the block under the chest; this will facilitate the dissection of the region offering better access (**Fig. 4.2**).
2. Reflect the trapezius upwards with its cervical fascial attachment left intact.
3. Remove the fascia over the *deltoid* and clear its borders. Trace the muscle to its proximal attachment, to the spine and acromion of the scapula and also the lateral third of the clavicle.
4. Note the distal attachment of the deltoid to the deltoid tuberosity of the humerus.
5. Using a scalpel, detach the deltoid from its proximal attachment. Let your cut be close to the bone. Leave the muscle distally attached to the deltoid tuberosity.
6. Reflect the deltoid laterally to expose the underlying vessels and nerve, avoiding damage to them.

   https://www.winkingskull.com/dissector/V1/video.aspx?vid=84

7. Note the *axillary nerve* and *posterior circumflex humeral artery* on the deep surface of the deltoid muscle. Using a probe, clean the nerve and vessels. Trace them around the surgical neck of the humerus.
8. Note the branches of the axillary nerve to the deltoid and teres minor muscles.
9. Push your finger parallel to the axillary nerve to trace the *axillary nerve* and the accompanying *posterior circumflex humeral vessels* through the *quadrangular space* bounded (**Fig 4.3**):
   - *Superiorly* by the inferior border of the teres minor
   - *Medially* by the long head of the triceps brachii
   - *Inferiorly* by the upper border of the teres major
   - *Laterally* by the surgical neck of the humerus
10. Identify the *long head of the triceps brachii* and note that it passes anterior to the teres minor but posterior to the teres major.

    https://www.winkingskull.com/dissector/V1/video.aspx?vid=248

11. Define the borders of the *teres minor muscle*. Trace its medial attachment along the lateral border of the scapula and lateral attachment to the greater tubercle of the humerus.
12. Clean and define the borders of the *teres major muscle*. Medially, it is attached to the facet along the inferior angle of the scapula. Laterally, it is attached to the medial lip of the intertubercular sulcus in front of the humerus.

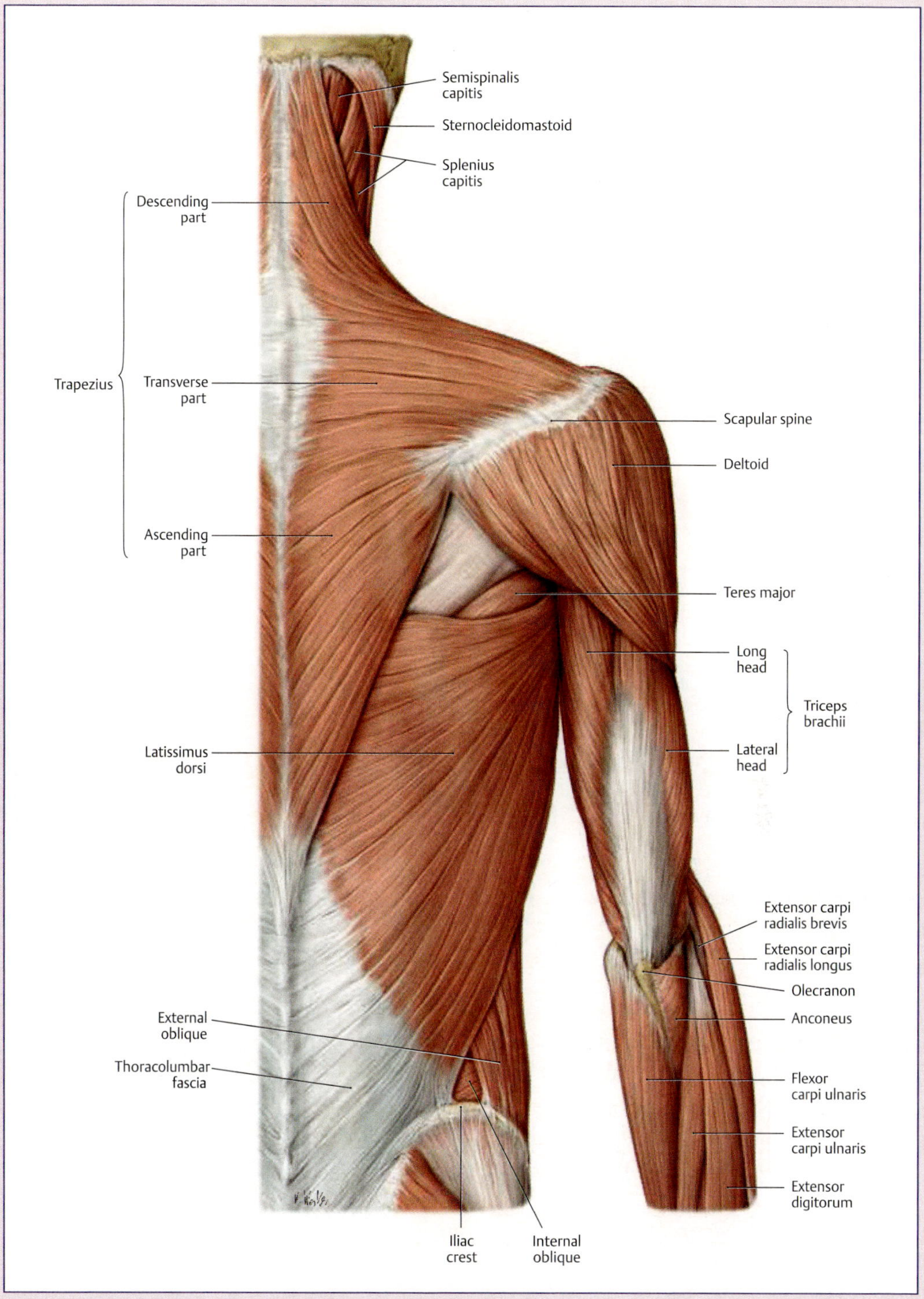

Fig. 4.2 Posterior muscles of the shoulder and arm (right side, posterior view).

Note the two triangular spaces in the region.

The *upper triangular space* is bounded (**Fig. 4.3**):

1. *Medially* by the teres minor
2. *Laterally* by the long head of triceps
3. *Inferiorly* by the teres major

Circumflex scapular artery passes through this space and anastomoses with the suprascapular artery.

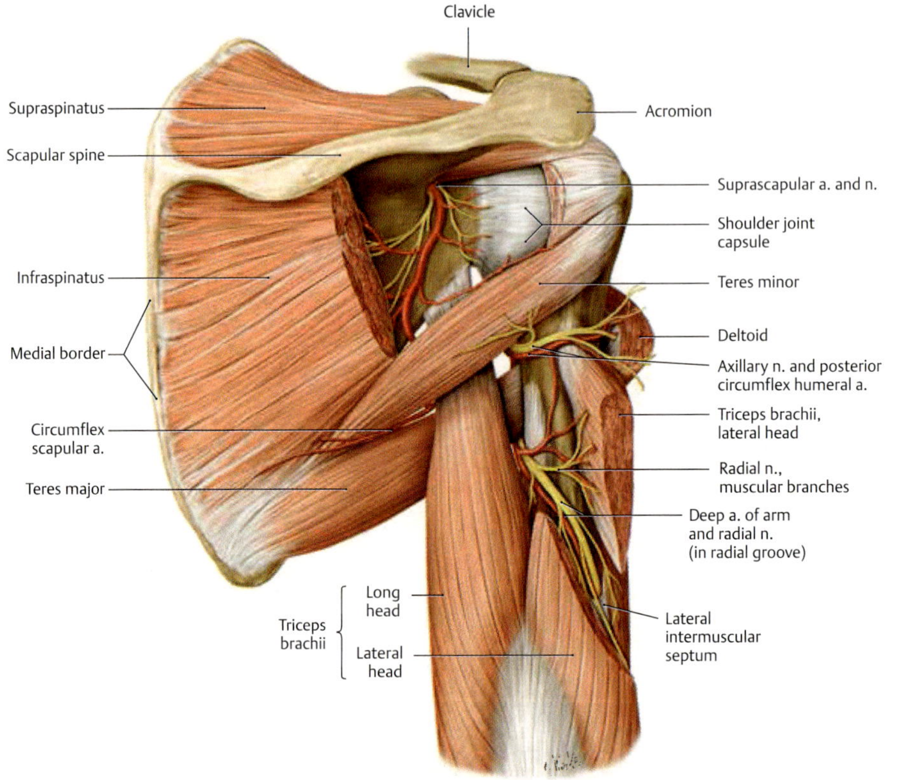

Fig. 4.3 Deep dissection of right shoulder (posterior view) showing quadrangular and triangular spaces.

The *lower triangular space* is bounded (**Fig. 4.3**):

1. *Medially* by the long head of the triceps brachii
2. *Laterally* by the shaft of the humerus
3. *Superiorly* by the teres major

Through this space, the *radial nerve* and *profunda brachii* vessels enter the radial/spiral groove.

Dissection and Identification

1. Now clean the surface of the *supraspinatus muscle* and observe its medial attachment to the supraspinous fossa and lateral to the highest facet on the greater tubercle of the humerus.

   https://www.winkingskull.com/dissector/V1/video.aspx?vid=251

2. Using a probe, define the attachment of the *infraspinatus muscle*. Trace its medial attachment to the infraspinous fossa of the scapula and lateral to the greater tubercle of the humerus.
3. Reflect the supraspinatus after transecting it about 5 cm lateral to the superior angle of the scapula and medial to the suprascapular notch.
4. By blunt dissection, loosen the supraspinatus from the supraspinous fossa and reflect it laterally towards its humeral attachment.
5. Now identify the *suprascapular artery* and *nerve*. Note that the artery passes above and the nerve passes below the *suprascapular ligament* (**Fig. 4.3**).
6. Transect the infraspinatus about 5 cm lateral to the vertebral border of the scapula; using blunt dissection, loosen the muscle from the infraspinous fossa and reflect it laterally.
7. Follow the suprascapular artery and nerve as they enter the infraspinatus fossa passing through the spinoglenoid notch.

   https://www.winkingskull.com/dissector/V1/video.aspx?vid=133

8. Note that the suprascapular artery contributes to the *scapular anastomosis* along with the circumflex scapular artery and deep branch of the transverse cervical artery.

https://www.winkingskull.com/dissector/V1/video.aspx?vid=252

Rotator Cuff/Musculotendinous Cuff

It consists of four muscles: (a) *supraspinatus*, (b) *infraspinatus*, (c) *teres minor* and (d) *subscapularis* (**Fig. 4.4**). At this stage, we have seen three of them. The subscapularis has already been studied during the dissection of the axilla (Chapter 2).

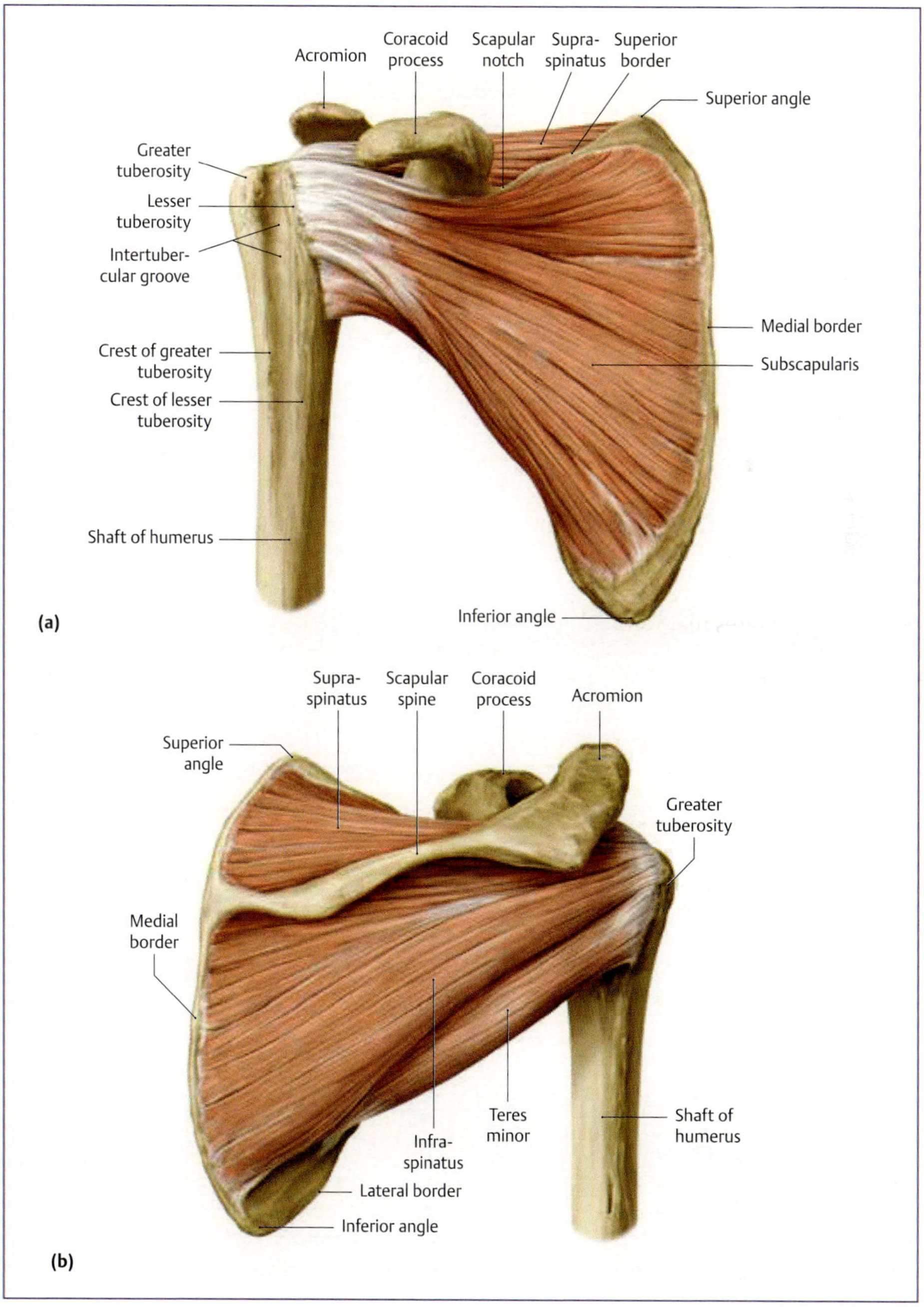

Fig. 4.4 Rotator cuff/musculotendinous cuff: **(a)** Anterior view and **(b)** posterior view. *(continued)*

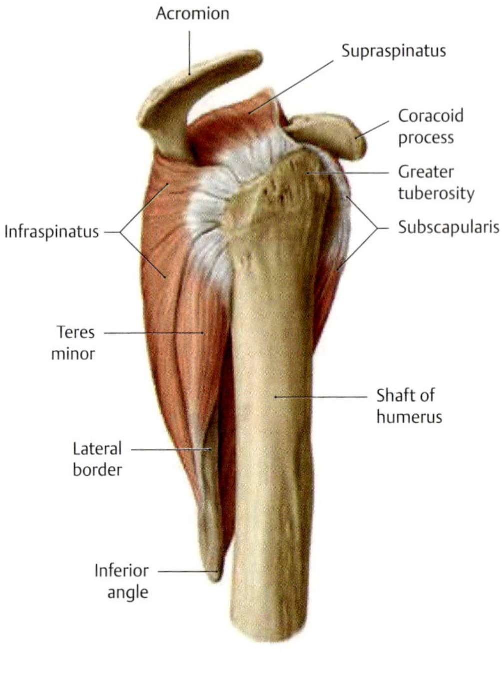

Fig. 4.4 *(continued)* Rotator cuff/musculotendinous cuff: **(c)** lateral view.

Overview of the muscles of the scapular region is given in **Table 4.1** (**Fig. 4.4**).

Table 4.1 Muscles of the scapular region

Name of muscle	Origin	Insertion	Nerve supply	Action/Function
Deltoid (**Fig. 4.5**)	Lateral third of the clavicle, lateral border of the acromion and spine of the scapula	Deltoid tuberosity of the humerus	Axillary nerve	Flexion and medial rotation, extension, lateral rotation and abduction
Supraspinatus (**Fig. 4.4b**)	Medial three-fourths of the supraspinous fossa of the scapula	Superior part of the greater tubercle of the humerus	Suprascapular nerve	Initiation of abduction at the shoulder joint with the deltoid and action along with the rotator cuff muscles
Infraspinatus (**Fig. 4.4b**)	Medial three-fourths of the infraspinous fossa of the scapula	Middle part of the greater tubercle of the humerus	Suprascapular nerve	Lateral rotation at the shoulder joint and action along with the rotator cuff muscles
Teres minor (**Fig. 4.3**)	Middle third of the posterior surface of the lateral border of the scapula	Inferior part of the greater tubercle of the humerus	Axillary nerve	Lateral rotation at the shoulder joint and action along with the rotator cuff muscles
Teres major (**Fig. 4.3**)	Inferolateral along the lateral border on posterior surface of the scapula	Medial lip of the bicipital groove of the humerus	Inferior subscapular nerve	Adduction and medial rotation at the shoulder joint

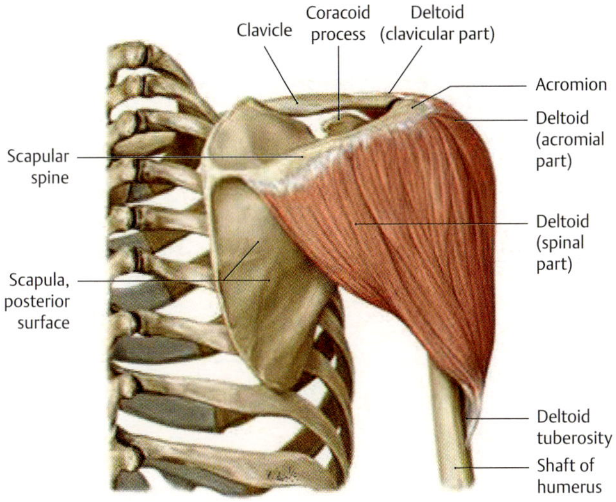

Fig. 4.5 Deltoid muscle (posterior view).

Clinical Notes

1. *Subacromial bursitis*: Pressure over the deltoid below the acromion causes pain; however, pressure over the same point does not cause pain when the arm is abducted because the bursa moves under the acromion. It is referred to as the *Dawbarn's sign*.
2. *Supraspinatus tendinitis*: It is the inflammation of supraspinatus tendon. The inflammatory changes are usually associated with calcification.
3. *Damage to the axillary nerve* may occur in the inferior dislocation (subglenoid) of the shoulder or in fracture involving surgical neck of the humerus. The deltoid is paralyzed and may undergo disuse atrophy leading to loss of rounded contour of the shoulder.
4. *Scapular anastomosis* provides collateral circulation if the distal part of the subclavian or proximal part of the axillary artery is blocked.

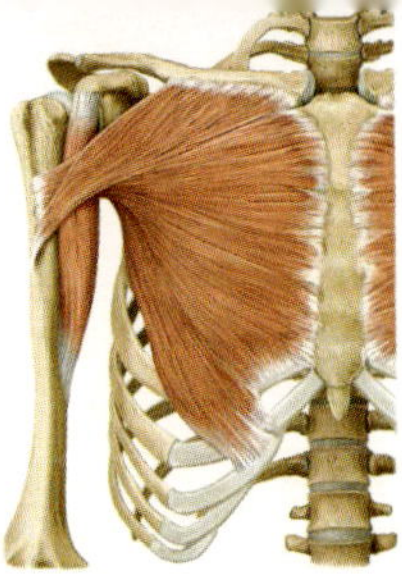

CHAPTER 5

Anterior Compartment of the Arm and Cubital Fossa

Learning Objectives

At the end of the dissection of the anterior compartment of the arm, students should be able to identify the following:

- *Muscles*: Biceps brachii, brachialis, coracobrachialis, muscles bounding the cubital fossa.
- *Nerves*: Musculocutaneous, median, radial, ulnar and their branches.
- *Vessels*: Brachial artery and its branches.
- *Cubital fossa* (Latin: cubitus = elbow).
- Clinical correlation associated with the structures.

Anterior Compartment of the Arm

Introduction

The arm is enclosed by a thick sleeve of deep fascia called *brachial fascia*. Proximally, it is continuous with the pectoral and axillary fascia and distally with the *antebrachial fascia* (i.e., the deep fascia of the forearm). From the deep surface of the brachial fascia, the *medial* and *lateral intermuscular septa* reach the humerus, thus forming the anterior and posterior compartments of the arm.

The anterior compartment contains *three* muscles, namely *biceps brachii, brachialis and coracobrachialis*. They are supplied by the *musculocutaneous nerve*. The posterior compartment has *two* muscles, the *triceps brachii* and *anconeus*. They are supplied by the radial nerve.

Surface Landmarks (Fig. 5.1)

1. *Upper end of the humerus*: Feel for the greater and lesser tubercles.
2. *Medial and lateral epicondyles* of the humerus can be felt at the lower end on their respective sides (refer to **Fig. 1.3**).
3. *Ulnar nerve* can be palpated *behind the medial epicondyle* of the humerus.
4. *Radial head* can be palpated in a depression on the lateral side of the back of the extended elbow. It can be rolled between the fingers keeping one in the depression and the other in front of the forearm with an alternate pronation and supination.
5. *The tip of the olecranon* process can be prominently seen and felt on the flexion of the elbow.
6. The olecranon process of the ulna and medial and lateral epicondyles of the humerus form an *equilateral triangle* in a fully flexed elbow.
7. Median cubital vein connects cephalic with basilic vein.

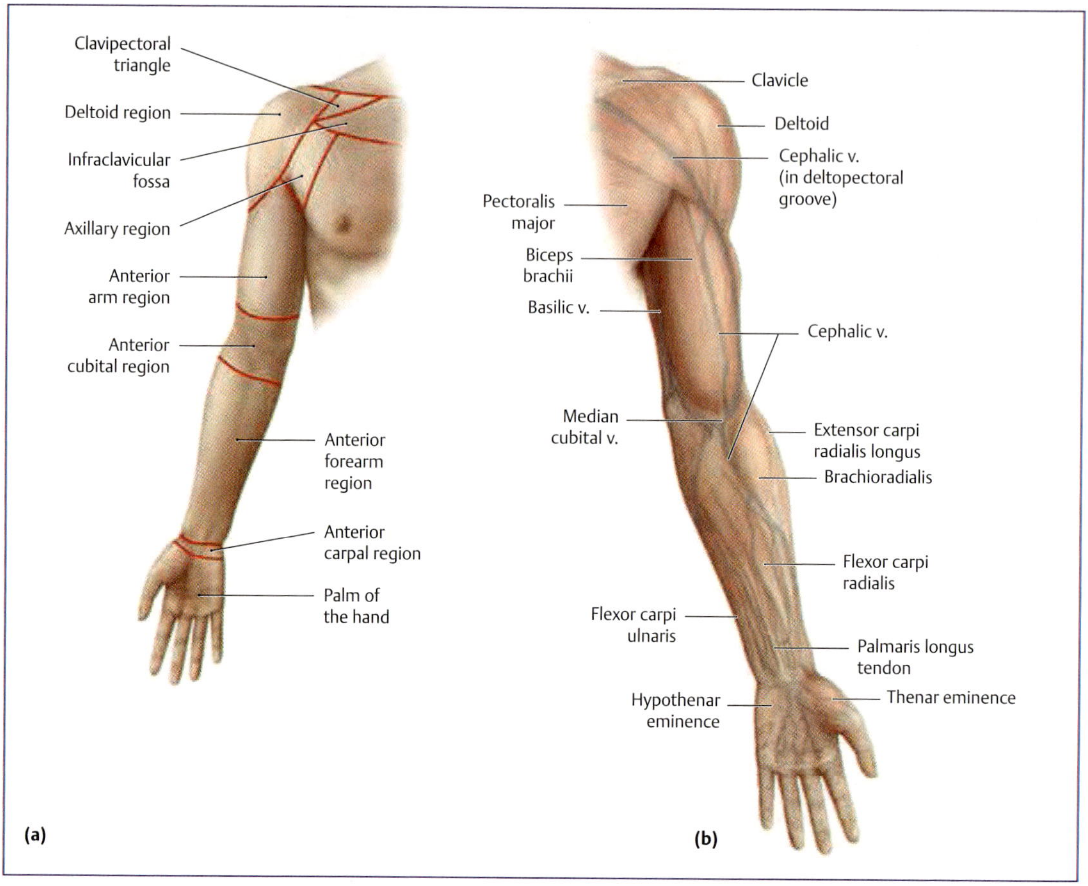

Fig. 5.1 Surface landmarks, anterior compartment of the arm and cubital fossa. **(a)** Regions of the upper limb (right limb, anterior view). **(b)** Palpable musculature of the upper limb (right limb, anterior view).

Dissection and Identification

Skin Incisions

Let the incision C along the anterior axillary fold reaching the arm be continued subsequently along the midline of the arm and then the forearm (refer to **Fig. 2.1**).

1. Remove the brachial fascia over the underlying muscles. Note the presence of the *medial and lateral intermuscular septa.*
2. Use your fingers to separate the three muscles in the anterior/flexor compartment of the arm. These are the coracobrachialis, biceps brachii and brachialis (**Fig. 5.2**).

   https://www.winkingskull.com/dissector/V1/video.aspx?vid=254
3. The biceps brachii has two heads: short and long. *Its short head* arises from the coracoid process of the scapula, while its *long head* arises from the supraglenoid tubercle of the scapula.
4. The long head of the biceps brachii is tendinous. It courses through the intertubercular sulcus, under the *transverse humeral ligament*. At this stage, do not trace it to the scapular attachment.
5. Identify the biceps tendon at the elbow. It is attached to the radial tuberosity. Biceps brachii is a powerful supinator of the forearm and flexor of the elbow joint.
6. *Bicipital aponeurosis*: Identify it as a broad extension from the medial side of the biceps tendon which blends with the deep fascia of the forearm.
7. Find the *musculocutaneous nerve* in the axilla (**Fig. 5.3**). Follow it as it pierces the *coracobrachialis muscle*. Note that the musculocutaneous nerve supplies the three muscles of the anterior compartment of the arm.
8. Use your finger to trace the proximal attachment of the coracobrachialis to the coracoid process and the distal attachment to the medial aspect of the shaft of the humerus.

   https://www.winkingskull.com/dissector/V1/video.aspx?vid=256

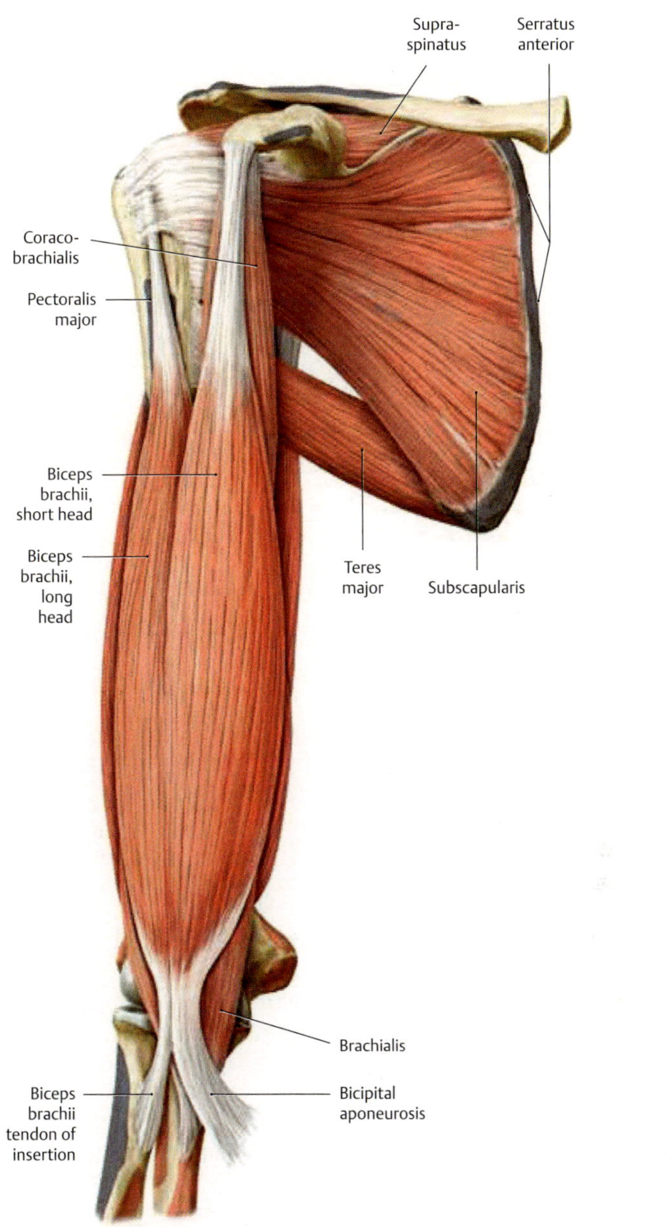

Fig. 5.2 Muscles of the anterior/flexor compartment of the arm.

9. Now follow the musculocutaneous nerve as it emerges from the coracobrachialis. It then passes between the biceps brachii and brachialis, supplying both muscles (pays the tax of passing through them).
10. Beyond this, the musculocutaneous nerve continues as the *lateral cutaneous nerve* of the forearm. In the cubital fossa, it emerges on the lateral side, proximal to the tendon of the biceps brachii.
11. At this stage, transect the biceps brachii about 5 cm above the elbow using a pair of scissors, saving the musculocutaneous nerve. Reflect the two parts of the biceps.
12. Note the *brachialis* muscle deep to the biceps brachii muscle. It arises from the anterior aspect of the lower half of the humerus and is attached distally to the coronoid process of the ulna.

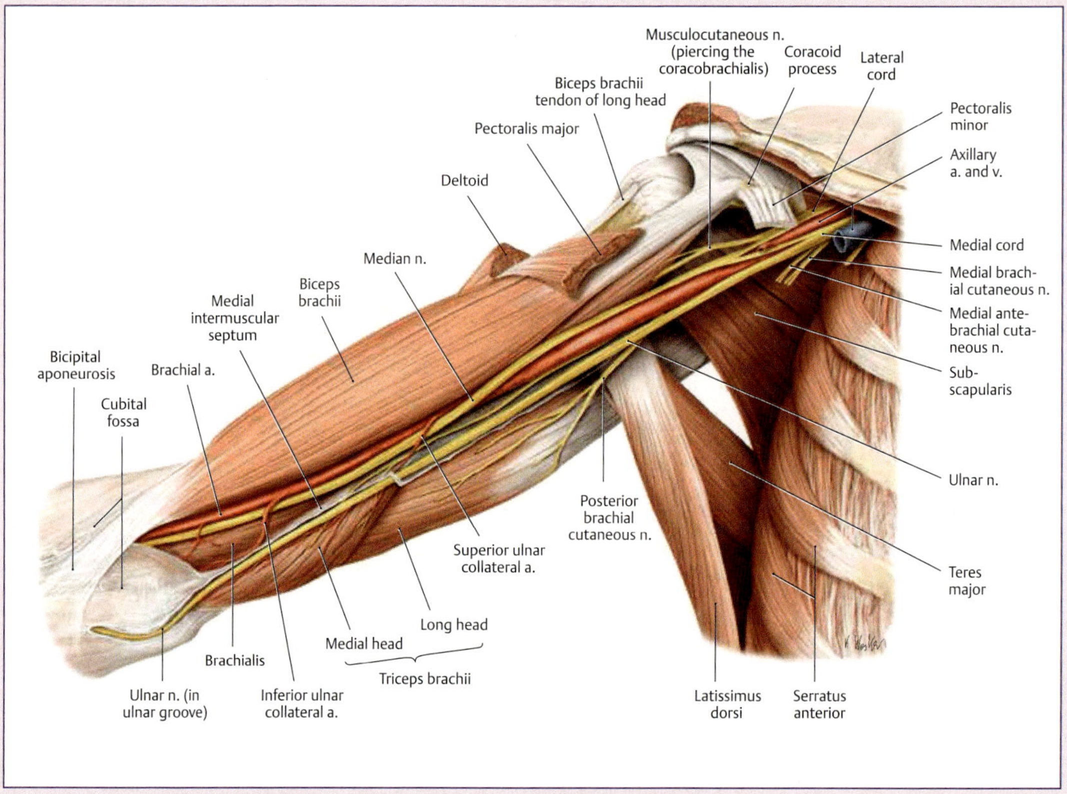

Fig. 5.3 Topography of the right arm (anterior view) and cubital fossa.

13. Trace the *medial cutaneous nerve* of the forearm from the axilla to the elbow. Note its proximity to the basilic vein.
14. Follow the *median nerve* where it arises from the union of the medial and lateral roots; trace it to the cubital fossa (**Fig. 5.3**).
15. Using blunt dissection, trace the *ulnar nerve* from the medial cord of the brachial plexus to the back of the medial epicondyle of the humerus. At the midarm level, the ulnar nerve pierces the medial intermuscular septum to enter the posterior compartment. It can be felt in a living being behind the medial epicondyle of the humerus.
16. Follow the *brachial artery* as it begins (as a continuation of the axillary artery) at the inferior border of the teres major muscle (**Fig. 5.4**). It terminates at the elbow by dividing into its two terminal branches, the *ulnar artery* and *radial artery*. Note the relationship of the median nerve with the brachial artery. The median nerve crosses in front of the artery from the lateral to the medial side.

   https://www.winkingskull.com/dissector/V1/video.aspx?vid=255
17. Trace the branches of the brachial artery. There are three branches: (a) *profunda brachii artery*, (b) *superior ulnar collateral artery* and (c) *inferior ulnar collateral artery*. In addition, there are numerous muscular branches.
18. In the upper part, trace the *profunda brachii artery* arising from the brachial artery. It soon courses to the posterior side in company with the radial nerve in the *spiral/radial groove*. We will learn about it when we deal with the posterior compartment of the arm.
19. The *superior ulnar collateral artery* arises from the brachial artery at the midarm level, then courses with the ulnar nerve passing behind the medial epicondyle of the humerus. It anastomoses with the *posterior ulnar recurrent artery*.
20. Follow the *inferior ulnar collateral artery* arising from the brachial artery about 3 cm above the medial epicondyle of the humerus. It then passes anterior to the medial epicondyle and anastomoses with the *anterior ulnar recurrent artery*.

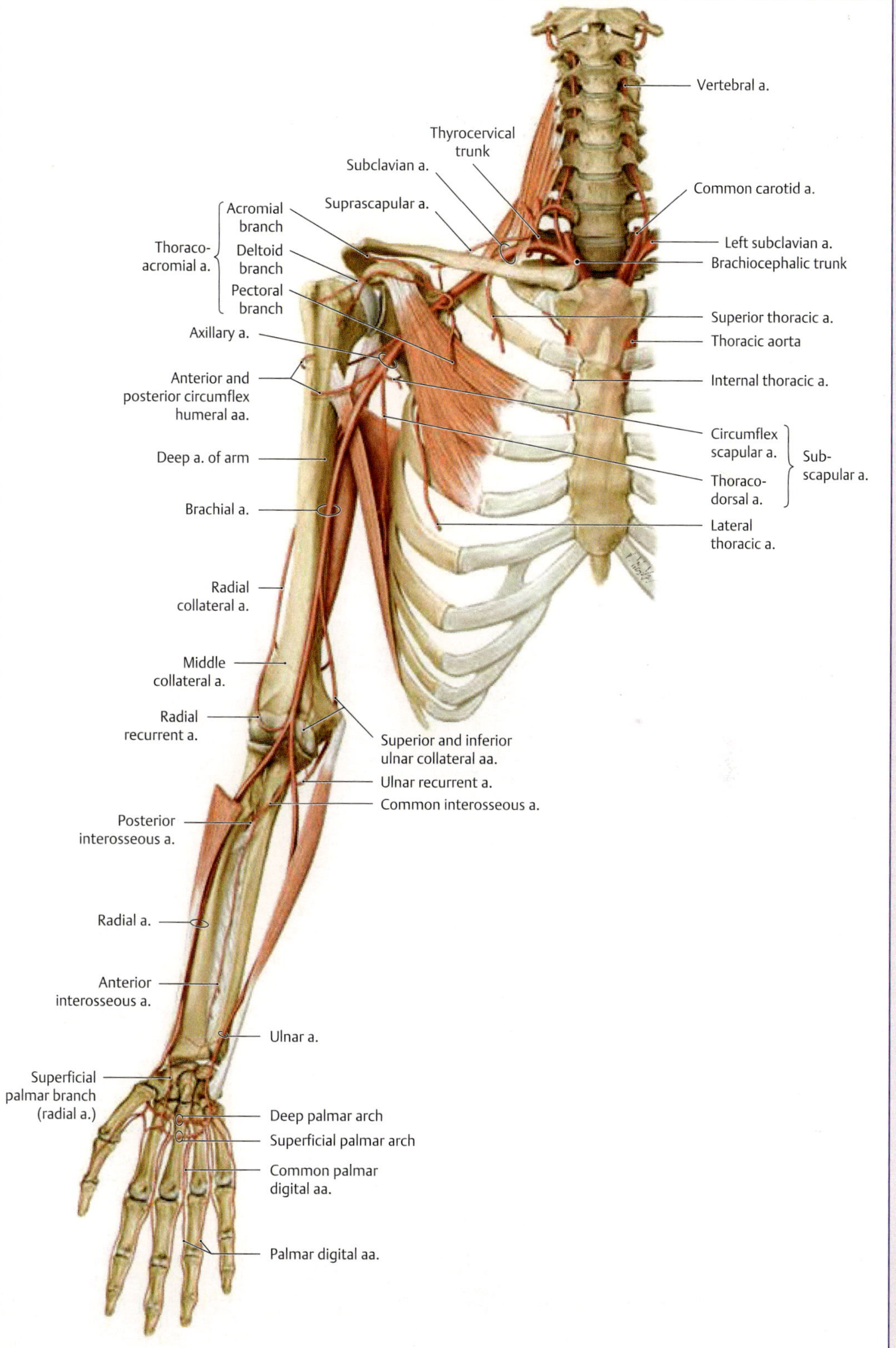

Fig. 5.4 Arteries of the upper limb.

Muscles of the Anterior Compartment of the Arm

An overview of the muscles of the anterior compartment of the arm is given in **Table 5.1** (**Figs. 5.5–5.7**).

Table 5.1 Muscles of the anterior compartment of the arm

Name of muscle	Origin	Insertion	Nerve supply	Main action
Biceps brachii (**Fig. 5.5**)	*Long head:* Supraglenoid tubercle *Short head:* Tip of the coracoid process	Radial tuberosity and bicipital aponeurosis to the forearm fascia	Musculocutaneous nerve	Supination at the radioulnar joint, flexion at the elbow joint
Coracobrachialis (**Fig. 5.6**)	Tip of the coracoid process	Medial surface of the humerus in the middle portion	Musculocutaneous nerve	Flexion and adduction at the shoulder joint
Brachialis (**Fig. 5.7**)	Lower part of the anterior surface of the humerus	Coronoid process and ulnar tuberosity	Musculocutaneous nerve and radial nerve	Flexion at the elbow joint

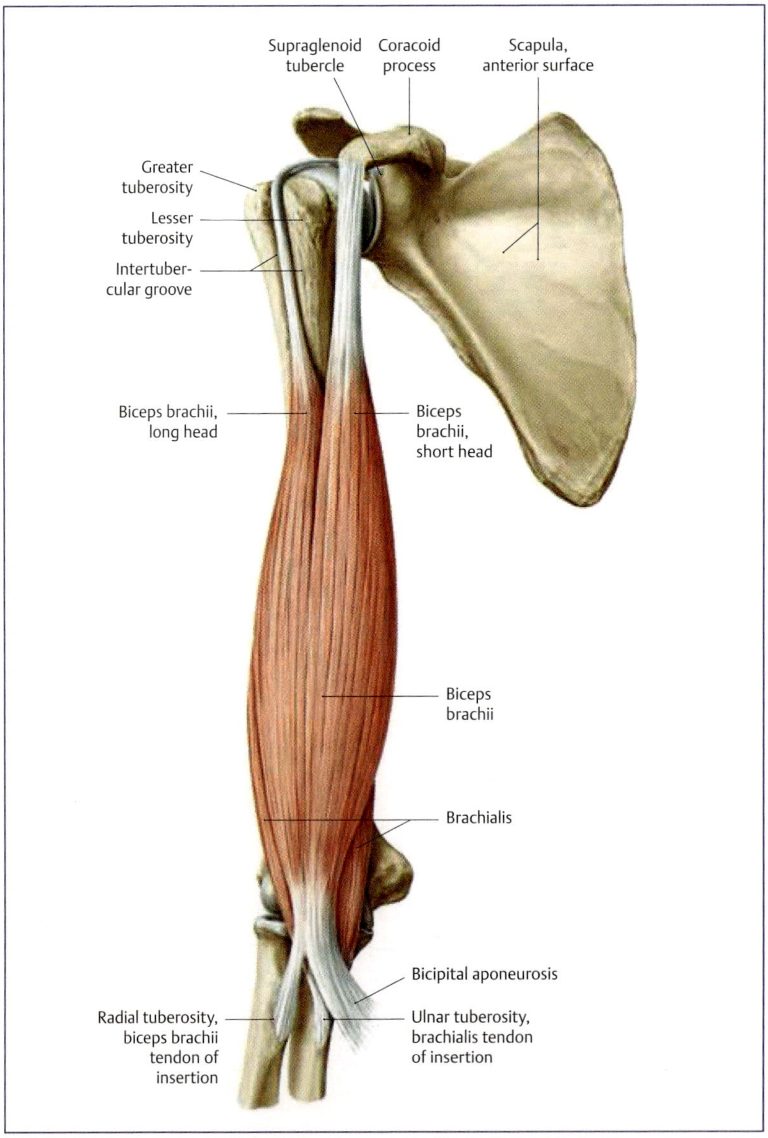

Fig. 5.5 Biceps brachii.

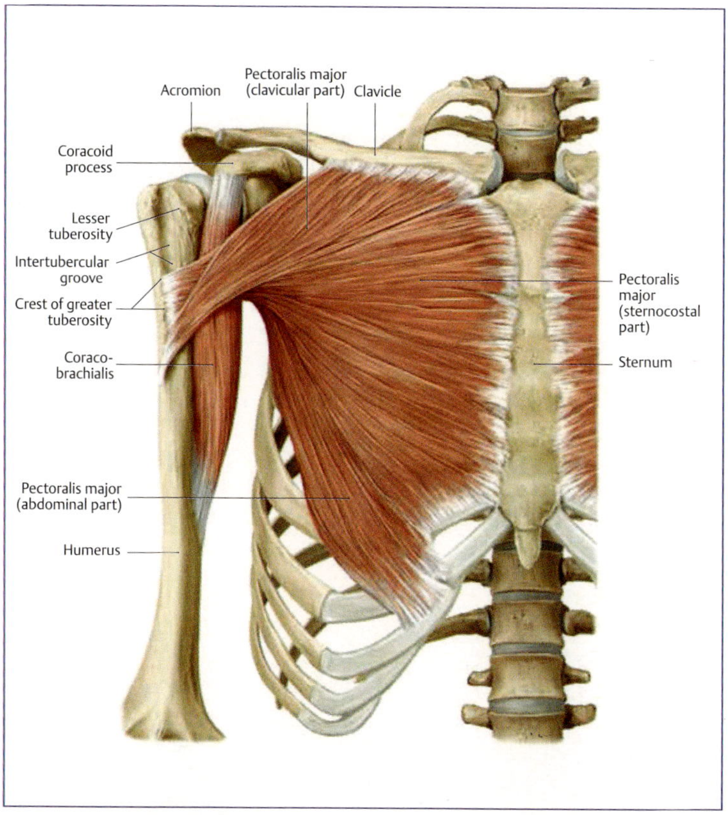

Fig. 5.6 Coracobrachialis.

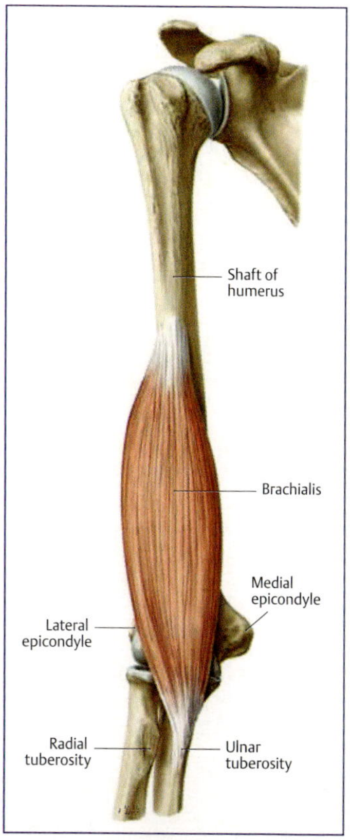

Fig. 5.7 Brachialis.

Arteries of the Anterior Compartment of the Arm

The origin and course of the arteries of the anterior compartment of the arm is summarized in **Table 5.2** (refer to **Fig. 5.4**).

Table 5.2 Arteries of the anterior compartment of the arm

Artery	Origin	Course
Profunda brachii	Brachial artery	Runs in the radial groove of the humerus along with the radial nerve
Superior ulnar collateral	Brachial artery	Anastomoses with the posterior ulnar recurrent artery on the dorsal aspect of the medial epicondyle
Inferior ulnar collateral	Brachial artery	Anastomoses with the anterior ulnar recurrent artery in front of the medial epicondyle

Nerves of the Anterior Compartment of the Arm

The nerves of the anterior compartment of the arm are given in **Table 5.3** (refer to **Fig. 5.3**).

Table 5.3 Nerves of the anterior compartment of the arm

Name of nerve	Source with root value	Course	Distribution
Musculocutaneous	Lateral cord of the brachial plexus, C5–C7	Enters the arm by piercing the coracobrachialis followed by course between the biceps brachii and brachialis muscles, finally continues as the lateral cutaneous nerve of the forearm	Coracobrachialis, biceps brachii, brachialis and lateral forearm skin
Medial cutaneous nerve of the arm	Medial cord of the brachial plexus (C8, T1)	It runs along the axillary artery	Skin of the medial side of the arm

Cubital Fossa

Introduction

The cubital fossa is a triangular depression on the anterior aspect of the elbow. It is clinically significant because it contains superficial veins which are used for venipuncture. It also has significant nerves and vessels in it. The brachial artery in cubital fossa is used for recording blood pressure.

Dissection and Identification

https://www.winkingskull.com/dissector/V1/video.aspx?vid=257

1. Note the positions of the cephalic and basilic veins and the interconnecting *median cubital vein*. In order to have better access to the contents of the cubital fossa, if necessary, cut the median cubital vein and retract the cut ends medially and laterally. Identify/define the boundaries of the cubital fossa (**Figs. 5.8a–c**).

   https://www.winkingskull.com/dissector/V1/video.aspx?vid=258

   - *Medial boundary*: Pronator teres muscle.
   - *Lateral boundary*: Brachioradialis muscle.
   - *Superior boundary*: An imaginary line joining the medial and lateral epicondyles of the humerus.
2. *Roof*: The skin, superficial fascia and deep fascia. The latter is reinforced by the bicipital aponeurosis.
3. *Floor*: Brachialis and supinator muscles.
4. Identify the tendon of the biceps brachii in the fossa.
5. Cut the bicipital aponeurosis close to the tendon and reflect it medially. Avoid injury to the brachial artery as it lies deep to the bicipital aponeurosis.
6. Trace the *median nerve* and *brachial artery* from the arm to the cubital fossa.

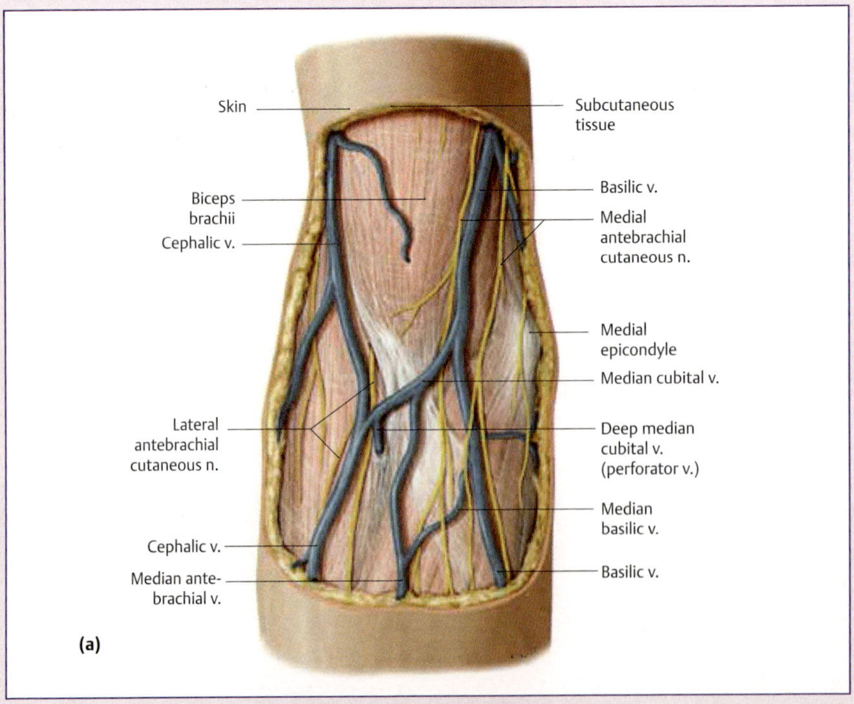

Fig. 5.8 Cubital fossa. **(a)** Cutaneous neurovascular structures in the cubital fossa.

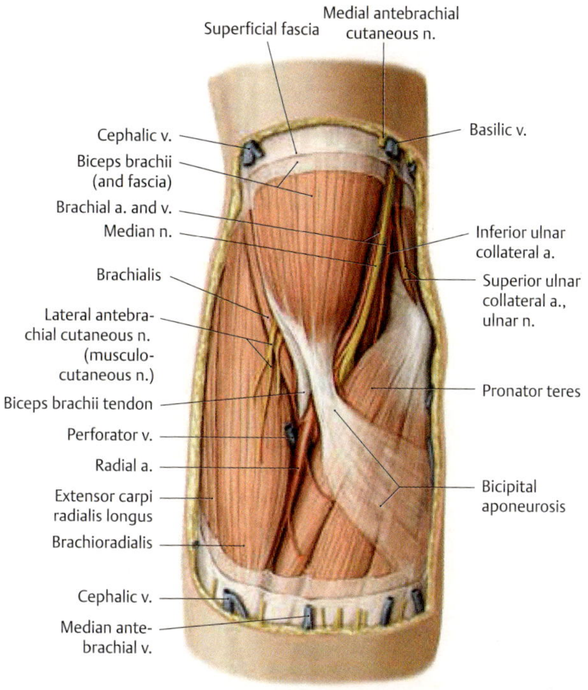

(b)

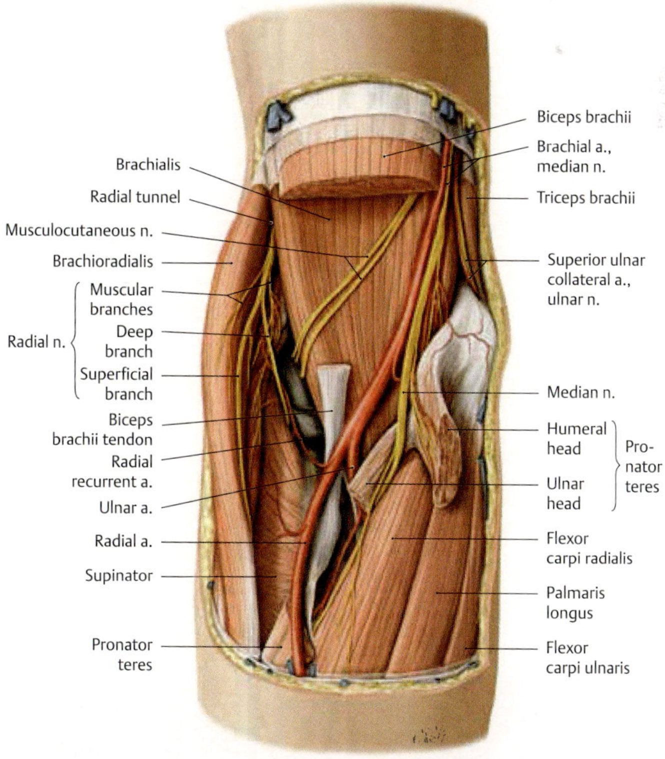

(c)

Fig. 5.8 Cubital fossa. **(b)** Superficial cubital fossa. **(c)** Deep cubital fossa.

10. Note the relationship of the three important structures from the *lateral to the medial* side. These are as follows:

    https://www.winkingskull.com/dissector/V1/video.aspx?vid=259

    - Tendon of the biceps brachii (lateral)
    - Brachial artery (intermediate)
    - Median nerve (medial)
11. Note that the bicipital aponeurosis passes superficial to the brachial artery and median nerve but deep to the *median cubital vein*. The median cubital vein is supported by the aponeurosis.

Clinical Notes

1. The median cubital vein is used for venipuncture and for giving intravenous injections.
2. The brachial artery is used for recording blood pressure.
3. The ulnar nerve can be palpated behind the medial epicondyle of the humerus and is thickened in *leprosy*.

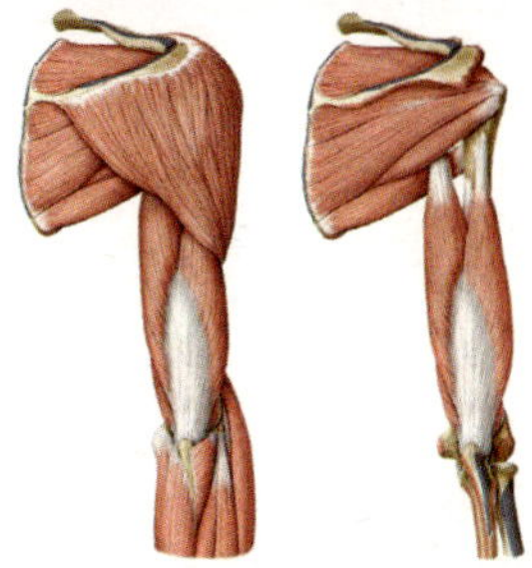

CHAPTER 6

Posterior Compartment of the Arm

Learning Objectives

At the end of the dissection of the posterior compartment of the arm, students should be able to identify the following:

- *Muscles*: Triceps brachii and anconeus.
- *Vessels*: Profunda brachii artery.
- *Nerves*: Radial nerve and ulnar nerve.

Introduction

Posterior compartment of the arm is located on the back of the humerus and is occupied by the muscle bulk of triceps brachii accompanied by the small anconeus muscle. Both are extensors of the elbow joint, the former being the chief extensor and the latter being the weak extensor (anconeus). The radial nerve accompanied by the profunda brachii vessels runs in the spiral groove on the back of the humerus placed between the lateral and medial heads of the triceps brachii muscle to which it supplies.

Surface Landmarks (Fig. 6.1)

1. *Triceps brachii*: The prominence of the muscle bulk of the three heads of the triceps can be seen to olecranon.
2. *Olecranon process of the ulna* presents as a bony prominence at the lower end of the back of the arm.

Dissection and Identification

1. Place the body in prone position with the arm medially rotated to have a better access.
2. *Incision*: With the help of a pair of scissors, open the posterior compartment by giving a longitudinal cut through the deep fascia of the arm from the olecranon of the ulna to the distal attachment of the teres minor muscle (back of the greater tubercle of the humerus). Detach the fascia from the medial and lateral intermuscular septa.
3. Observe the three heads of the *triceps brachii*. The *long head* descends from the infraglenoid tubercle of the scapula to which it is attached. The *lateral head* is attached to the back of the

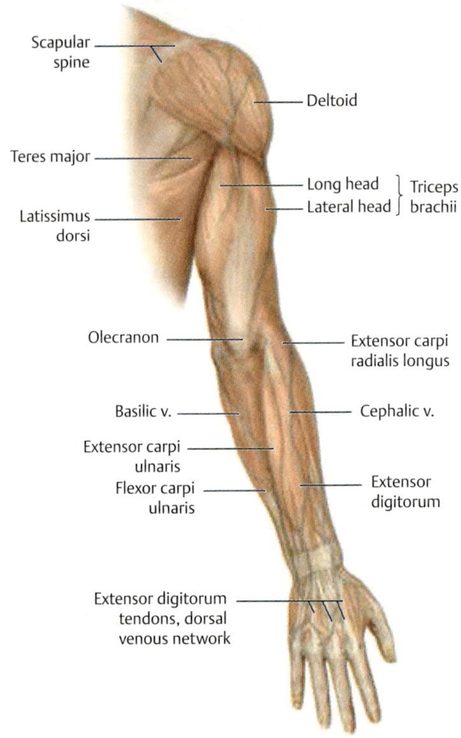

Fig. 6.1 Palpable musculature of the upper limb (right limb, posterior view).

humerus just outside the spiral groove. The *medial head* has an extensive attachment along the back of the humerus medial to the spiral groove and the area below (**Figs. 6.2** and **6.3**).

https://www.winkingskull.com/dissector/V1/video.aspx?vid=253

4. Trace the distal attachment of the triceps to the top of the olecranon process of the ulna.
5. Using your fingers, separate the long head of the triceps from the lateral head. Note that the teres major crosses anteriorly to the long head of the triceps.
6. Note that below the inferior border of the teres major is an opening between the long and lateral heads of the triceps (the triangular space). With the help of a probe, widen this opening and identify the *radial nerve* and the *profunda brachii artery* (refer to **Fig. 4.3**).
7. Negotiate the probe along the course of the radial nerve. It now lies between the lateral head of the triceps and the underlying humerus.
8. Transect the lateral head of the triceps brachii over the probe. This separates the lateral head from the medial head of the triceps. This reveals the contents of the radial/spiral groove, that is, the radial nerve and profunda brachii artery.
9. Using the probe, clean the radial nerve and profunda brachii artery. Both structures are in direct contact with the bone.
10. Trace the radial nerve towards the elbow. Now turn your attention to the lateral boundary of the cubital fossa. Locate the brachioradialis forming this boundary. Put your finger between the brachioradialis and brachialis; embedded in the connective tissue between these muscles is the radial nerve. Trace it proximally towards the lower end of the spiral/radial groove.
11. Note that at the level of the elbow, the radial nerve is placed on the flexor side and is accompanied by the *radial recurrent artery*.
12. Now identify the *anconeus muscle* arising from the back of the lateral epicondyle of the humerus, passing obliquely downwards and medially to be attached to the lateral surface of the olecranon process of the ulna. It is the weak extensor of the elbow joint.

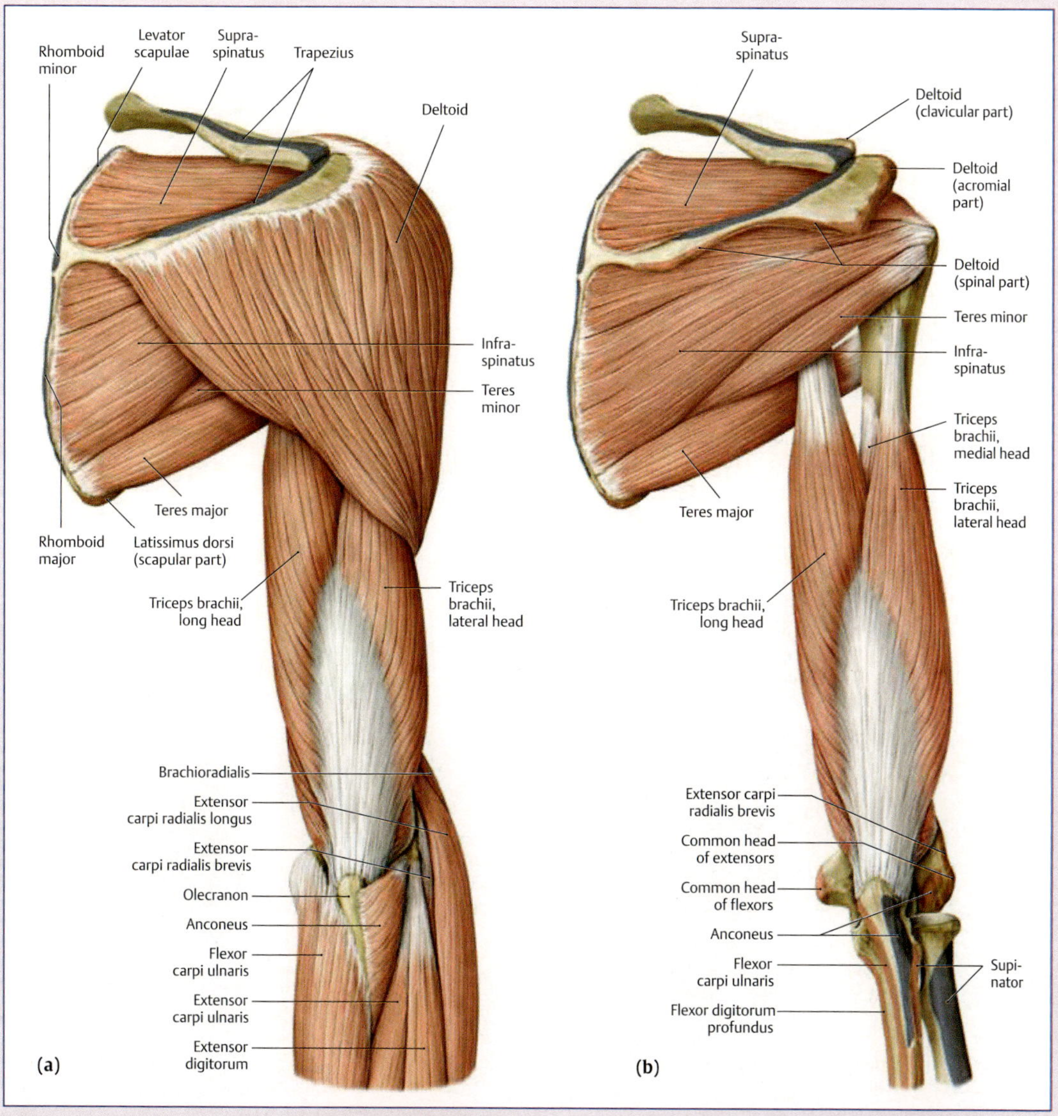

Fig. 6.2 Posterior muscles of the shoulder and posterior compartment of the arm. **(a)** *Removed*: Rhomboids major and minor, serratus anterior and levator scapulae. **(b)** *Removed*: Deltoid and forearm muscles.

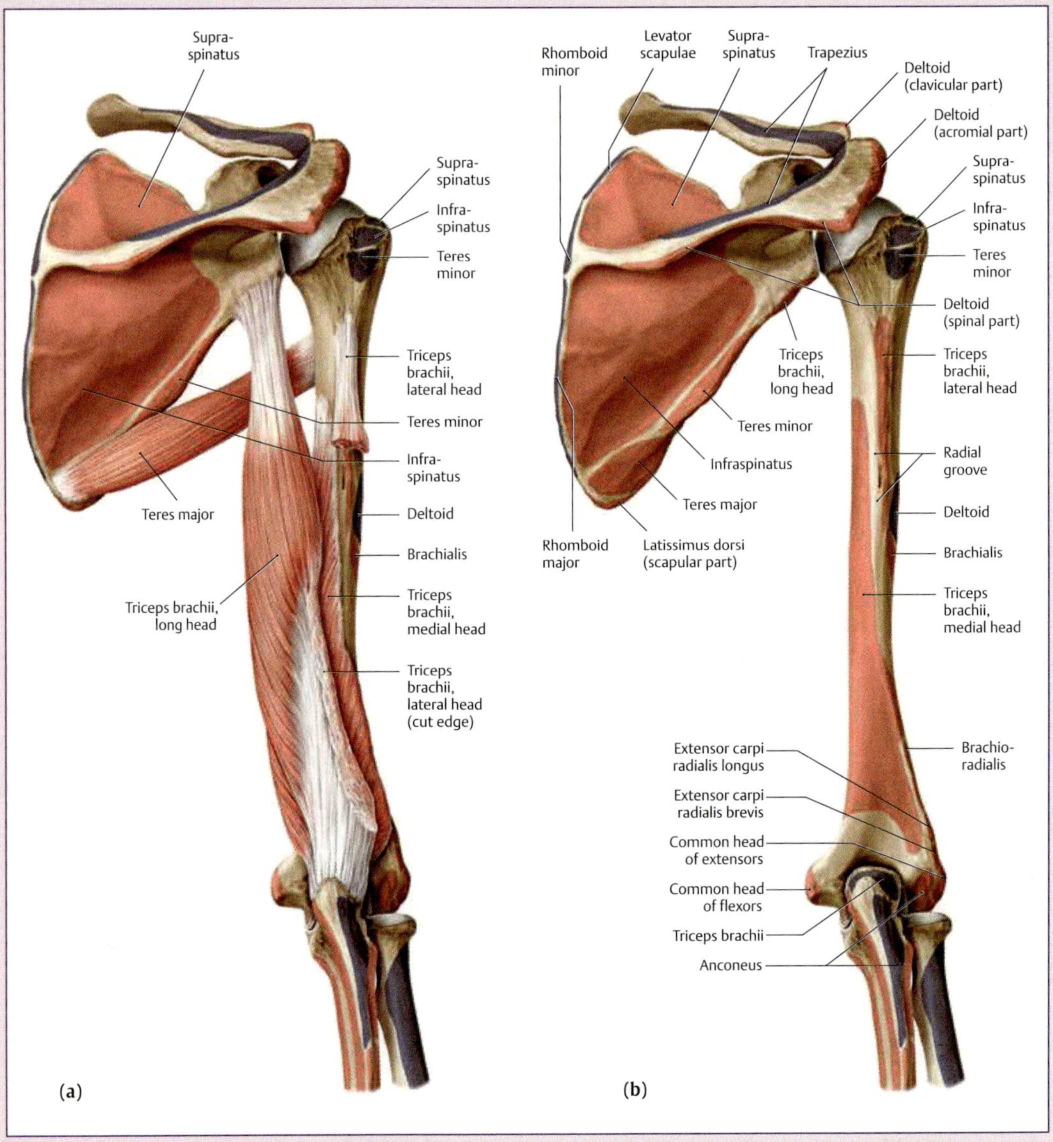

Fig. 6.3 Muscles of the posterior compartment of the arm. **(a)** Lateral head of triceps brachii removed to expose the medial head. **(b)** Bony attachment of the three heads of triceps brachii.

Muscles of the Posterior Compartment of the Arm

Table 6.1 provides an overview of the muscles of the posterior compartment of the arm (**Fig. 6.3**).

Table 6.1 Muscles of the posterior compartment of the arm

Name of muscle	Origin	Insertion	Nerve supply	Action/Function
Triceps brachii	*Long head*: Infraglenoid tubercle of the scapula *Lateral head*: Posterior surface of the humerus above the radial groove *Medial head:* Posterior surface of the humerus below the radial groove	Upper end of the olecranon process of the ulna	Radial nerve	Extension at the elbow joint
Anconeus	Lateral epicondyle of the humerus	Olecranon process of the ulna extending to the upper part of the ulna	Radial nerve	Extension at the elbow joint

Nerves of the Posterior Compartment of the Arm

Table 6.2 provides an overview of the nerves of the posterior compartment of the arm.

Table 6.2 Nerves of the posterior compartment of the arm

Name of nerve	Source with root value	Course	Distribution
Radial nerve	Branch of the posterior cord (C5–T1)	First passes posterior to the axillary artery, enters the posterior compartment of the arm with the profunda brachii artery in the radial groove, pierces the lateral intermuscular septum and enters cubital fossa and terminates into deep and superficial radial nerves	Muscles of the posterior compartment of the arm and forearm Cutaneous branches: Posterior and inferolateral parts of the arm, posterior forearm and lateral part of the dorsum of the hand up to the axial line of the fourth digit

Vessels of the Posterior Compartment of the Arm

Table 6.3 provides an overview of the vessels of the posterior compartment of the arm.

Table 6.3 Vessels of the posterior compartment of the arm (refer to **Fig. 4.3**)

Artery	Origin	Course
Profunda brachii artery	Brachial artery	Runs over the radial groove of the humerus along with the radial nerve

Clinical Notes

1. The radial nerve may be damaged in the midshaft fracture involving the humerus, leading to wrist drop.
2. The ulnar nerve can be palpated behind the medial epicondyle of the humerus.
3. The intramuscular injections can be given in the triceps.

CHAPTER 7

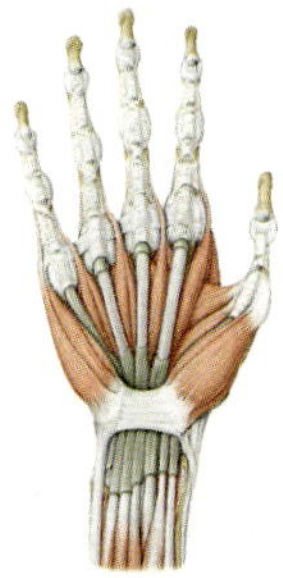

Flexor Compartment of the Forearm and Palm

Learning Objectives

At the end of the dissection of the flexor compartment of the forearm and palm, students should be able to identify, understand and correlate the following:

Muscles

- *Superficial group*: Pronator teres, flexor carpi radialis, palmaris longus and flexor carpi ulnaris.
- *Intermediate group*: Flexor digitorum superficialis.
- *Deep group*: Flexor pollicis longus, flexor digitorum profundus and pronator quadratus.
- *Nerves*: Median nerve and its branches, ulnar nerve and its branches, anterior interosseous nerve and cutaneous nerves (medial and lateral cutaneous nerves of the forearm).
- *Vessels*: Radial artery and its branches, ulnar artery and its branches, cephalic vein and basilic vein.

Introduction

The forearm extends from the elbow to the wrist. It has two bones, the radius laterally and the ulna medially. The deep fascia in this region (antebrachial fascia) forms an envelope around the muscles and sends in intermuscular septa that reach the radius and ulna. Between these two bones runs an interosseous membrane. Anterior to it is the *anterior or flexor compartment* and posterior to it is the *posterior* or *extensor compartment of the forearm.*

The muscles in the anterior compartment are grouped as follows:

1. Superficial group
2. Intermediate group
3. Deep group of muscles

These muscles are supplied by median and *ulnar* nerves. Vessels in this compartment are the *radial artery*, *ulnar artery* and *anterior interosseous artery*. These arteries supply the structures in the flexor compartment.

Surface Landmarks (refer to Fig. 5.1)

1. Medial and lateral epicondyles of the humerus (refer to **Figs. 1.3** and **1.4**)
2. Radial head
3. Ulnar head at the lower end

4. Styloid processes of the radius and ulna
5. Tendon of the flexor carpi radialis (lateral to which the radial arterial pulsations can be felt in a living subject)

Dissection and Identification

1. Remove the superficial and deep fascia along the anterior side of the forearm, preserving the cephalic and basilic veins. After an initial cut, separate the fascia from the underlying muscles by using your fingers, that is, blunt dissection.
2. Identify the *four* muscles of the superficial group (**Fig. 7.1**):

   https://www.winkingskull.com/dissector/V1/video.aspx?vid=260

   - *Pronator teres* runs obliquely from its attachment to the lower part of the humerus and upper end of the ulna towards the radius midway down the shaft. The *median nerve* enters the forearm between the *two heads of the pronator teres muscle.*
3. Identify the *common flexor tendon* arising from the medial epicondyle of the humerus. This is the common origin (proximal attachment) of the superficial group of muscles.
   Let us identify the other muscles in the superficial group.
   - *Flexor carpi radialis* is attached distally to the base of the second metacarpal.
   - *Palmaris longus* is attached distally to the *palmar aponeurosis.* It is believed that the palmar aponeurosis is a flattened tendon of the palmaris longus.
   - *Flexor carpi ulnaris* is attached distally to the pisiform bone. Pisiform is regarded as a sesamoid bone in the tendon of the flexor carpi ulnaris muscle. Distal to pisiform, the pisohamate and pisometacarpal ligaments are believed to be the morphologically degenerated parts of the flexor carpi ulnaris muscle.

   The anterior aspect of the wrist shows the following structures (**Fig. 7.1**) from the lateral to the medial side:

1. Radial artery
2. Tendon of the flexor carpi radialis
3. Tendon of the palmaris longus
4. Tendons of the flexor digitorum superficialis
5. Ulnar artery
6. Ulnar nerve
7. Tendon of the flexor carpi ulnaris

Feel the pulsations of the radial artery on your wrist lateral to the tendon of the flexor carpi radialis. The ulnar nerve and artery can be palpated close to the pisiform bone.

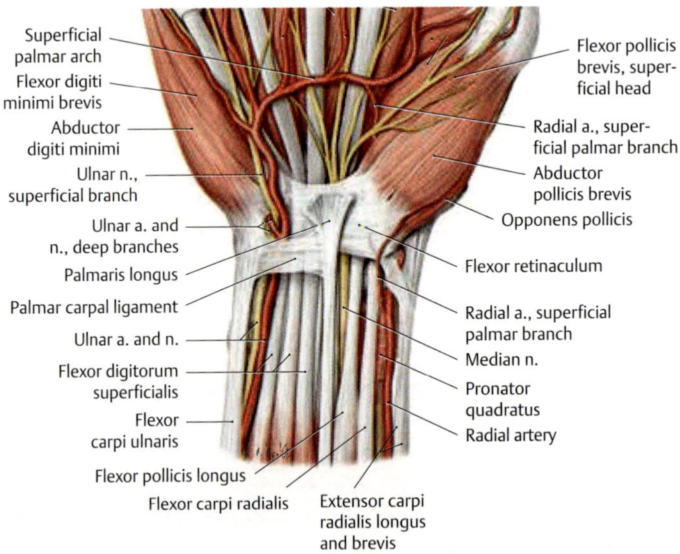

Fig. 7.1 Structures on the anterior aspect of the wrist.

Muscles of the Flexor Compartment of the Forearm

Superficial Layer

An overview of different muscles of the flexor compartment of the forearm is given in **Tables 7.1** to **7.3.**

Table 7.1 Muscles of the superficial layer of the forearm (**Fig. 7.2**)

Name of muscle	Origin	Insertion	Nerve supply	Action/Function
Pronator teres	*Humeral head*: Medial epicondyle of the humerus *Ulnar head*: Coronoid process	Middle of the lateral surface of the radius	Median nerve	Pronation and flexion at the elbow joint
Palmaris longus	Common flexor origin of the medial epicondyle of the humerus	Palmar aponeurosis	Median nerve	Weakly flexes the wrist and tightens the palmar aponeurosis
Flexor carpi radialis		Base of the second metacarpal	Median nerve	Flexion and abduction at the wrist joint
Flexor carpi ulnaris		Fifth metacarpal, hook of the hamate and pisiform bones	Ulnar nerve	Adduction and flexion at the wrist joint

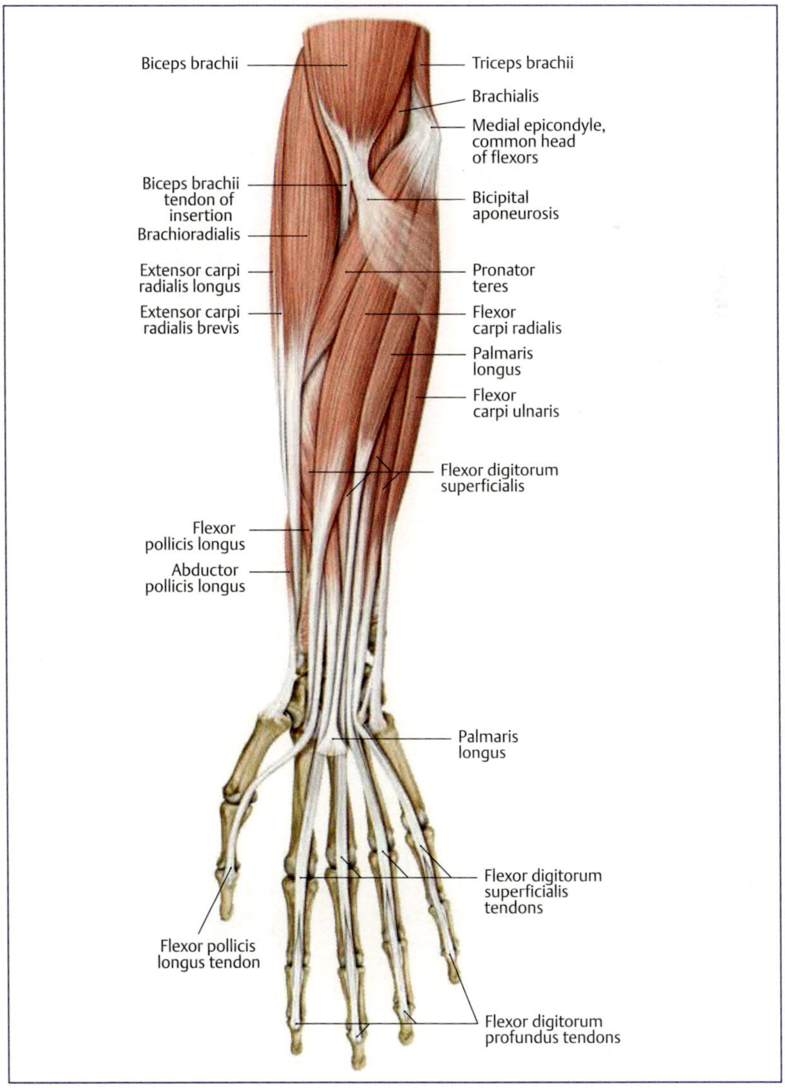

Fig. 7.2 Superficial layer of muscles of the flexor compartment of the forearm.

Dissection and Identification

The intermediate layer consists of *flexor digitorum superficialis* muscle. Reveal its tendons by using a pair of scissors (**Fig. 7.3**).

1. Cut the tendon of the *palmaris longus* about 5 cm above the wrist and reflect it upwards.
2. Cut across the tendon of the *flexor carpi radialis* about 5 cm above the wrist and reflect it upwards.

The flexor digitorum superficialis is attached proximally to the following:

1. Humerus via the common flexor origin.
2. Ulna at the upper end.
3. Linear attachment to an anterior oblique line of the radius. These attachments form a fibrous arch deep to which the ulnar artery and median nerve can be seen. The distal attachment of the four tendons is to the middle phalanges of two to five digits and shall be studied in Chapter 8.

Note the positions of the tendons of the *flexor digitorum superficialis at the wrist* with the *median nerve laterally and ulnar artery and nerve medially*.

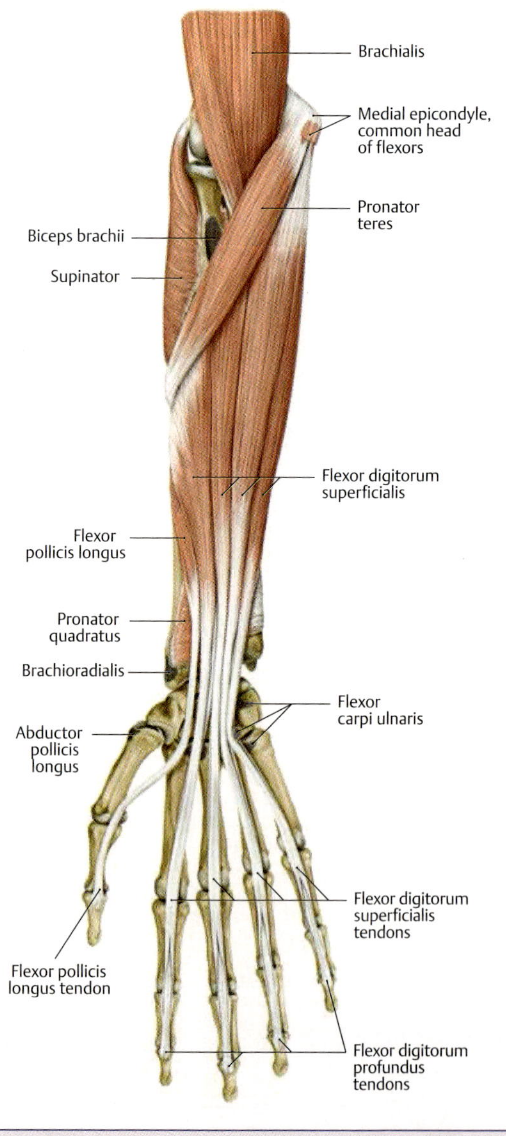

Fig. 7.3 Intermediate muscle layer of the flexor compartment of the forearm (pronator teres is also seen).

Intermediate Layer

An overview of flexor digitorum superficialis muscle is given in **Table 7.2**.

Table 7.2 Muscles of the intermediate layer of the forearm (**Fig. 7.3**)

Name of muscle	Origin	Insertion	Nerve supply	Action/Function
Flexor digitorum superficialis	*Radial head:* Anterior border (superior part) *Humeroulnar head*: Common flexor origin on the medial epicondyle and coronoid process	Middle phalanges of the medial four digits	Median nerve	Flexion at the proximal interphalangeal and metacarpophalangeal joints of the medial four digits

The muscles of the deep layer of the forearm are given in **Table 7.3**. To explore deep group of muscles, the flexor digitorum superficialis is removed, the steps towards this are given in following text.

Table 7.3 Muscles of the deep layer of the forearm (**Fig. 7.4**)

Name of muscle	Origin	Insertion	Nerve supply	Action/Function
Flexor digitorum profundus	Proximal three-fourths of the anterior and medial surfaces of the ulna along with the interosseous membrane	*Lateral part*: Bases of the distal phalanges of the second and third digits *Medial part:* Bases of the distal phalanges of the fourth and fifth digits	*Lateral part:* Anterior interosseous nerve from the median nerve *Medial part:* Ulnar nerve	*Lateral part:* Flexion at the second and third distal interphalangeal joints *Medial part:* Flexion at the fourth and fifth distal interphalangeal joints
Flexor pollicis longus	Anterior surface of the radius and interosseous membrane	Distal phalanx of the first digit (on the base of the thumb)	Anterior interosseous nerve from the median nerve	Flexion at the joints of the thumb
Pronator quadratus	Lower fourth of the ulna at the anterior surface	Lower fourth of the radius at the anterior surface	Anterior interosseous nerve from the median nerve	Pronation at the radioulnar joints

Dissection and Identification

Nerves and vessels in the flexor compartment of the forearm (**Fig. 7.5**):

https://www.winkingskull.com/dissector/V1/video.aspx?vid=262

1. *Superficial division (sensory) of the radial nerve*: To find this, identify the *brachioradialis* on the lateral side of the upper part of the forearm. Reach the point where the *pronator teres passes deep to this muscle.* Insert your finger to clear the connective tissue at this intermuscular plane to find the *superficial division of the radial nerve.* Trace it distally as it courses deep to the brachioradialis.
2. Identify the *brachial artery* in the cubital fossa. Trace it downwards as it bifurcates into the *radial* and *ulnar artery.*

Now using a probe and blunt dissection, trace the radial artery up to the wrist. The radial artery gives many unnamed branches to the muscles of the forearm.

3. *Radial recurrent artery*: It arises from the radial artery and takes a recurrent course, that is, passes upwards between the brachioradialis and brachialis. It anastomoses with the radial collateral branch of the profunda brachii artery, thus forming a part of the cubital anastomosis.
4. *Median nerve*: In the cubital fossa, we have seen the median nerve medial to the brachial artery. It enters the flexor compartment of the forearm between the two heads of the pronator teres. It then courses deep to the flexor digitorum superficialis muscle.

5. To trace the median nerve further, the *flexor digitorum superficialis* is retracted medially after cutting the tendons of this muscle with a pair of scissors, little above the wrist and detaching the muscle from the anterior oblique line of the radius.
6. Use a probe to clean the median nerve from the loose connective tissue as the nerve is traced distally. Trace the *muscular branches* to the (a) pronator teres, (b) palmaris longus, (c) flexor carpi radialis and (d) flexor digitorum superficialis muscles.
7. Identify the *anterior interosseous nerve* from the median nerve, which supplies the deep group of muscles of the flexor compartment.
8. Identify the *ulnar artery* in the cubital fossa. Observe that the artery passes posterior to the deep head of the pronator teres. To trace the artery, cut the deep head of the pronator teres with a pair of scissors protecting the artery. Clean the artery from the cubital fossa to the wrist.

Ulnar artery:

1. It passes posterior to the median nerve in the cubital fossa.
2. In the upper part of the forearm, it lies between the flexor digitorum superficialis and flexor digitorum profundus.

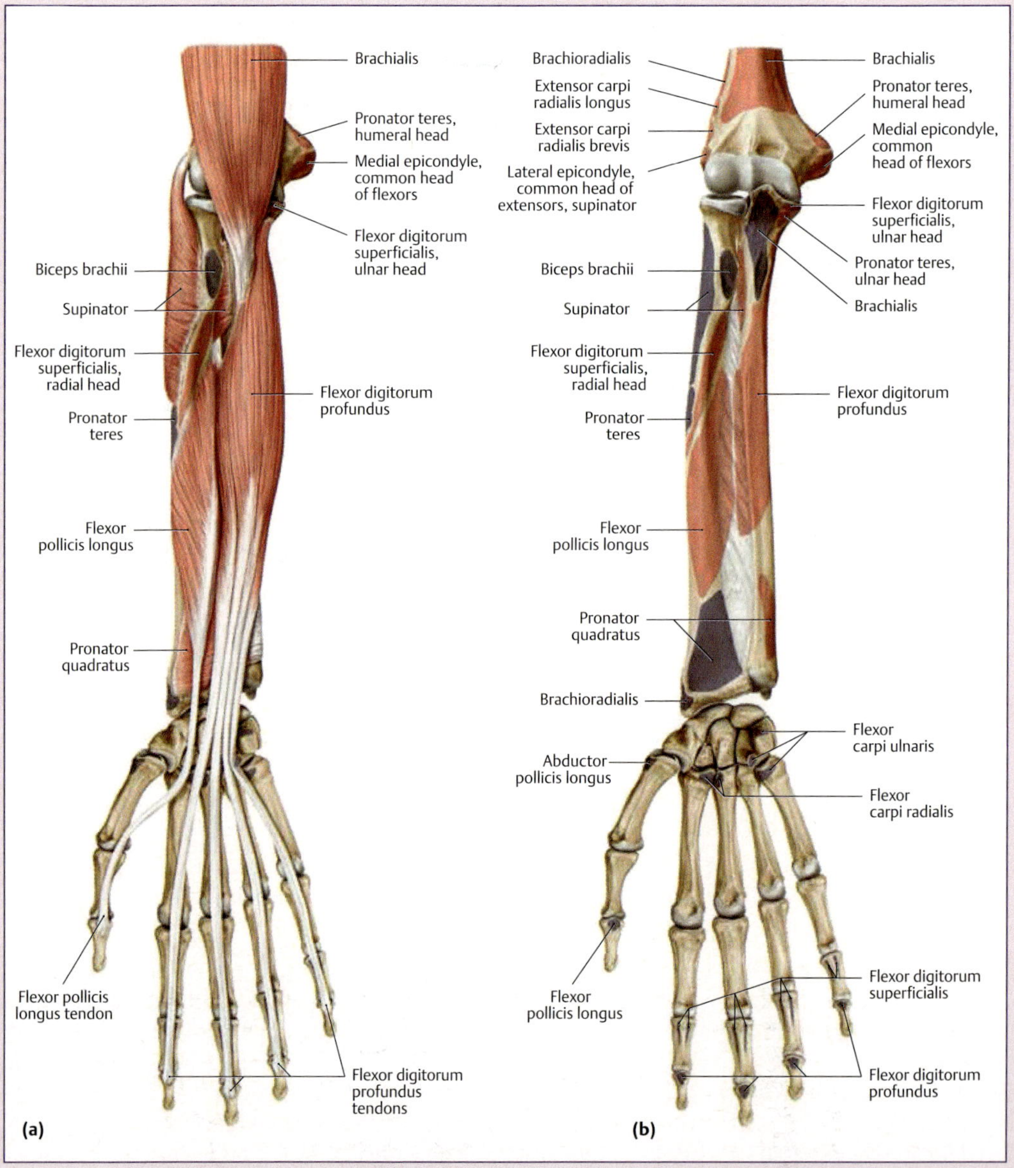

Fig. 7.4 **(a)** Muscles of the deep layer of the forearm. **(b)** Areas of bony attachments of the muscles of the deep layer of the forearm.

3. About one-third way down the forearm, it is joined by the ulnar nerve.
4. Both the ulnar artery and nerve lie deep to the flexor carpi ulnaris.
5. Both ulnar artery and nerve pass anterior to the flexor retinaculum (**Fig. 7.5**).

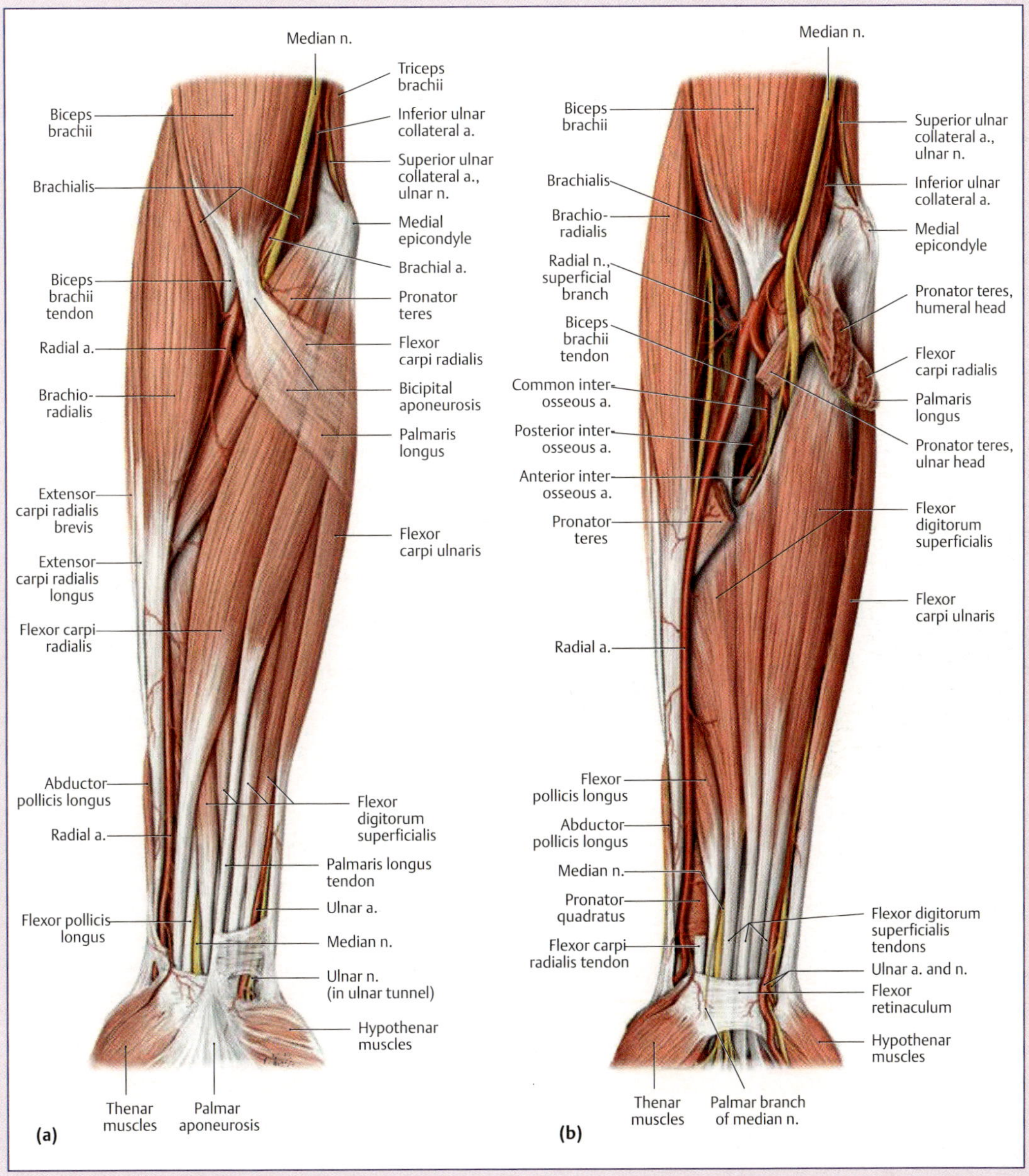

Fig. 7.5 Nerves and vessels of the forearm: **(a)** With muscles of the superficial layer intact and **(b)** with muscles of the intermediate layer intact.

Branches:

1. *Common interosseous artery*: It arises from the ulnar artery about 3 cm below its origin from brachial artery. Soon, it divides into the *anterior interosseous artery* and *posterior interosseous artery*. They pass on respective sides of the interosseous membrane. Trace the anterior interosseous artery with the anterior interosseous nerve between the flexor digitorum profundus (medial) and flexor pollicis longus (laterally) muscles. The posterior interosseous artery passes into the posterior compartment to supply the muscles in that compartment. At this stage, do not follow it.
2. *Anterior ulnar recurrent artery:* It arises from the ulnar artery in the upper part of the forearm and then takes recurrent course; passing upwards, it anastomoses with the inferior ulnar collateral artery, a branch of the brachial artery.

3. *Posterior ulnar recurrent artery*: It arises from the ulnar artery and passes upwards and anastomoses with the superior ulnar collateral artery, branch of the brachial artery.
4. *Muscular branches*: There are several muscular branches supplying the muscles of the flexor compartment.
5. *Ulnar nerve*: Passing behind the medial epicondyle of the humerus, the ulnar nerve enters the forearm piercing the flexor carpi ulnaris, and runs under the muscle. It supplies the flexor carpi ulnaris and medial (ulnar) half of the flexor digitorum profundus muscle. It passes anterior/superficial to the flexor retinaculum accompanied by the ulnar artery lateral to it. It supplies majority of the intrinsic muscles in the hand.

Nerves of the Forearm

Nerves of the forearm are summarized in **Table 7.4**.

Table 7.4 Nerves of the forearm

Name of nerve	Source with root value	Course in forearm
Median	By union of the medial and lateral roots from medial and lateral cords (C8–T1 and C6–C7, respectively)	Lies medial to the brachial artery at the elbow, descends down between the two heads of the pronator teres, then between the flexor digitorum superficialis and profundus, at the wrist joint traverses carpal tunnel
Anterior interosseous	Median nerve	Runs in the anterior aspect of the forearm between the flexor digitorum profundus and flexor pollicis longus
Palmar cutaneous branch (median)	Median nerve	Crosses over the flexor retinaculum at the wrist and supplies the palmar skin in the centre
Ulnar	Terminal branch of the medial cord (C8–T1, often C7)	Passes between the heads of the flexor carpi ulnaris, passing posterior to the medial epicondyle of the humerus, after traversing between the flexor carpi ulnaris and flexor digitorum profundus becomes superficial
Palmar cutaneous (ulnar)	Ulnar nerve	Runs down accompanying the ulnar artery and supplies medial one and half digit on palmar aspect
Dorsal cutaneous branch of the ulnar nerve	Ulnar nerve	Descends between the flexor carpi ulnaris and ulna, subcutaneous supplying the dorsal skin of medial one and half digit
Radial	Terminal branch of the posterior cord (C5–C8)	Gives terminal branches superficial and deep at the lateral humeral epicondyle anteriorly
Posterior cutaneous nerve of the forearm	Radial nerve	Runs down on the lateral side of the arm followed by the posterior side of the arm and subsequently the wrist
Superficial branch of the radial nerve	Terminal branch of the radial nerve	Passes between the brachioradialis and pronator teres, crosses over the anatomical snuff box and supplies the lateral three and half digits on the dorsum of the hand
Posterior interosseous nerve	Deep terminal branch of the radial nerve	Passes over the neck of the radius, enters the posterior compartment of the forearm piercing the supinator muscle and runs down over the interosseous membrane with the accompanying artery
Lateral cutaneous nerve of the forearm	Musculocutaneous nerve	Emerging between the brachialis and biceps brachii, accompanies the cephalic vein, runs down over the lateral aspect of the forearm
Medial cutaneous nerve of the forearm	Medial cord (C8–T1)	Becomes subcutaneous above the elbow, descends to the medial border of the forearm with the basilic vein

Clinical Notes

1. Pulsations of the radial artery can be palpated in front of the lower end of the radius just lateral to the tendon of the flexor carpi radialis muscle.
2. Pulsations of the ulnar artery can also be felt on careful palpation just lateral to the tendon of the flexor carpi ulnaris muscle.

Dissection of the Palm

Introduction

Deep to the skin of the palm, in the middle, the palmar fascia is thickened to form the *palmar aponeurosis*. It is thin over the *thenar and hypothenar eminence* formed by the *thenar* and *hypothenar muscles*, respectively. Deep to the palmar aponeurosis are tendons of the *flexor digitorum superficialis* and *profundus*. These muscles cause flexion of the digits. Deep to these are muscles causing adduction and abduction of the digits (interossei muscles).

Blood supply to the palm is furnished by two arterial arches, the *superficial palmar arch*, formed mainly by the ulnar artery, and the *deep palmar arch*, mainly derived from the radial artery. Nerves in this region are branches of the ulnar and median nerves.

Dissection and Identification (Figs. 7.6 and 7.7)

Skin incision (refer to **Fig. 2.1**):

1. In most cadavers, the hand is clenched. Make efforts to forcefully open it.
2. Make a vertical incision from the middle of the wrist to the base of the middle finger (incision E).
3. Take the transverse incision across bases of all the digits from the index to the little finger (incision F).
4. Make longitudinal incisions along the palmar surfaces of other digits, that is, from the index to the little fingers (incision G).
5. Remove the skin carefully from the palm and digits.
6. Immediately deep to the skin, there are digital vessels, nerves and fibrous digital sheaths.
7. Clean the fat over the palmar aponeurosis. Distally, it leads to *four longitudinal bands*. They blend with the fibrous digital sheaths at the proximal phalanx of each digit from the second to the fifth.
8. Observe the thin palmar fascia over the hypothenar eminence and *palmaris brevis* muscle superficial to it. It stretches from the medial edge of the palmar aponeurosis to the skin of the hypothenar eminence.
9. Detach the palmaris brevis from the palmar aponeurosis and retract it medially.
10. Trace the palmaris longus tendon from the forearm to the palmar aponeurosis.
11. Detach the palmar aponeurosis carefully from the proximal to the distal side avoiding injury to the deeper structures. During this, use the palmaris longus tendon to pull the palmar aponeurosis and complete the removal. Avoid injury to the superficial palmar arch which is immediately deep to the aponeurosis. Preserve the branch of the median nerve to the supplying thenar muscles.

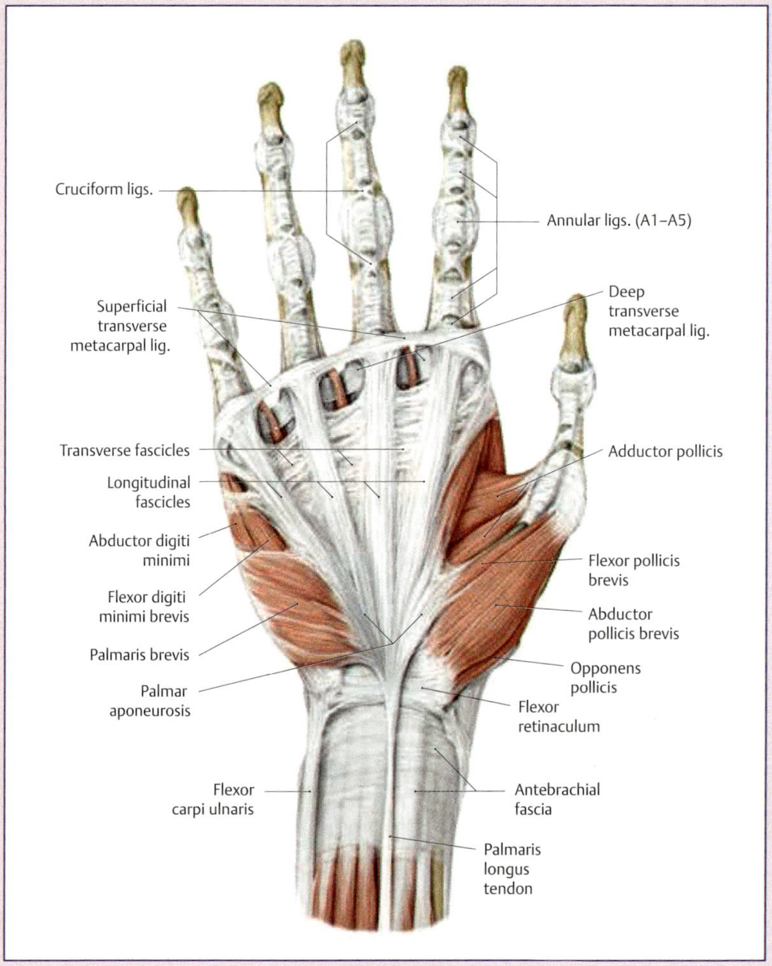

Fig. 7.6 Palmar aponeurosis.

Dissection and Identification

1. Trace the *ulnar artery* from the forearm into the palm using a probe as it passes lateral to the pisiform with the ulnar nerve. The *ulnar nerve* divides into the *superficial palmar branch* and *deep branch.*
2. The ulnar artery gives superficial palmar branch that crosses from the medial to the lateral side to form the *superficial palmar arch* along with the superficial palmar branch of the radial artery.
3. *Common palmar digital arteries*: They arise from the convexity of the superficial palmar arch, pass towards the webs between fingers and each then divides into *two palmar digital arteries* to supply adjacent sides of two digits. Trace the common palmar digital artery distally in proper digital arteries.
4. Trace the *ulnar nerve* lateral to the pisiform, using a probe. Dissect its *superficial branch* supplying the medial one and a half digits, that is, the medial side of little finger and adjacent side of little and ring fingers.
5. The *deep branch of the ulnar nerve* dips between the muscles of the hypothenar muscles (abductor and flexor of digit five). Do not trace it at this stage.

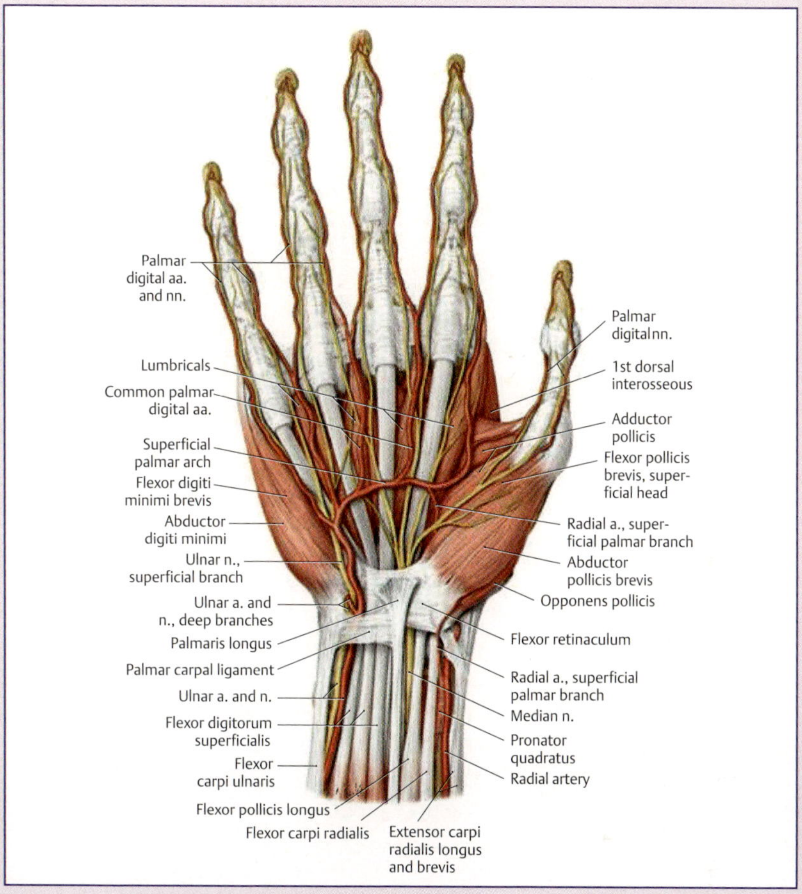

Fig. 7.7 Superficial palmar arch.

Carpal Tunnel

1. It is an osseofibrous tunnel formed by the *flexor retinaculum* anteriorly and the *carpal bones* posteriorly (**Fig. 7.8**).

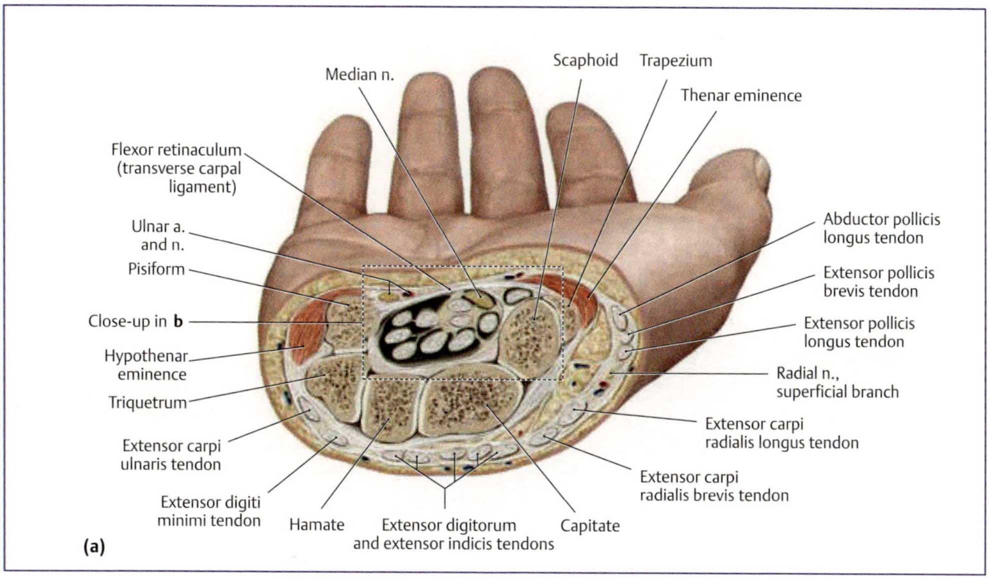

Fig. 7.8 Carpal tunnel: **(a)** Cross section through the right wrist.

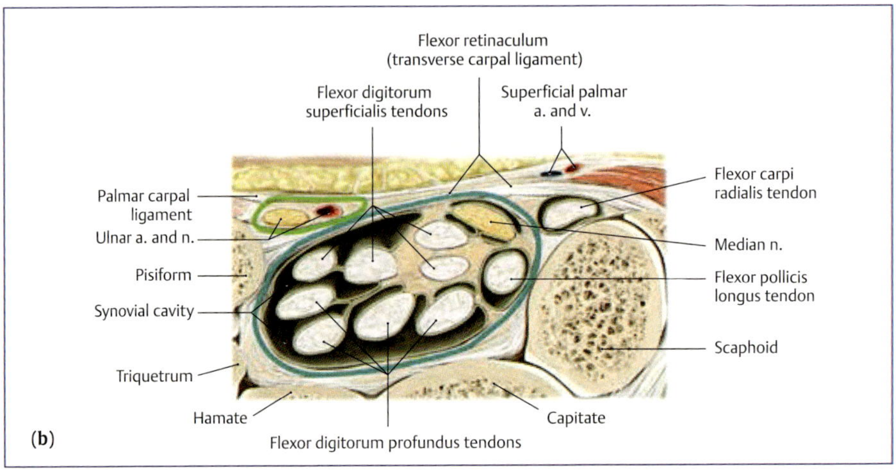

Fig. 7.8 Carpal tunnel: **(b)** Structures in the ulnar tunnel (green) and carpal tunnel (blue).

2. Note the attachment of the flexor retinaculum to the *tubercle of the scaphoid* and *crest of the trapezium* laterally and *pisiform bone* and *hook of the hamate* medially. It allows passage of the tendons of the long digital flexors, flexor pollicis longus along with the median nerve into the palm.

Dissection and Identification

1. Note the attachment of the flexor retinaculum (**Fig. 7.9**).
2. Insert a probe under the flexor retinaculum from the proximal to the distal side. Cut the retinaculum over the probe to open the carpal tunnel.

https://www.winkingskull.com/dissector/V1/video.aspx?vid=87

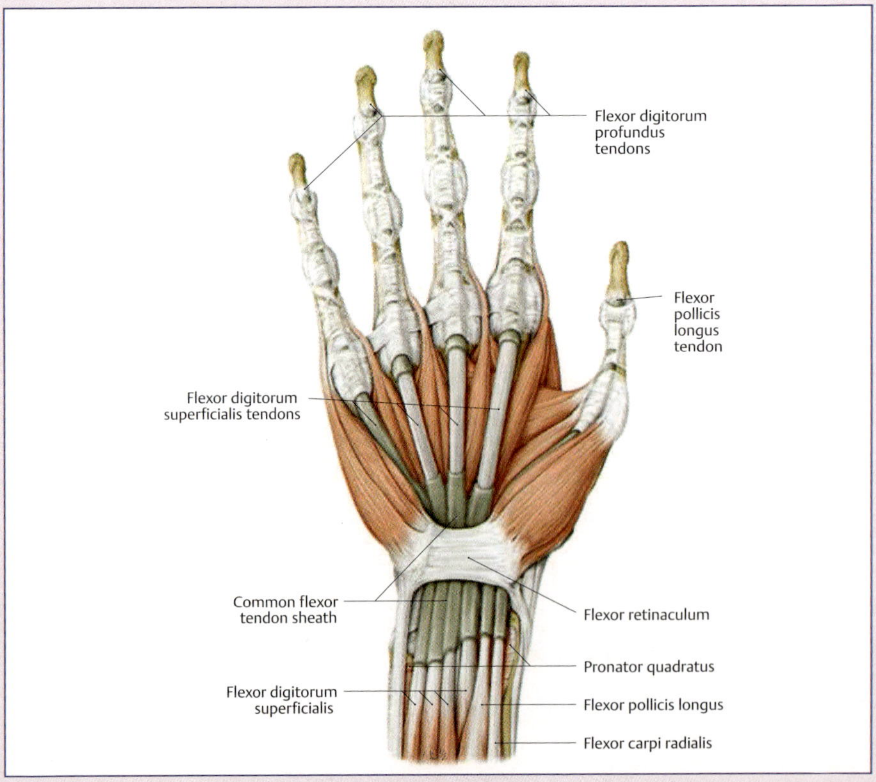

Fig. 7.9 Flexor retinaculum with carpal and digital tendon sheaths. ***Removed***: Palmar aponeurosis, palmaris longus, antebrachial fascia and palmaris brevis.

3. Identify the contents of the carpal tunnel. They are (a) the *median nerve*, (b) four tendons of the *flexor digitorum superficialis*, (c) four tendons of the *flexor digitorum profundus* and (d) the tendon of the *flexor pollicis longus*.
4. Follow the median nerve through the carpal tunnel and identify the *recurrent branch of the median nerve* that supplies the three thenar muscles and lateral two lumbricals.

   https://www.winkingskull.com/dissector/V1/video.aspx?vid=271

5. Now trace the *common palmar digital branches* of the median nerve. The median nerve supplies the lateral three and a half digits. Each common palmar digital nerve divides into *two proper palmar digital nerves*. Study this cutaneous distribution of the median nerve using an illustration.
6. Follow the long flexor tendons passing through the carpal tunnel. In the hand, they pass posterior to the superficial palmar arch and digital nerve. They then enter the fibrous digital sheaths in the digits.
7. The flexor tendons are surrounded by the synovial sheaths described as follows:
   - *Ulnar bursa*: It surrounds the tendons of the flexor digitorum superficialis and profundus.
   - *Radial bursa*: It envelops the tendon of the flexor pollicis longus.
   - Three separate *digital synovial sheaths* for digits two to four.
8. To trace the flexor tendons further, cut the superficial palmar arch in midline and retract the digital branches of the median and ulnar nerves on the respective sides. Make a longitudinal incision on the palmar surface of the fibrous digital sheath of digits two to five. Now reflect the tendons of the flexor digitorum superficialis distally.
9. In the palm, follow the tendons of the flexor digitorum profundus and identify the lumbricals associated with these tendons (**Fig. 7.10**). The lateral two lumbricals are unipennate and supplied by the median nerve while the medial two are bipennate and supplied by the deep branch of the ulnar nerve. All the lumbricals are distally attached to the extensor expansion.

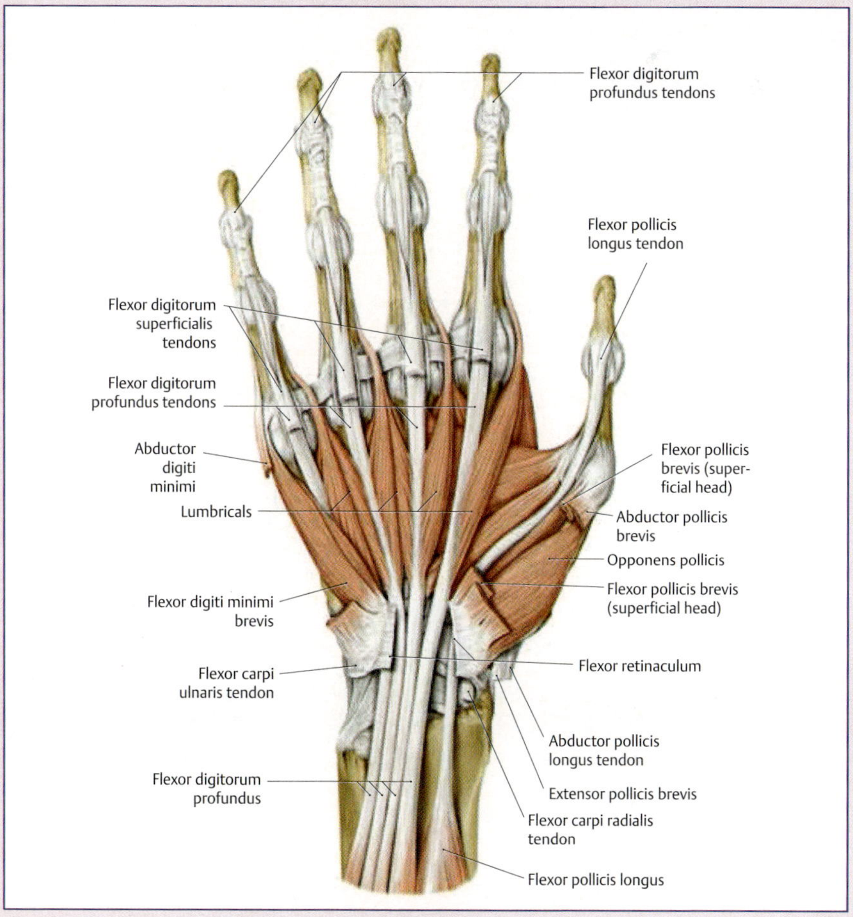

Fig. 7.10 Tendons of flexor digitorum profundus and lumbricals.

All of them cause flexion of the metacarpophalangeal joints and extension at the interphalangeal joints.

10. Note the distal attachments of the flexor digitorum profundus and superficialis. In digits two to five, the superficialis tendons split to permit the profundus tendon to pass through. The *superficialis* splits and is attached to the *sides of the middle phalanx*, while the *profundus tendon is attached* to the palmar surface of the *base of the distal phalanx* in each digit.
11. Trace the tendon of the *flexor pollicis longus* from the forearm through the carpal tunnel into the palm. It is distally attached to the distal phalanx of the thumb. Pull the tendon to confirm its distal attachment.

Thenar muscles:

1. Using blunt dissection, remove the thin fascia over the thenar eminence to expose the thenar muscles.

There are three muscles:

- *Abductor pollicis brevis*: It stretches from the tubercle of the scaphoid to the lateral side of the proximal phalanx of the thumb. It is abductor of the thumb.
- *Flexor pollicis brevis*: It stretches from the crest of the trapezium to the lateral side of the proximal phalanx of the thumb. It is medial to the abductor pollicis and causes flexion of the thumb.
- *Opponens pollicis*: It lies deep to the other two muscles and stretches from the crest of the trapezium to the lateral side of the shaft of the first metacarpal bone. It causes opposition movement.

2. All the three muscles are supplied by the *recurrent branch of the median nerve*. Identify it passing across the flexor pollicis and disappearing under the abductor pollicis brevis. It can be traced by separating the abductor from the flexor pollicis using a probe.
3. Now elevate the abductor pollicis and cut it with a pair of scissors to expose the opponens pollicis. Note the attachment of the opponens pollicis to the first metacarpal (**Fig. 7.10**).

Hypothenar muscles:

https://www.winkingskull.com/dissector/V1/video.aspx?vid=270

1. Using blunt dissection, remove the thin fascia over the hypothenar muscles. Among the three muscles of this group, the abductor and flexor digiti minimi brevis lie superficial with the abductor being medial to the flexor digiti minimi. The opponens digiti minimi lies deep to these two muscles.
2. *Abductor digiti minimi brevis*: It is attached proximally to the pisiform and distally to the medial side of the proximal phalanx of little finger. It abducts the little finger.
3. *Flexor digiti minimi brevis*: It is proximally attached to the hook of the hamate; the muscle gains its distal attachment to the medial aspect of the base of the proximal phalanx of the little finger. It lies lateral to the abductor digiti minimi. It flexes the little finger.
4. *Opponens digiti minimi*: Proximally, it is attached to the hook of the hamate and distally to the medial border of the shaft of the fifth metacarpal bone.
5. Separate the abductor digiti minimi from the flexor digiti minimi using a probe. Trace them to their distal attachments and reflect the muscle distally. In the attempt, avoid damage to the deep branches of both the ulnar nerve and ulnar artery.

Palm:

1. To expose the deep structures of the palm, transect the flexor digitorum profundus in the lower forearm and reflect its tendons.
2. Identify and follow the *deep branch of the ulnar nerve* and the *deep palmar branch of the ulnar artery*, as they dip between the abductor and flexor digiti minimi. The deep branch of the ulnar nerve then pierces the opponens digiti minimi.
3. To trace the deep branch of the ulnar nerve, insert a probe between the flexor and abductor digiti minimi. Push it parallel to the nerve laterally and using a scalpel cut down to the probe to expose the nerve. Clean the nerve by blunt dissection.
4. The deep branch of the ulnar nerve passes over the interossei muscles and ends into the adductor pollicis muscle. It supplies all the interossei muscles (palmar as well as dorsal) and the adductor pollicis muscle.

5. Note the *deep palmar arch* that courses with the deep palmar branch of the ulnar nerve. It is formed by the *radial artery* as it enters the palm from the lateral side and completed by the deep palmar branch of the ulnar artery (**Fig. 7.11**).

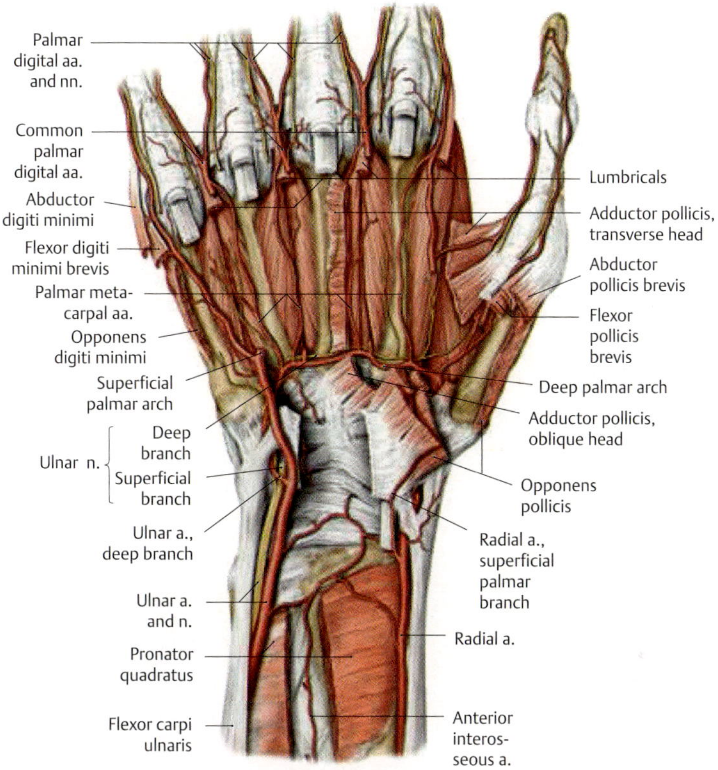

Fig. 7.11 Deep palmar arch.

Adductor pollicis muscle: Identify the *adductor pollicis muscle* and define its borders by blunt dissection. The muscle has two heads, oblique and transverse. The *oblique head* arises from the bases of the second and third metacarpals and adjacent carpals. The *transverse head* arises from the palmar surface of the shaft of the third metacarpal. Both heads unite and attach to the medial side base of the proximal phalanx of the thumb. The adductor pollicis is supplied by the deep branch of the ulnar nerve and causes adduction of the thumb.

Palmar interossei muscles: They are unipennate and are attached to the shaft of metacarpals: one and two on the ulnar side and four and five on the lateral side. Distally, they attach to the bases of the proximal phalanx and extensor expansion of the respective digit. They adduct the fingers. The first palmar interosseus is thin because the thumb is provided with adductor pollicis (**Fig. 7.12a**).

Dorsal interossei muscles (**Fig. 7.12b**): They are four in number. They are bipennate. They are numbered from the lateral to the medial side. They are attached to the adjacent sides of the metacarpals. Distally, they are attached to the bases of the proximal phalanx and extensor expansion of digits two, three and four. They cause abduction of the fingers.

All the interossei palmar and the dorsal muscles are supplied by the deep branch of the ulnar nerve. In addition, it also supplies the hypothenar muscles, medial two lumbricals and adductor pollicis. The lateral two lumbricals and thenar muscles are supplied by the median nerve.

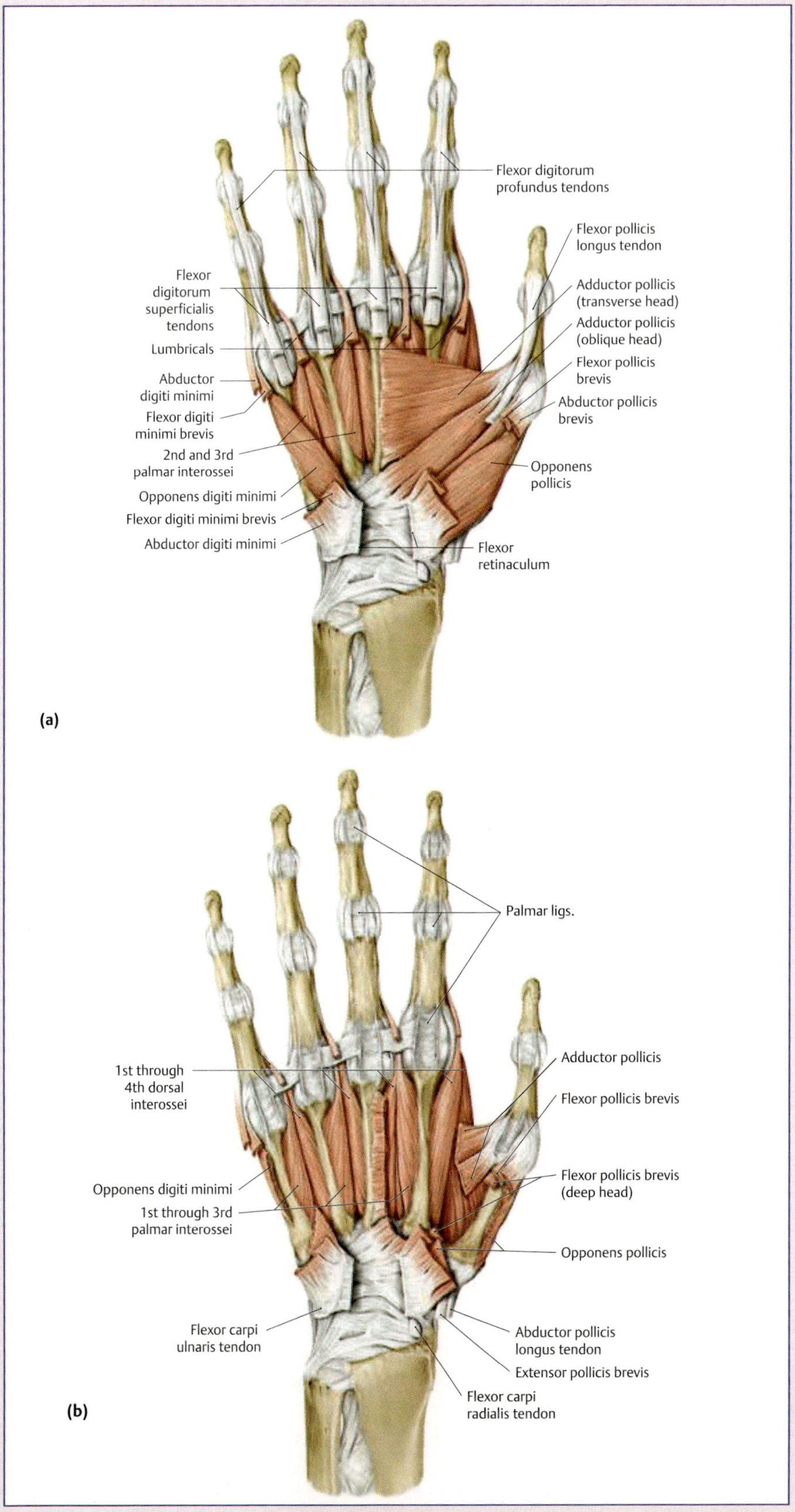

Fig. 7.12 Deep dissection of palm: **(a)** Middle layer of muscles in the hand. **(b)** Heads of adductor pollicis removed to show deeper structures clearly.

Fascial Spaces in the Hand

The fascia in this region (along with the septae) is so displayed that it encloses the spaces. These are surgically important. The spaces may be infected and with the accumulation of pus these may warrant surgical intervention. According to their placement, they can be grouped as follows:

1. *Palmar space*: (a) Midpalmar space, (b) thenar space, (c) adductor space and (d) pulp spaces of the fingers
2. *Dorsal spaces*: (a) Subcutaneous space and (b) subaponeurotic space
3. *Parona space* (in the forearm)

Midpalmar Space

Under the palmar aponeurosis on the medial side of the palm is the midpalmar space. Proximally, it extends up to the flexor retinaculum and communicates with the Parona space in the lower part of the forearm. Distally, it continues into the lumbrical canals (housing the second, third and fourth lumbrical muscles).

Boundaries

1. Anterior: Palmar aponeurosis
2. Posterior: Interossei muscles and third to fifth metacarpals
3. Medial: Medial palmar septum
4. Lateral: Intermediate palmar septum

Contents

1. Superficial palmar arch
2. Digital vessels and nerves for the third to fifth fingers
3. Flexor digitorum superficialis and profundus tendons to the third to fifth fingers
4. Lumbricals (second, third and fourth)

The midpalmar space may be infected because of tenosynovitis of the middle or ring finger or as a sequel to infection of the web spreading through the lumbrical canal. The palmar concavity is lost and the swelling spreads even to the dorsum of the hand.

Treatment: The midpalmar space can be drained by an incision in the third or fourth web.

Thenar Space

It is roughly triangular and located at the outer part of the palmar hollow. Proximally, it extends up to the distal borders of the flexor retinaculum and communicates with the forearm space. Distally, it communicates with the subcutaneous space of the first web through the lumbrical canal.

Boundaries:

1. Anterior: Palmar aponeurosis
2. Posterior: Fascia covering the transverse head of the adductor pollicis and the first dorsal interosseous muscle
3. Medial: Intermediate palmar septum
4. Lateral: Lateral palmar septum

Contents:

1. Long flexor tendons (flexor digitorum superficialis and flexor digitorum profundus) to the index finger
2. The first lumbrical muscle
3. The digital vessels and nerve to the thumb as well as the radial side of the index finger

Clinical Anatomy

The thenar space may be infected due to the spread of infection from the thumb or the index finger. It is characterized by a marked swelling in the first web. The thenar spaces can be drained by an incision in the first web.

Pulp Space

It is situated at the tip of the fingers and thumb. At the tips of the fingers and thumb, the subcutaneous fat is disposed in a compartment formed by the fibrous septae stretching from the skin to the periosteum of the terminal phalanx. The infection involving the pulp space is called *whitlow*. It leads to a throbbing pain owing to the unyielding nature of the fibrous tissue in this region. If not treated promptly by incision and drainage, it may lead to the necrosis of the terminal phalanx due to the occlusion of vessels. However, the basal part of the phalanx is retained because the artery supplying this portion is not occluded, due to the attachment of the flexor digitorum profundus tendon.

Synovial Sheaths in the Hand

The tendons destined to this region are surrounded by the synovial sheaths to a variable extent and infections involving these need surgical intervention, hence warrant attention. They are described in the following paragraphs.

Ulnar bursa: It surrounds the tendons of the flexor digitorum superficialis and profundus. It extends upwards for about 2 inches in the lower part of the forearm deep to the flexor retinaculum. Its lower extent is up to the middle of the metacarpals. At the lower end, it is continuous with the digital synovial sheath of the little finger. Usually the infection of the ulnar bursa is secondary to the infection involving the little finger. This may spread upwards to the space of Parona in the lower part of the forearm and give rise to an hourglass swelling, that is, the swelling in the forearm and palm with the constriction in the middle caused by the flexor retinaculum. The bursa (infection) can be drained by an incision along the lateral margin of the hypothenar eminence.

Radial bursa: It surrounds the tendon of the flexor pollicis longus. It also extends into the lower part of the forearm, like the ulnar bursa. Distally, it extends up to the distal phalanx of the thumb. The infection of the thumb may spread to the radial bursa and then to the ulnar bursa because they communicate with each other behind the flexor retinaculum in some individuals. The radial bursa can be drained by an incision along the medial side of the thenar eminence. During this, one has to be careful because the branch of the median nerve to the thenar muscles is close to this site.

Digital synovial sheaths: They enclose long flexor tendons to the fingers. Note that the digital sheath of the little finger is continuous with the ulnar bursa. The digital sheaths of the index, middle and ring fingers are, however, separate. They proximally end at the heads of the metacarpals. The digital synovial sheaths are drained by two transverse incisions, one at the crease of the distal interphalangeal joint and the other at the distal palmar crease, thus opening the digital sheath at both ends.

Parona space: This space is in the lower part of the forearm and clinically it is relevant to discuss it with the hand. It lies deep to the flexor tendons in front of the pronator quadratus. Proximally, it extends up to the origin of the flexor digitorum superficialis muscle. Distally, it extends till the upper border of the flexor retinaculum.

Clinical Notes

The *Parona space* may be infected by the spread of an infection involving the ulnar bursa leading to an hourglass swelling with constriction caused by the flexor retinaculum. The space can be drained by an incision along the medial and lateral borders of the lower part of the forearm.

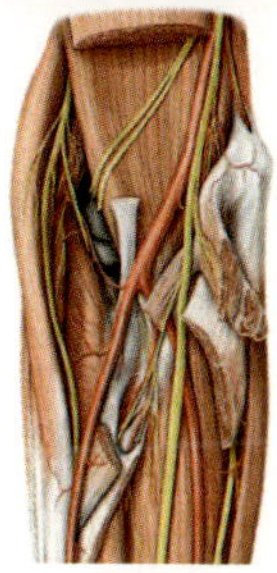

CHAPTER 8

Extensor Compartment of the Forearm and Dorsum of the Hand

Learning Objectives

At the end of this dissection, students should be able to identify the following two layers of muscles of the extensor (posterior) compartment of the forearm:

Muscles

- *Superficial layer*: Brachioradialis, extensor carpi radialis longus (ECRL), extensor carpi radialis brevis, extensor digitorum, extensor digiti minimi and extensor carpi ulnaris.
- *Deep layer*: Supinator, abductor pollicis longus, extensor pollicis brevis, extensor pollicis longus and extensor indicis.

Introduction

The posterior compartment of the forearm contains extensors of the wrist joint and digits. They are arranged in two layers: (a) *superficial* and (b) *deep*. The superficial layer contains six muscles which cause extension of the wrist and metacarpophalangeal joints. The muscles of the deep layer, especially supinator, cause supination of the forearm, extension of the index finger and extension as well as abduction of the thumb. All the extensor compartment muscles are supplied by the posterior interosseous nerve (i.e., deep branch of the radial nerve).

Surface Landmarks (refer to Figs. 1.3 and 1.4)

1. Medial and lateral epicondyles of the humerus
2. Radial head
3. Ulnar head at the lower end
4. Styloid process of the radius and ulna

Dissection and Identification

1. Remove the superficial fascia from the posterior compartment of the forearm and dorsum of the hand, taking care to preserve the *dorsal venous arch* (**Fig. 8.1**).
2. Observe the *extensor retinaculum*, define its margins and use a pair of scissors to remove the antebrachial fascia from the olecranon down to the extensor retinaculum. Using blunt dissection, separate it from the underlying muscles (**Fig. 8.2**). Now detach the fascia from its attachments to the radius and ulna.

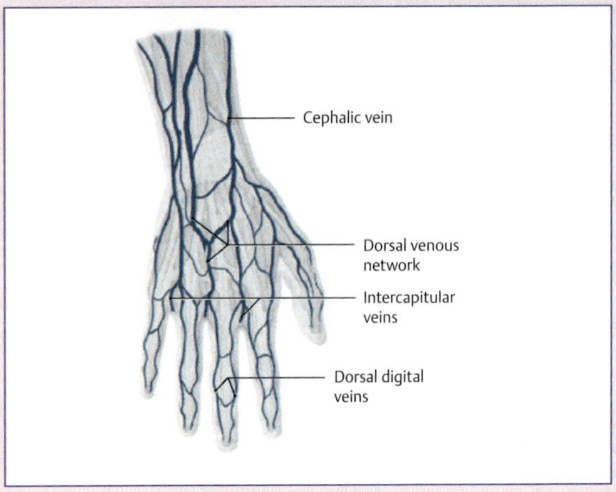

Fig. 8.1 Superficial veins of the dorsum of the right hand. Note the formation of the dorsal venous network/arch.

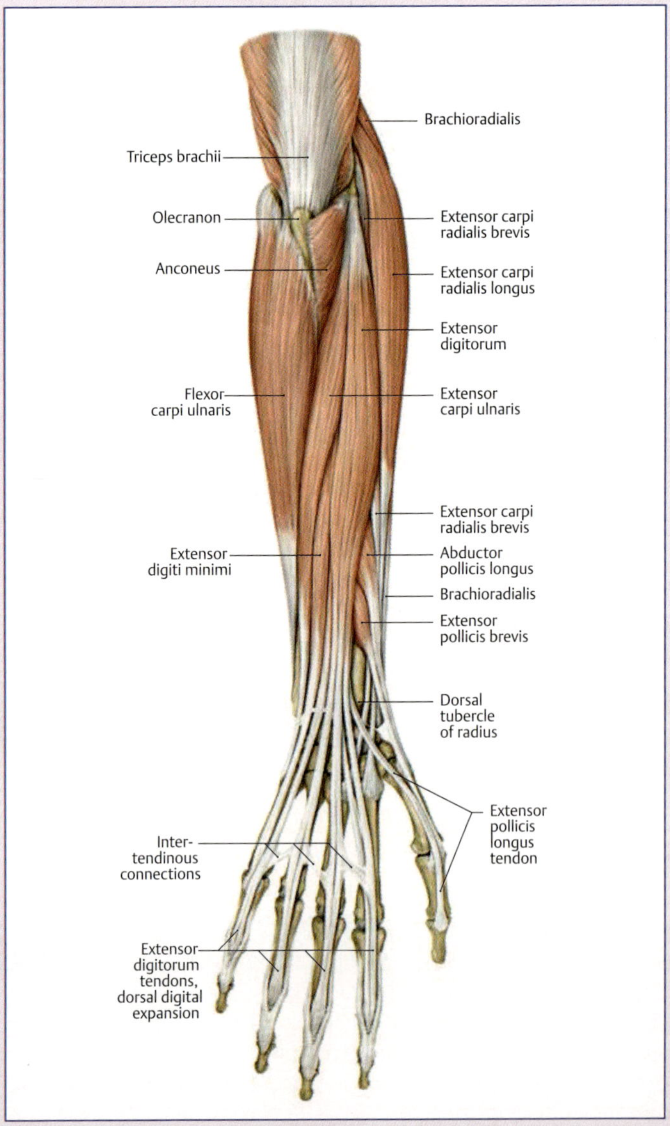

Fig. 8.2 Muscles of the posterior compartment of the forearm: dissection (right forearm, posterior view).

3. This exposes *six* muscles of superficial layer (**Figs. 8.2** and **8.3**).

   https://www.winkingskull.com/dissector/V1/video.aspx?vid=263

   Brachioradialis and extensor carpi radialis longus (ECRL): These are attached proximally to the lateral supracondylar ridge of the humerus.

   Trace them distally. The brachioradialis is attached distally to the lateral surface of the lower end of the radius. ECRL is distally attached to the base of the second metacarpal.

   - Rest of the *four muscles* of the superficial layer, that is, the extensor carpi radialis brevis, extensor digitorum, extensor digiti minimi and extensor carpi ulnaris arise from the *common extensor tendon* attached to the lateral epicondyle of the humerus.
   - Now trace these muscles to their distal attachments.
   - *Extensor carpi radialis brevis* is attached to the base of the third metacarpal.
   - *Extensor digitorum* terminates in the *extensor expansion* (dorsal digital expansion).
   - *Extensor digiti minimi* is attached to the base of the fifth metacarpal.

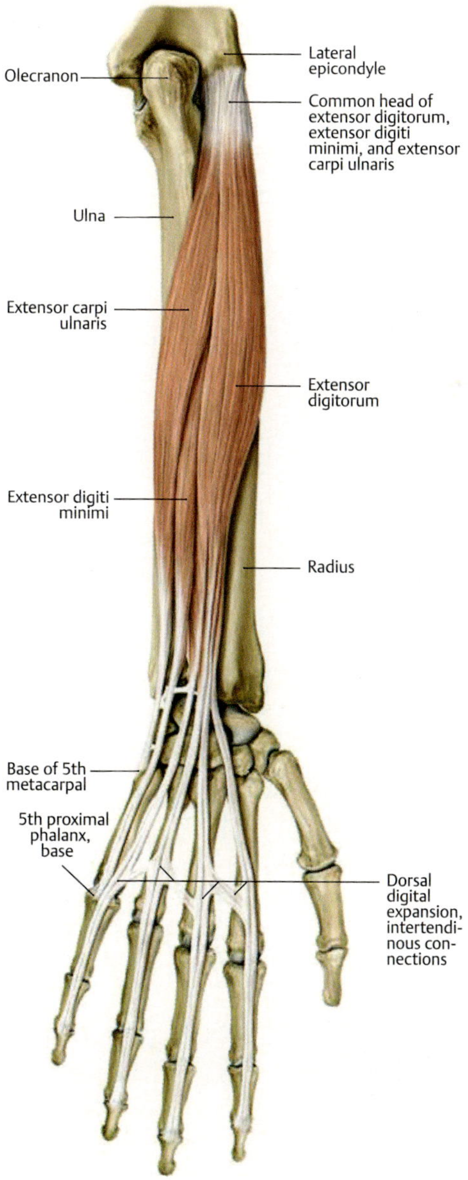

Fig. 8.3 Superficial long extensors.

4. *Extensor expansion/dorsal digital expansion:.*
As you try to trace the tendons of the extensor digitorum distally, it flattens at the head of the metacarpal bone and proximal phalanx. The lumbrical and interosseous tendons join the extensor expansion and then *divide into three slips*: the *central slip* is attached to the dorsal surface of the base of the middle phalanx, while the *two collateral slips* are attached to the dorsal surface of the base of the distal phalanx.

https://www.winkingskull.com/dissector/V1/video.aspx?vid=266

5. The deep layer contains five muscles (**Fig. 8.4**): supinator, abductor pollicis longus, extensor pollicis brevis, extensor pollicis longus and extensor indicis muscles.

https://www.winkingskull.com/dissector/V1/video.aspx?vid=264

6. To expose the deep group of muscles, cut through the extensor retinaculum and retract the tendons of the extensor digitorum.

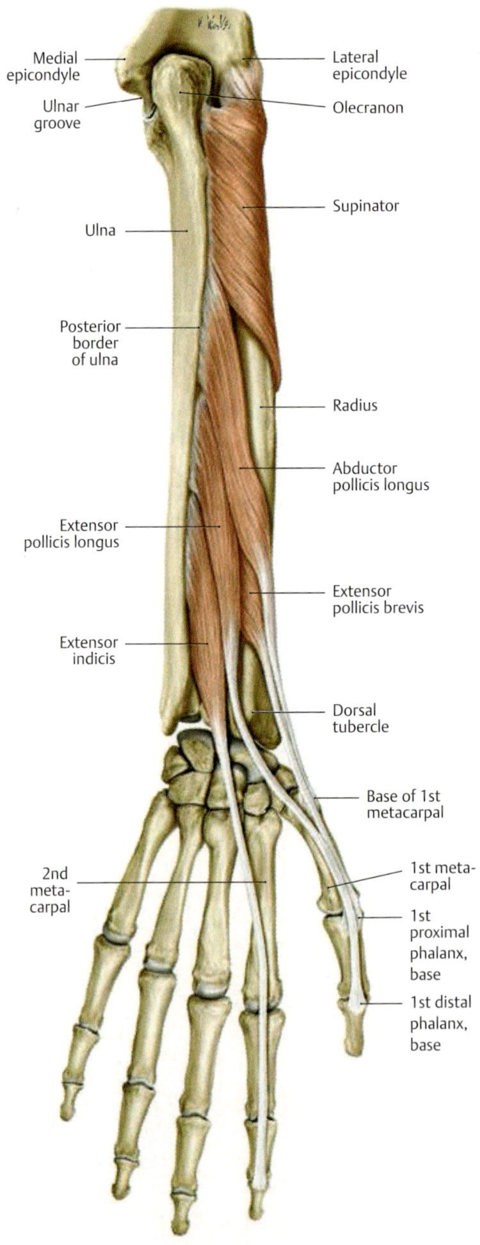

Fig. 8.4 Deep muscles (extensors) of the posterior compartment of the forearm.

7. The deep layer muscles have their proximal attachments (origin) from the posterior surfaces of the radius, ulna and the interosseous membrane. Their distal attachments (insertion) are as follows:
   - *Abductor pollicis longus*: To the base of the first metacarpal.
   - *Extensor pollicis brevis*: To the base of the proximal phalanx of the thumb.
   - *Extensor pollicis longus*: To the base of the distal phalanx of the thumb.
   - *Extensor indicis*: It blends with the extensor expansion of the index finger.
8. Identify the *anatomical snuffbox* and its boundaries (**Fig. 8.5**). It is bounded anteriorly by the abductor pollicis longus and extensor pollicis brevis and posteriorly by the extensor pollicis longus.
   It contains *radial artery*. Trace it distally as it dips between two heads of the first dorsal interosseous muscle. Note its dorsal carpal branch forming the *dorsal carpal arch* with a similar branch of the ulnar artery.

   https://www.winkingskull.com/dissector/V1/video.aspx?vid=265

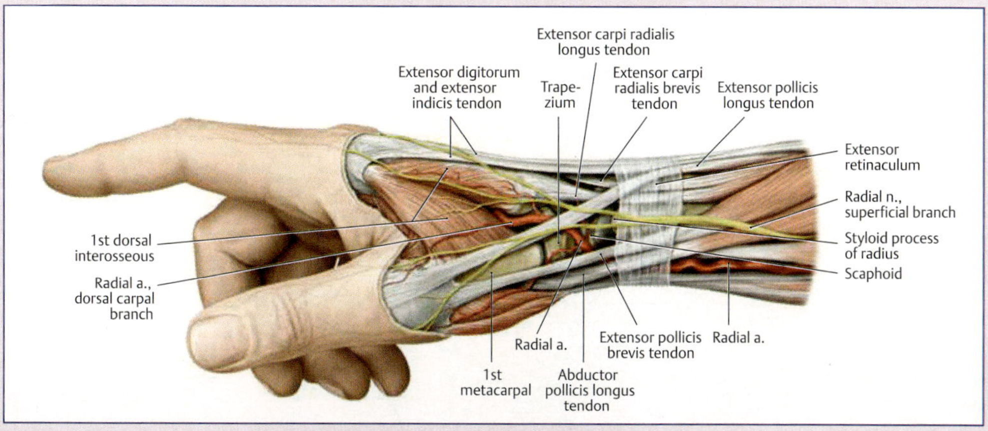

Fig. 8.5 Boundaries and contents of anatomical snuffbox.

9. At the elbow, using your fingers, retract the brachioradialis to identify the *supinator muscle*. The supinator has a proximal attachment at the lateral epicondyle of the humerus, annular and radial collateral ligaments of the elbow and lateral aspect of the ulna. The distal attachment (insertion) of the supinator is to the upper third of the radius.
10. Once again back to the elbow, find the *radial nerve* in the intermuscular plane between the brachialis and brachioradialis (**Fig. 8.6**). Note that it divides into *superficial* and *deep branches (posterior interosseous)*. The deep branch enters the supinator muscle.

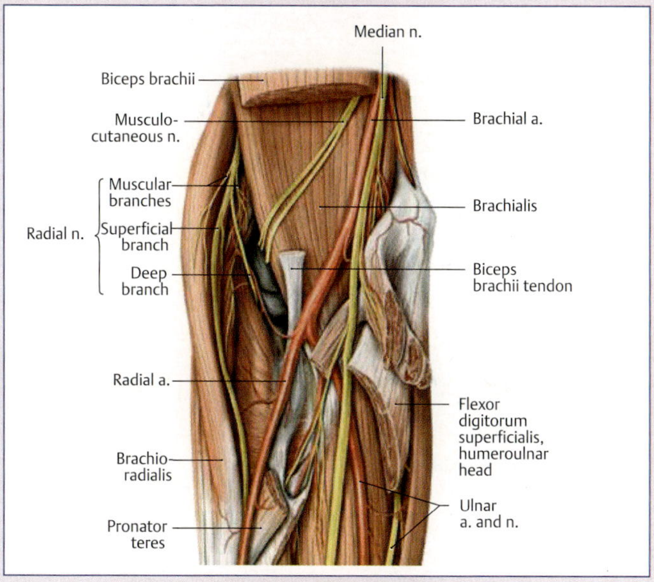

Fig. 8.6 Exposure of terminal branches of radial nerve.

11. At the distal border of the supinator, the posterior interosseous nerve gives branches to supply the extensors of the forearm.
12. Note the *posterior interosseous artery* accompanying the posterior interosseous nerve (**Fig. 8.7**).
13. Expose the neurovascular structures of the dorsum of the hand (**Fig. 8.8**).

Note that the radial nerve (posterior interosseous n.) innervates all the muscles of the extensor (posterior) compartment of the forearm. There is no intrinsic muscle in the dorsum of the hand.

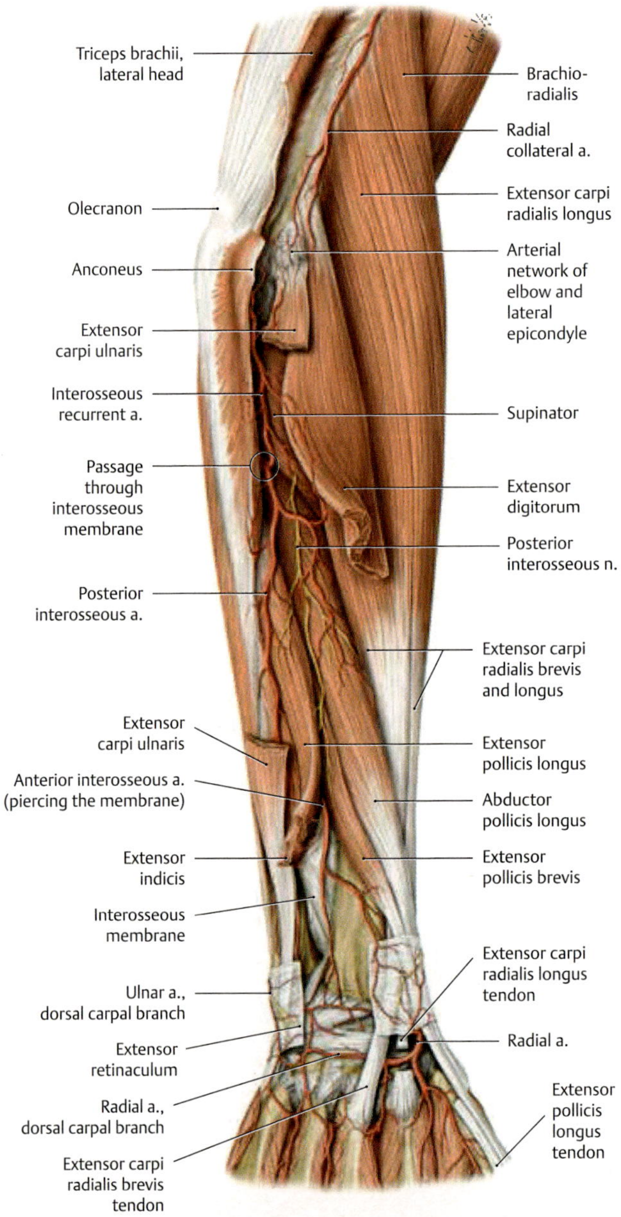

Fig. 8.7 Exposure of posterior interosseous nerve and artery.

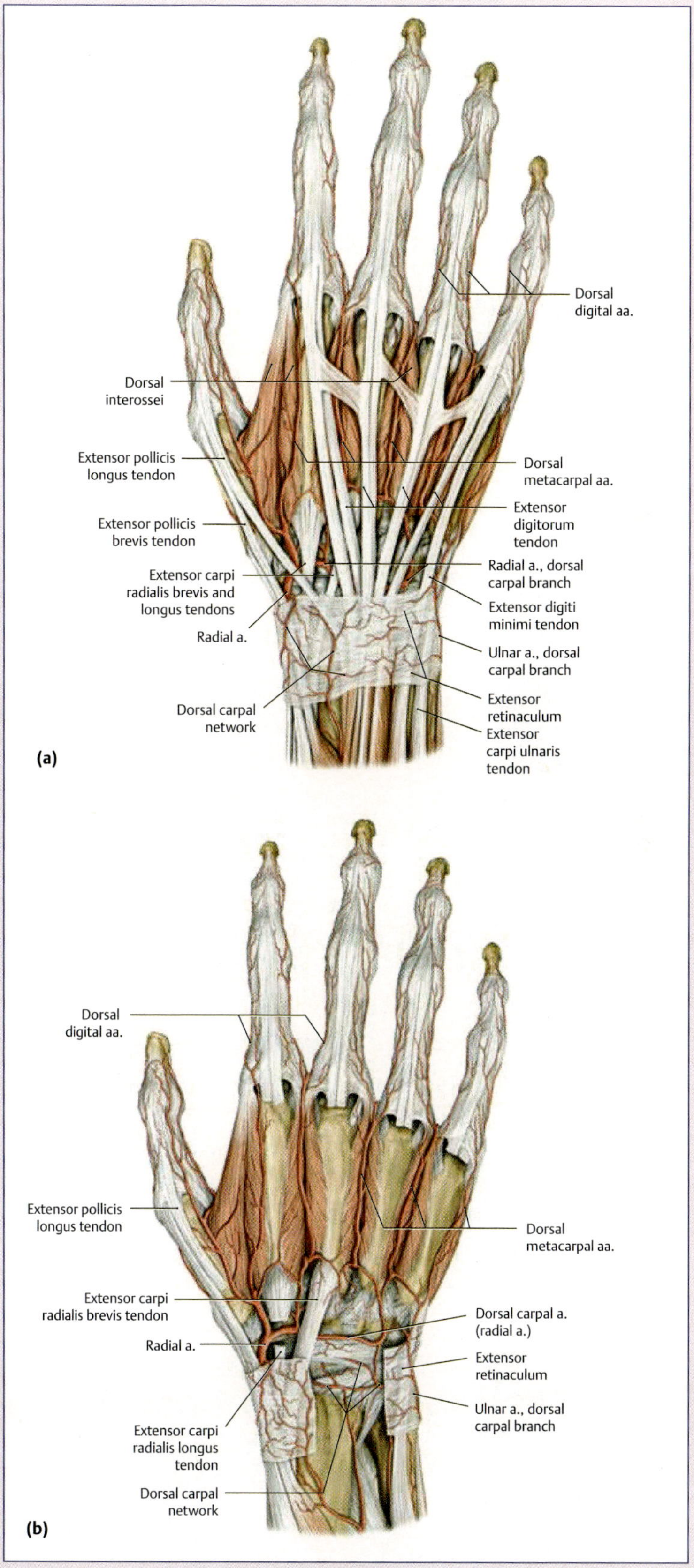

Fig. 8.8 **(a, b)** Neurovascular structures of the dorsum of the hand.

Clinical Notes

Wrist drop: Damage to the radial nerve above the elbow leads to the loss of extension of wrist joint, called wrist drop.

Radial pulse: It can be felt against the lower end of radius lateral to the tendon of flexor carpi radialis. It is of immense value in peripheral vascular disease such as Raynaud's syndrome.

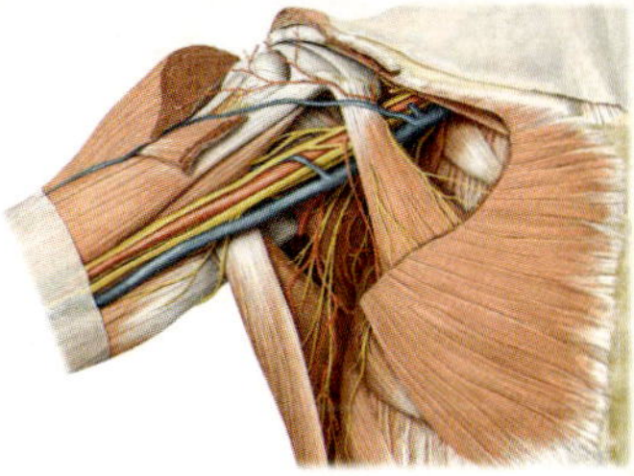

CHAPTER 9

Nerves of the Upper Limb

Learning Objectives

At the end of this dissection, students should be able to identify the following:

- Nerves of the upper limb (axillary, musculocutaneous and radial).
- Effect of the damage to these nerves.

Introduction

The nerves of the upper limb are derived from brachial plexus in the axilla. The major ones are axillary nerve, musculocutaneous nerve, radial nerve, median nerve and ulnar nerve (**Fig. 9.1**).

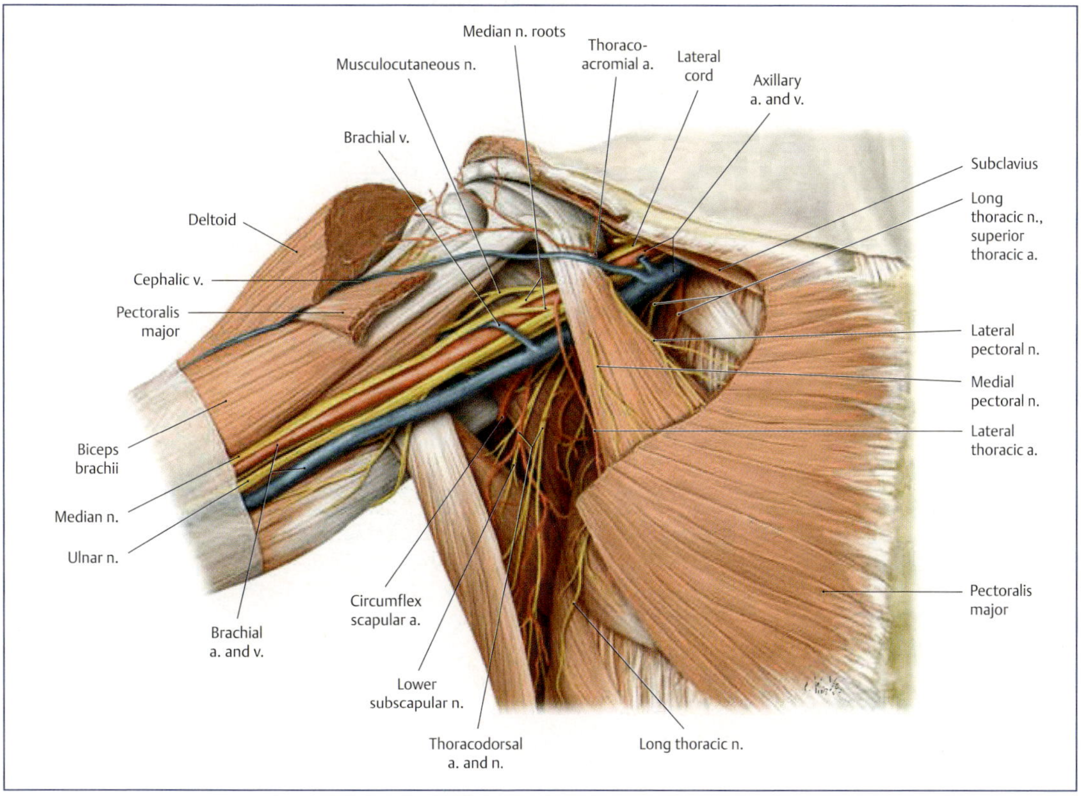

Fig. 9.1 Axilla: Dissection to show the nerves and vessels (right shoulder region).

Axillary Nerve

Axillary nerve is a branch of the posterior cord of the brachial plexus, root value C5, 6 (**Fig. 4.3**).

Course and Relations

In the axilla: It lies behind the third part of the axillary artery between it and the subscapularis. Winding around the lower border of the subscapularis, it leaves the axilla and enters the quadrangular space. Here, it is accompanied by the posterior circumflex vessels related to the subscapularis *superiorly*, teres major *inferiorly*, long head of the triceps *medially* and surgical neck of the humerus *laterally*.

Within the quadrangular space, the nerve divides into anterior and posterior branches. The *anterior branch* runs along with the posterior circumflex vessel around the surgical neck of the humerus deep to the deltoid muscle. It innervates the deltoid and skin over the lower half of the deltoid muscle (**Fig. 9.2**).

The *posterior branch* supplies the posterior part of the deltoid and teres minor. The branch to the teres minor has a pseudoganglion associated with it. The posterior branch pierces the deep fascia close to the posterior border of the deltoid and continues as the *upper lateral cutaneous nerve of the arm* (**Fig. 9.2**).

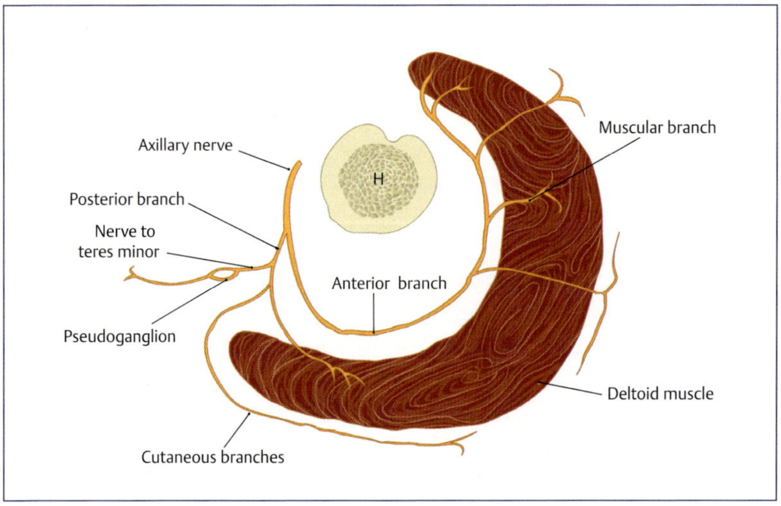

Fig. 9.2 Axillary nerve. H, neck of humerus.

Branches

1. *Muscular branches*: To the deltoid and teres minor.
2. *Cutaneous branches*: Upper lateral cutaneous nerve of the arm.
3. *Vascular branch*: To the posterior circumflex humeral artery.

Clinical Notes

Axillary nerve may be damaged due to the following:

1. Inferior/subglenoid dislocation of the shoulder joint.
2. Fracture involving surgical neck of the humerus.

The effects of this injury are as follows:

1. Deltoid is paralyzed and the abduction at the shoulder joint is lost.
2. Loss of rounded contour of the shoulder owing to disuse atrophy of the deltoid.
3. Anaesthesia of the skin over the lower half of the deltoid.

Musculocutaneous Nerve

It is a branch of the *lateral cord* of the brachial plexus (**Fig. 9.3**). It is the main nerve supplying the flexor/anterior compartment of the arm. Beyond the elbow, it continues as the *lateral cutaneous nerve of the forearm.* It has *root value* C5, C6 and C7.

Course and Relations

In the axilla: It lies lateral to the third part of the axillary artery sandwiched between it and the coracobrachialis. Then in the arm, it runs between the biceps brachii (superficial) and the brachialis muscle (deep) supplying both the muscles. A couple of centimetres above the elbow, it pierces the deep fascia to continue as the lateral cutaneous nerve of the forearm.

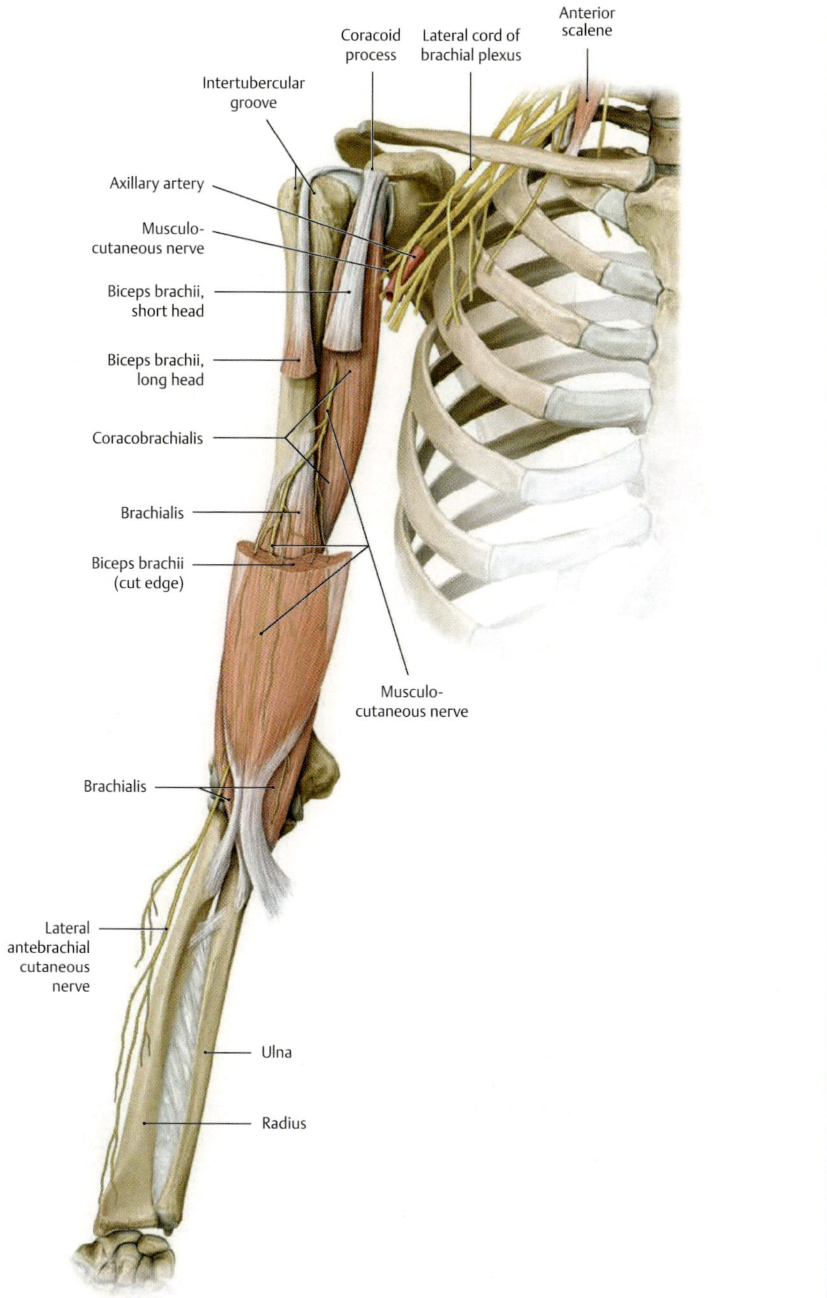

Fig. 9.3 Origin, course and branches of musculocutaneous nerve.

Branches

1. *Muscular branches*: To coracobrachialis, brachialis and biceps brachii.
2. *Cutaneous branch*: Lateral cutaneous nerve of the forearm.
3. *Articular branches*: To elbow joint, through branch to the brachialis muscle and to the humerus.
4. *Communicating branches*: With superficial branch of the radial nerve, posterior cutaneous nerve of the forearm and palmar cutaneous branch of the median nerve.

Radial Nerve

It is the largest branch of the posterior cord of the brachial plexus (**Fig. 9.4**). It has root value of C5, C6, C7, C8 and T1. It supplies the muscles in the extensor compartment of the arm and forearm. Its cutaneous distribution is also along the back of the arm, forearm and dorsum of the hand.

Course and Relations

In the axilla: It lies posterior to the third part of the axillary artery and crosses anterior to the posterior axillary wall muscles, that is, the subscapularis, latissimus dorsi and teres major. Laterally, it is related to the axillary nerve and coracobrachialis.

In the arm: It continues behind the brachial artery and passes through the lower triangular space below the teres major muscle to enter the spiral/radial groove (behind the humerus) in company with the profunda brachii. At the lower (lateral) end of the radial groove, it pierces the lateral intermuscular septum and enters the anterior/flexor compartment of the arm. Here it lies in a muscular gutter formed by the brachialis muscle medially and the brachioradialis and extensor carpi radialis longus laterally.

At elbow: It divides into superficial (sensory) and deep branches (motor). The deep branch is also called the posterior interosseous nerve. It passes to the extensor side and supplies the muscles of the extensor compartment of the forearm. *The superficial division of the radial nerve* is sensory; it crosses the anatomical snuffbox and supplies the skin over the dorsum of the hand and lateral three and half digits on the dorsal side.

Branches

1. *Muscular branches*
   - *In the axilla*: To the long and medial heads of the triceps brachii.
   - *In the spiral groove*: To the lateral and medial heads of the triceps brachii and anconeus muscle.
   - *In the flexor compartment of the arm*: To the brachialis, brachioradialis and extensor carpi radialis longus muscle.
2. *Cutaneous branches*
   - Above the spiral groove: Posterior cutaneous nerve of the arm.
   - In the spiral groove: Lower lateral cutaneous nerve of the arm and posterior cutaneous nerve of the forearm.
3. *Articular branch* to the elbow joint.
4. *Terminal branches*: (a) Superficial terminal branch (sensory) and (b) deep terminal branch (motor). This division occurs at the level of the head of the radius.
   - The superficial terminal branch travels on the anterolateral aspect of forearm underneath the brachioradialis with radial nerve being on its medial side. About 7 cm above the wrist, it passes deep to the tendon of brachioradialis and turns dorsally towards the anatomical snuffbox.
   - Deep terminal branch/posterior interosseous nerve

   It is a terminal branch of the radial nerve. It arises in the cubital fossa and then it passes between the two strata of the supinator muscle to enter the extensor compartment of the forearm. It then runs on the posterior surface of the interosseous membrane. At the wrist, it enlarges to form a pseudoganglion and terminates by supplying the wrist and carpal joints.

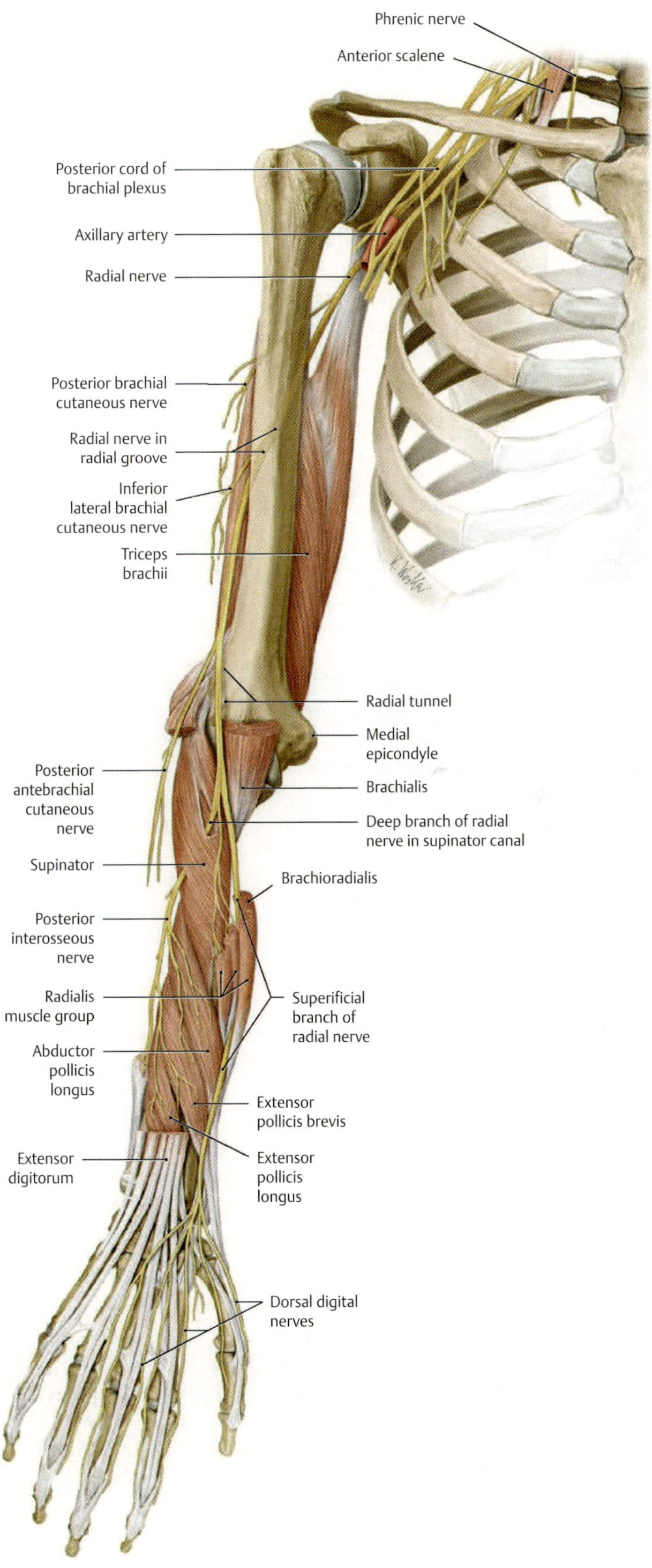

Fig. 9.4 Origin, course and branches of radial nerve.

Clinical Notes

1. *Saturday night palsy or crutch palsy*. In this condition, the radial nerve is damaged because of the pressure by crutches or against the back of chair in the axillary region. The effect being:
   - Loss of extension at the elbow (triceps brachii paralyzed).
   - *Wrist drop*: Extensors of the wrist are paralyzed.
   - *Sensory loss over* the back of the arm and forearm and lateral side of the dorsum of the hand.
2. At the midarm level, the damage to the radial nerve can be due to (a) *wrongly given intramuscular injection in* the triceps or (b) *midshaft fractures involving the humerus*. The effect of this is that the extension at the elbow is partly retained, because in the axilla the radial nerve issues a branch to the long head and one to the medial head of the triceps brachii.
3. Damage to the radial nerve at the elbow may occur because of the operative procedure involving the radial head. This does not lead to complete wrist drop because the extensor carpi radialis longus (one of the extensors of the wrist) is spared, being supplied already in the lower part of the arm.

Median Nerve

It is formed by the union of the *medial* and *lateral roots* derived from the respective cords of the brachial plexus (**Fig. 9.5**). It has a root value of C5, C6, C7, C8 and T1. The medial root crosses in front of the axillary artery and joins with the lateral root; thus initially the median nerve courses lateral to the axillary artery (third part) and then lateral to the brachial artery.

Course and relations: At the midarm level (insertion of the coracobrachialis), it crosses in front of the artery, and in the lower part of the arm and in the cubital fossa median nerve lies medial to the brachial artery.

The median nerve quits the cubital fossa and enters the flexor compartment of the forearm between the two heads of the pronator teres muscle. Here, it is immediately deep to the flexor digitorum superficialis and is accompanied by the median artery, a branch of the anterior interosseous artery. About 2 inches above the flexor retinaculum, the median nerve becomes superficial and lies between the flexor carpi radialis tendon laterally and the flexor digitorum superficialis tendon medially.

The median nerve enters the palm passing through the carpal tunnel, that is, under the flexor retinaculum. Immediately, it divides into medial and lateral divisions. The *lateral division* supplies the thenar muscles and gives three digital branches to lateral three and half fingers. The branch to the index finger also supplies the first lumbrical muscle. The medial division supplies the second lumbrical muscle and gives digital branches to the second and third clefts.

Branches

Note that the median nerve does not give any branch in the axilla or arm.

Muscular Branches

1. *In the forearm*: To the pronator teres, flexor carpi radialis, palmaris longus and flexor digitorum superficialis.
2. *Anterior interosseous nerve*: It is a branch of the median nerve given off when the nerve lies between the two heads of the pronator teres. The anterior interosseous nerve supplies the deep group muscles of the flexor compartment, namely (a) the flexor pollicis longus, (b) pronator quadratus and (c) lateral half of the flexor digitorum profundus.
3. *Palmar cutaneous branch*: It springs from the median nerve little above the flexor retinaculum and supplies the skin over the thenar eminence and central part of the palm (note that this branch is spared in the carpal tunnel syndrome).
   In the hand: Lateral division of the median nerve supplies
   - *Three thenar muscles*, that is, the abductor pollicis brevis, flexor pollicis brevis and opponens pollicis
   - First lumbrical muscle

   In the hand: Medial division of the median nerve supplies
   - Second lumbrical muscle

Cutaneous distribution in the hand: The median nerve supplies the lateral three and a half digits.

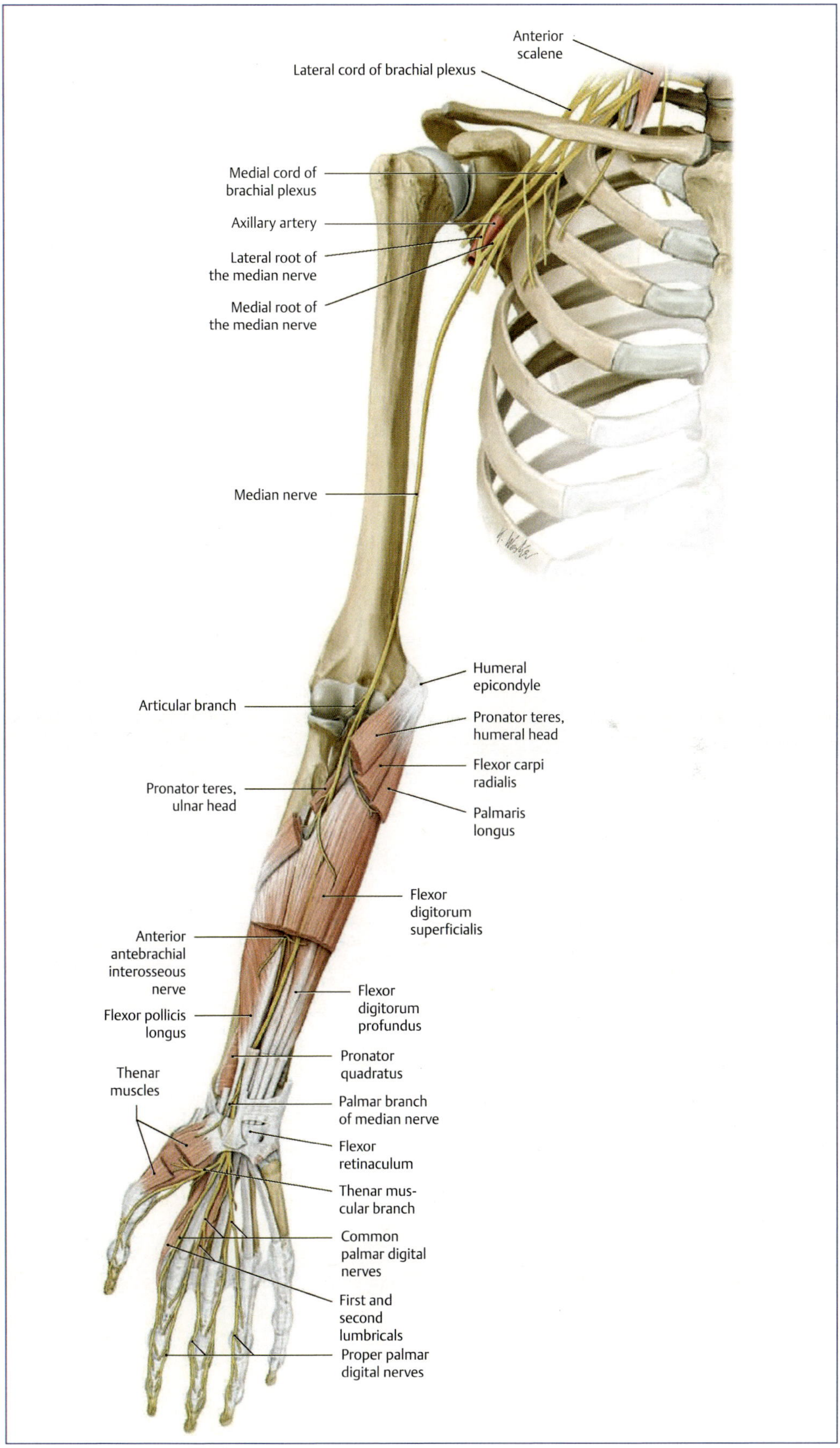

Fig. 9.5 Origin, course and branches of median nerve.

Articular branches: To the elbow joint, radioulnar joints and digital joints (metacarpophalangeal and interphalangeal joints).

Vascular branches to the radial and ulnar arteries.

Communication branches to the ulnar nerve.

Clinical Notes

1. Damage to the median nerve may follow the supracondylar fracture of the humerus at the elbow level or the nerve may be damaged at the wrist being superficial.
   Effects:
   - The forearm is supinated because the pronators are paralyzed.
   - The hand is adducted owing to the paralysis of the flexor carpi radialis.
   - Flexion is weak at the wrist and lost in the interphalangeal joints of the index and middle finger.
2. *Ape thumb deformity* results due to the paralysis of the thenar muscles.
   There is sensory loss over the skin of the central part of the palm, thenar eminence and lateral three and a half digits. Opposition of thumb is lost.
3. *Carpal tunnel syndrome*: It results from the compression of the median nerve in the carpal tunnel. It manifests with the sensory as well as the motor symptoms in the hand. The cause could be arthritis involving the wrist and carpal joints. The soft tissue involvement may be due to tenosynovitis, myxoedema, acromegaly, obesity, etc.

   It usually occurs in females of 40 to 70 years of age. Presents with intermittent attacks of pain at night along the distribution of the median nerve. Pain is relieved by splinting the wrist in slight dorsiflexion.

Ulnar Nerve

Ulnar nerve **(Fig. 9.6)** is the largest branch of the medial cord of the brachial plexus. It supplies one and a half muscle in the forearm and has its main distribution in hand where it supplies all the intrinsic muscles of the hand except three thenar muscles and lateral two lumbricals. It is often called the *musician nerve* because it controls the fine movements of the fingers.

Course and Relations

It is the largest branch of the medial cord of the brachial plexus and lies medial to the third part of the axillary artery sandwiched between the artery and the axillary vein. In the arm, it lies medial to the brachial artery in the upper part; however, at the midarm level, it pierces the medial intermuscular septum and enters the extensor or posterior compartment of the arm. *At the elbow*, it lies behind the medial epicondyle of the humerus. It then enters the forearm between the two heads of the flexor carpi ulnaris. In the forearm, it lies over the flexor digitorum profundus and is covered in the upper part of the forearm by the flexor carpi ulnaris. In the upper third of the forearm, it is away from the ulnar artery, but then in the rest of the forearm it is close to the artery lying medial to it. About 5 cm above the wrist, it gives off its *dorsal branch* and then it passes superficial to the flexor retinaculum lateral to the pisiform bone. On entering the palm, it divides into *superficial* and *deep terminal branches*.

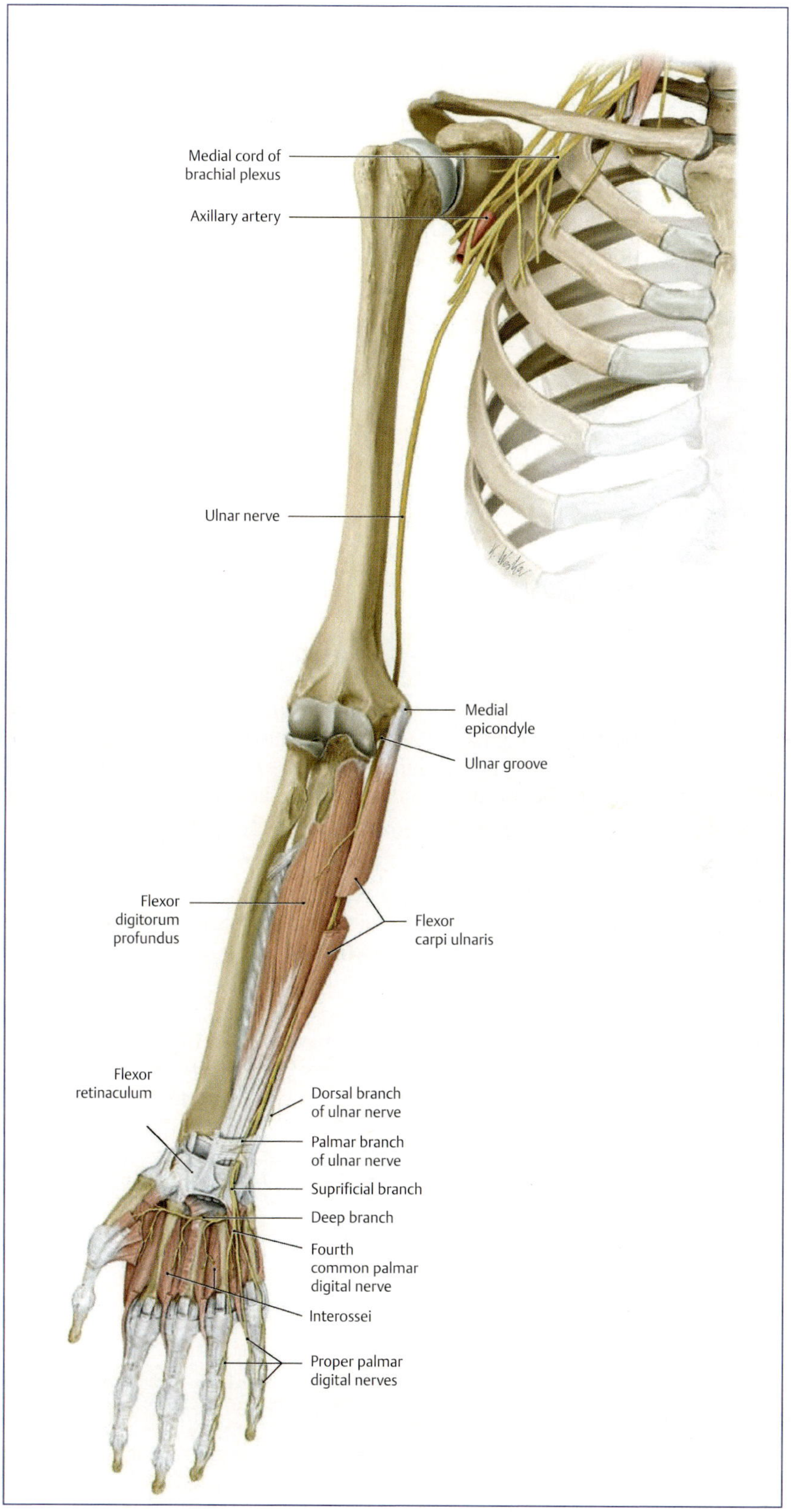

Fig. 9.6 Origin, course and branches of ulnar nerve.

Branches

1. *Muscular*: At the elbow, it gives a branch to the flexor carpi ulnaris and then to the ulnar half of the flexor digitorum profundus.
2. *Articular*: To the elbow joint.
3. *Palmar cutaneous branch*: It arises from the ulnar nerve at the midforearm level, ends in the palmar skin and communicates with the palmar cutaneous branch of the median nerve.
4. *Dorsal branch*: It arises about 5 cm proximal to the wrist, passes backwards and supplies the medial one and a half digits along the dorsal side.
5. *Superficial terminal branch*: It supplies the palmaris brevis, medial palmar skin and gives off two palmar digital branches that supply the medial one and a half digits, that is, the little finger and medial side of the ring finger.
6. *Deep terminal branch*: It passes between the abductor digiti minimi and flexor digiti minimi and then pierces the opponens digiti minimi to follow the deep palmar arch. On the way, it crosses the interossei muscles and supplies the following muscles: three hypothenar muscles, four palmar interossei, four dorsal interossei medial to the lumbricals and adductor pollicis.

Clinical Notes

1. Damage to the ulnar nerve at the *elbow level*, behind the medial epicondyle, leads to paralysis of the flexor carpi ulnaris as well as the medial/ulnar half of the flexor digitorum profundus.
   Effect of this is that the medial border of the forearm becomes flat. An attempt to flex the wrist produces abduction at the wrist. The terminal phalanges of the little and ring fingers cannot be flexed.
2. *Injury to the ulnar nerve at the wrist*: It leads to partial *claw hand*. The complete claw hand results when both the median and ulnar nerves are damaged.
3. *Claw hand deformity*: It presents with the hyperextension at the metacarpophalangeal joints and flexion at the interphalangeal joints of all the digits. This results from paralysis of the lumbricals and interossei muscles which normally cause flexion at the metacarpophalangeal joints and extension at the interphalangeal joints.
4. *Ulnar paradox*: Normally if the nerve is damaged at a more proximal point, one expects more damage and deformity, but in case of the ulnar nerve this does not hold true. Damage to the ulnar nerve at the elbow and wrist is considered. In this situation, when there is an injury at the elbow and we expect more damage and deformity than when the nerve is injured at the wrist. The paradox is that the flexion deformity in ring at little fingers is more when the nerve is injured at the wrist (this is caused by the flexor digitorum profundus). However, if the nerve is damaged at the elbow, even this flexor digitorum profundus (medial half) is paralyzed and hence flexion deformity is less pronounced.

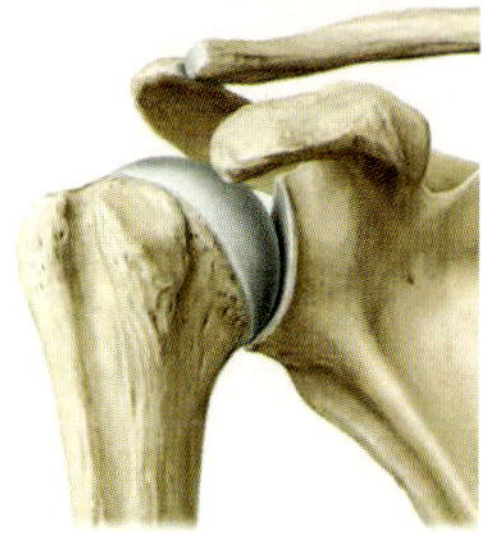

CHAPTER 10

Joints of the Upper Limb

Learning Objectives

At the end of the dissection of the joint, students should be able to answer and discuss the following:

- Type of joint
- Bones taking part
- Articular surfaces involved
- Ligaments associated with the joint
- Muscles involved in movement
- Clinical anatomy pertaining to the part/joint

Introduction

In order to understand the anatomy of the joints, dissect the joints of the upper limb, keeping the soft-tissue structures intact. During the course of dissection, the muscles will be removed; but before removing them, identify their attachments, innervations and actions.

Shoulder Joint (Glenohumeral Joint)

Shoulder joint is a *ball and socket type* of synovial joint with a wide range of movements. It is a *polyaxial diarthrodial* type of joint. A greater degree of movement is achieved through the shallow glenoid cavity and larger humeral head making small area of contact and lax capsular ligament (**Fig. 10.1**). However, it is duly strengthened by the *musculotendinous cuff/rotator cuff* formed by the four muscles (tendons) blending with the capsule (**Figs. 10.1** and **10.2**).

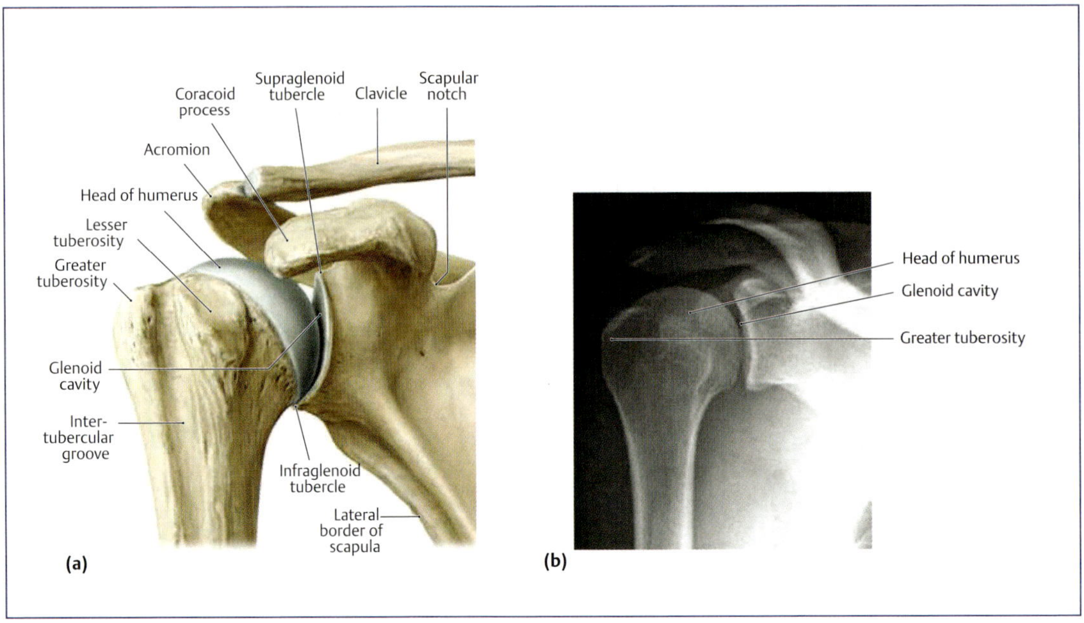

Fig. 10.1 Shoulder (glenohumeral) joint: **(a)** Bony elements. **(b)** Radiograph (anteroposterior view).

Dissection and Identification

1. Place the cadaver in a supine position.
2. Observe the following relevant bony features:
   - The glenoid cavity of the scapula
   - The head of the humerus (more than a hemisphere)
3. Expose the capsule by removing the muscles and tendons around it (**Figs. 10.2** and **10.3**). Define the proximal and distal attachments.

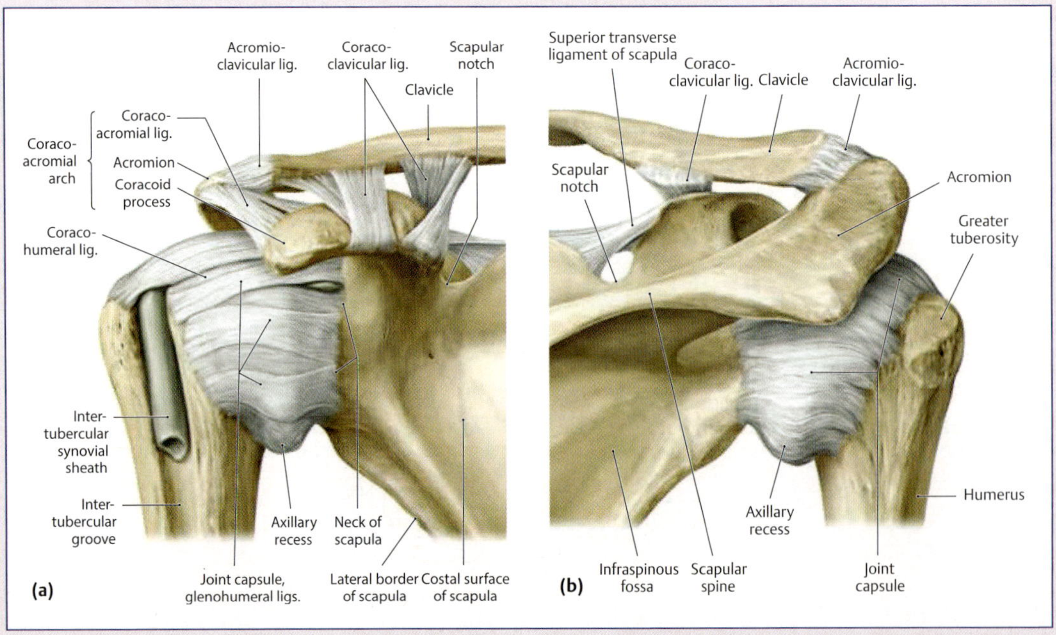

Fig. 10.2 Glenohumeral joint: capsule and ligaments (right shoulder). **(a)** Anterior view. **(b)** Posterior view.

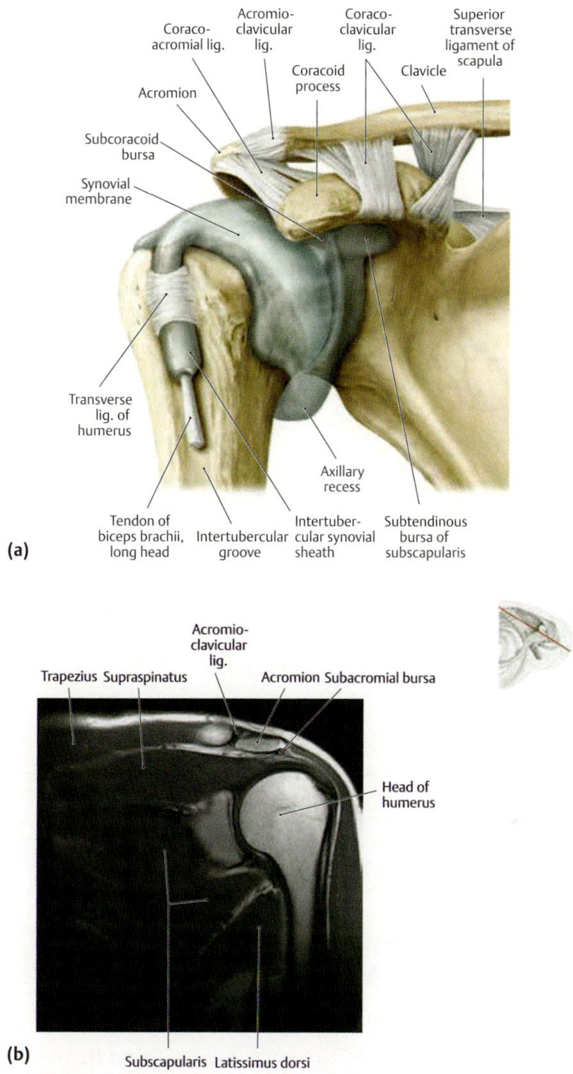

Fig. 10.3 **(a)** Glenohumeral joint cavity (anterior view). **(b)** MRI of the shoulder (coronal section, anterior view).

4. Remove the coracobrachialis and short head of the biceps, leaving the subscapularis intact.
5. Now turn the cadaver in a prone position and identify the tendons of the *supraspinatus*, *infraspinatus* and *teres minor* that blend with the capsule and remove them.
6. Detach the long head of the triceps.
7. Now the posterior surface of the capsule of the joint is exposed. Trace its attachment to the anatomical neck of the humerus.
8. Using a scalpel, cut through the posterior surface of the capsule.
9. Using a probe, explore the *glenoid cavity* of the scapula and observe the *glenoid labrum*. Try to identify the three *glenohumeral ligaments, superior, middle and inferior*, strengthening the anterior part of the capsule.
10. Observe the tendon of the *long head of the biceps brachii* attached to the supraglenoid tubercle of the scapula.
11. Define and clean the *coracoacromial ligament* that stretches from the coronoid process to the acromion (placing the cadaver in a supine position).
12. This ligament along with the two processes (coracoid and acromion) forms the *coracoacromial arch* which prevents superior displacement of the head of the humerus.

Movements

The movements at the shoulder joint are described in **Table 10.1**.

Table 10.1 Movements at the shoulder joint

Movement	Prime movers	Accessory muscles
Flexion	Pectoralis major (clavicular fibres) Anterior fibres of the deltoid	Coracobrachialis Short head of the biceps
Extension	Posterior fibres of the deltoid Latissimus dorsi	Teres major Long head of the triceps
Adduction	Pectoralis major Latissimus dorsi	Teres major Coracobrachialis
Abduction	Supraspinatus, first (15–20 degrees) Deltoid Serratus anterior Trapezius (Serratus anterior and trapezius help in overhead abduction)	
Medial rotation	Pectoralis major Deltoid (anterior fibres) Latissimus dorsi Teres major	Subscapularis
Lateral rotation	Deltoid (posterior fibres) Infraspinatus Teres minor	

Clinical Notes

1. *Dislocation*: Subglenoid dislocation (most common) may injure the axillary nerve.
2. *Shoulder tip pain*: It may be referred to as the pain due to lesion involving the diaphragm because C4 segment supplies both the skin over the shoulder and the diaphragm (phrenic nerve C3–5).
3. *Frozen shoulder*: It occurs due to adherence of the two layers of the synovial membrane. It involves middle age group, that is, 40 to 60 years.
4. *Subacromial bursitis*: Pain on abduction.
5. *Supraspinatus tendinitis*: Painful abduction.

Elbow and Superior Radioulnar Joints (Fig. 10.4)

Please review the bony features of the humerus (lower end), radius and ulna (upper ends). The elbow joint belongs to the *synovial, hinge, uniaxial* and *diarthrodial type* of joint. The *lower end of the humerus* presents the following:

1. *The trochlea* (pulley shaped) on the medial side and the *capitulum* (rounded) on the lateral side. Both have articular surfaces.
2. *The upper end of the radius* has a discoid *head* with concavity on the top, and it articulates with the capitulum.
3. The ulna presents a *trochlear notch* for the trochlea of the humerus. The notch is formed by the olecranon and coronoid processes of the ulna.

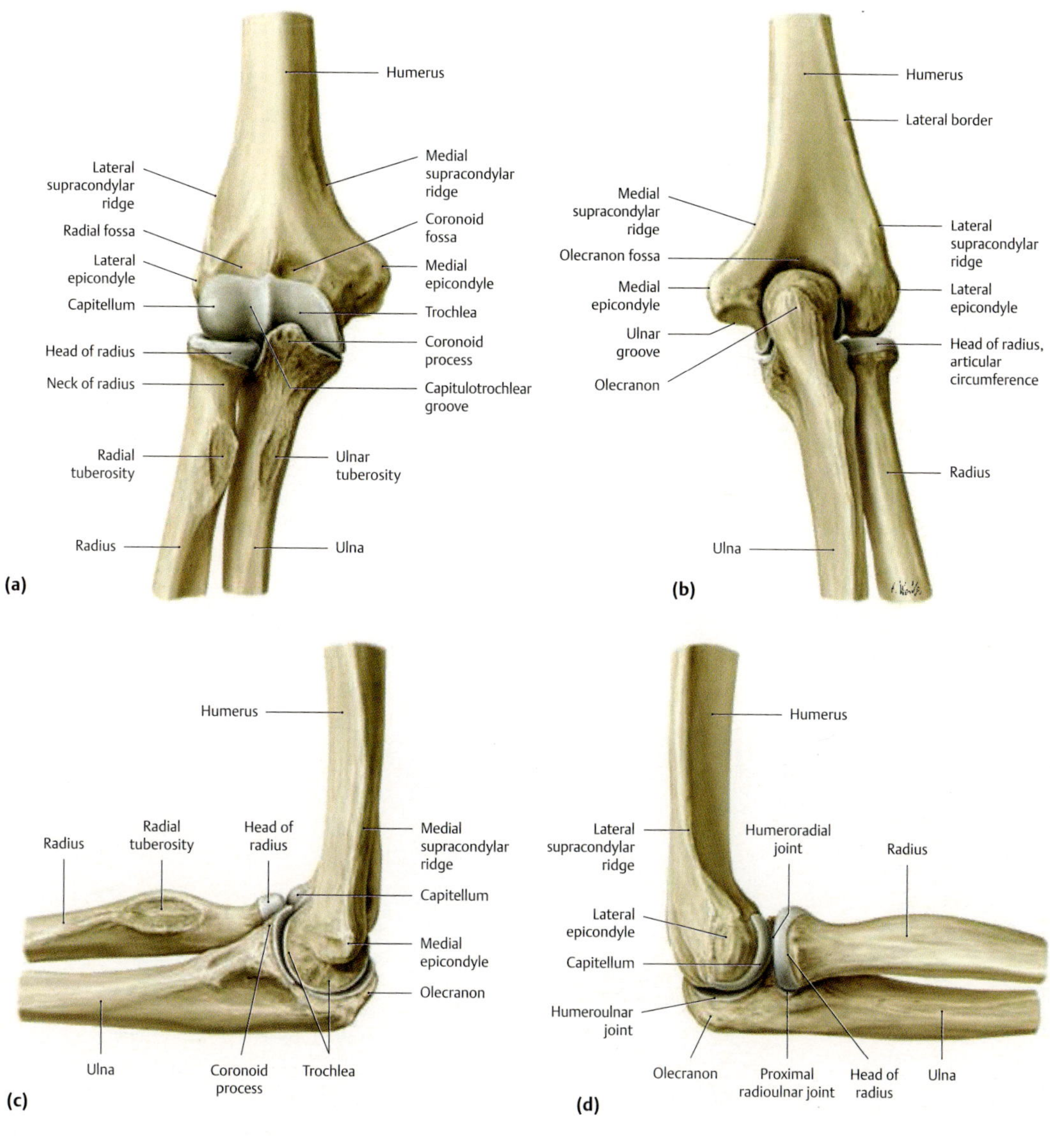

Fig. 10.4 Bones taking part and articular surfaces of the elbow joint: **(a)** Anterior view. **(b)** Posterior view. **(c)** Medial view. **(d)** Lateral view.

Dissection and Identification

To expose the elbow joint (**Fig. 10.5**):

1. Remove the brachialis covering the anterior aspect of the capsular ligament.
2. Detach the triceps brachii from the olecranon process and expose the posterior surface of the capsular ligament.
3. Detach the common flexor tendon (of the forearm superficial muscle) from the medial epicondyle of the humerus.
4. Identify the *ulnar collateral ligament* along the medial aspect of the elbow joint. It has three bands, the *anterior, posterior* and *oblique bands*.
5. Detach the superficial extensor muscles of the forearm from the lateral epicondyle of the humerus.
6. Next step is removal of the supinator muscle.
7. Now identify the *radial collateral ligament*. It fans out from the lateral epicondyle of the humerus and attaches to the upper edge of the *annular ligament* and radius.

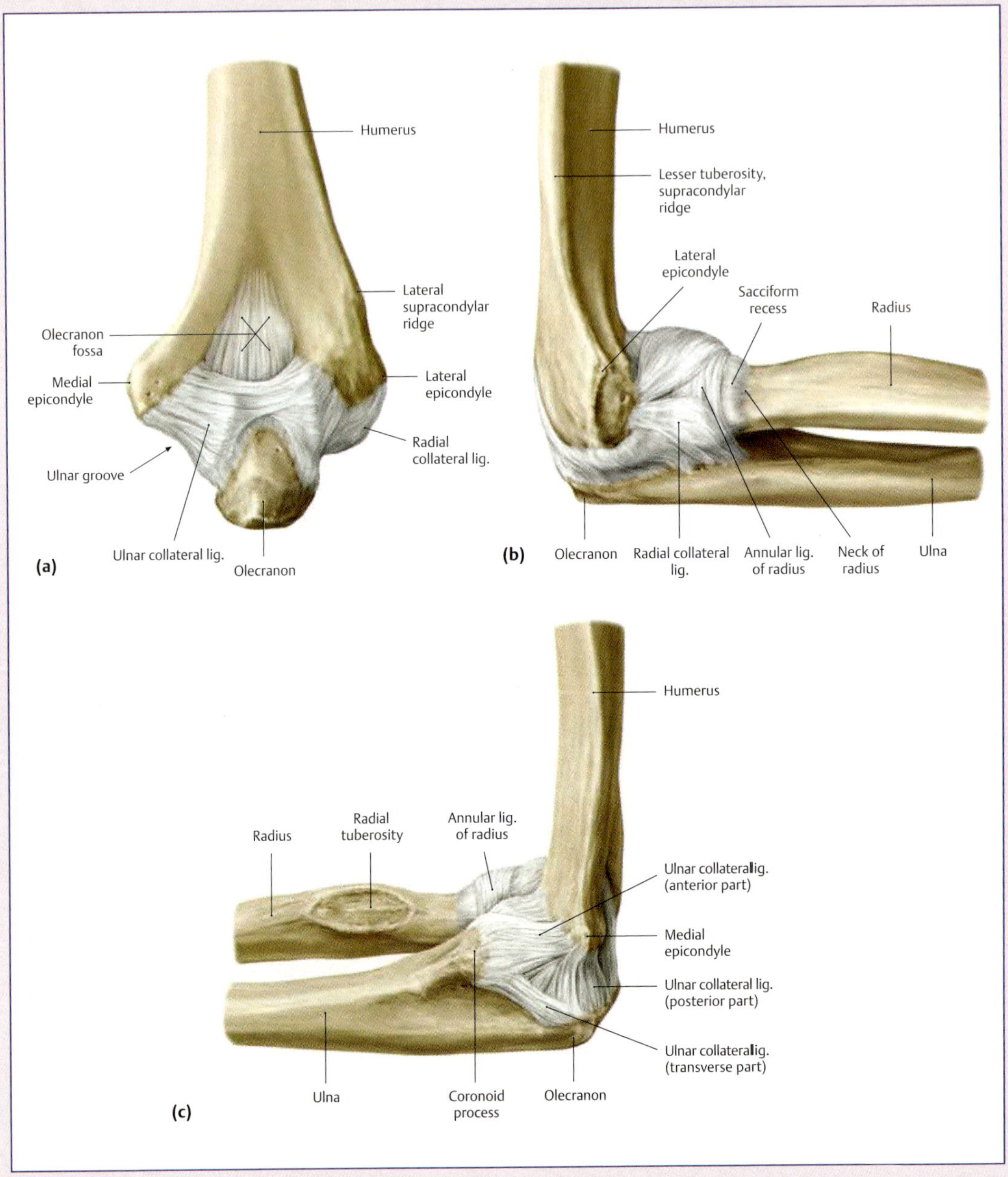

Fig. 10.5 Ligaments of the elbow joint (right elbow in flexion): **(a)** Posterior view. **(b)** Medial view. **(c)** Lateral view.

Movements

The movements at the elbow joint are given in **Table 10.2**.

Table 10.2 Movements at the elbow joint

Movement	Muscles causing movement
Flexion	Brachialis Biceps brachii Brachioradialis
Extension	Triceps brachii Anconeus

Clinical Notes

1. *Dislocation*: Usually it occurs posteriorly and is often associated with fracture.
2. *Subluxation of the radial head*: It occurs in children.
3. *Tennis elbow*: Sudden pronation leads to pain at the lateral epicondyle. It may be due to sprain of the radial collateral ligament or tearing of fibres of the extensor carpi radialis brevis.
4. *Student's (Minor's) elbow*: Effusion involving the subcutaneous bursa on the posterior surface of the olecranon process of the ulna.

Superior Radioulnar Joint (Fig. 10.6)

1. Superior radioulnar joint is a synovial *pivot type* of joint.
2. Its articular surfaces include the *radial notch of the ulna* articulating with the *rim of the discoid head of the radius.*
3. The radial head rotates freely within the annular socket formed by the annular ligament and the radial notch of the ulna. You can feel the rotation of the radial head putting the tip of the index finger in depression on the lateral side of the back of an extended elbow and thumb placed on the anterior side, during pronation and supination.

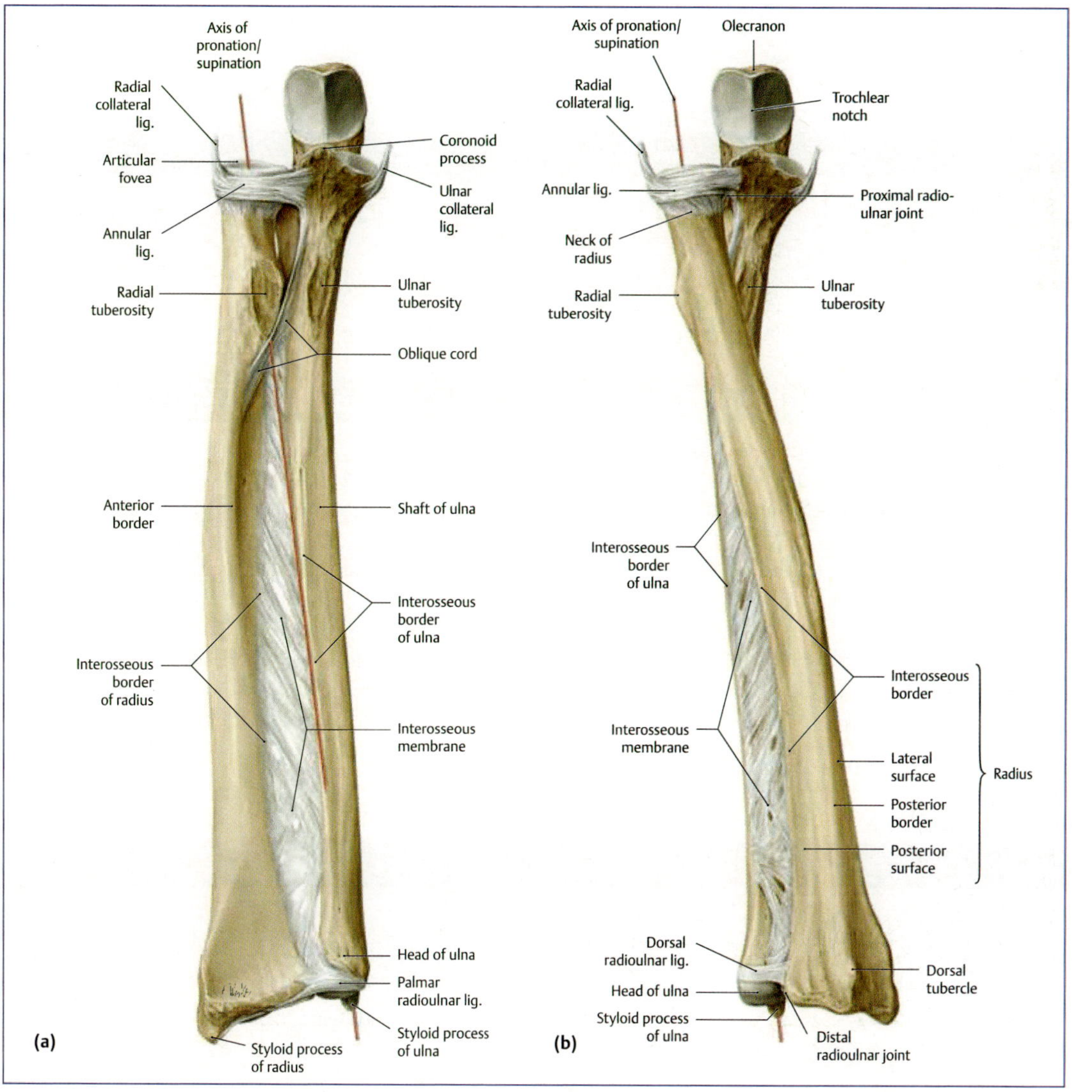

Fig. 10.6 Radioulnar joints: **(a)** As seen during supination. **(b)** As seen during pronation.

Dissection and Identification

1. Cut open the joint capsule with a transverse incision on the anterior side.
2. Using a probe, explore the joint cavity. Observe the articular surfaces of the humerus, radius and ulna.
3. Note that the synovial cavity of the elbow joint is continuous with the superior radioulnar joint.

Middle Radioulnar Joint (Fig. 10.6)

1. Middle radioulnar joint is a *fibrous* type of joint.
2. It is simply formed by the *interosseous membrane* that stretches between the interosseous borders of the radius and ulna.

Inferior Radioulnar Joint (Fig. 10.6)

1. Inferior radioulnar joint is a *synovial, pivot* type of joint.
2. Its articular surfaces include the *ulnar head* and *ulnar notch* on the medial aspect of the lower end of the radius.
3. Note that the *triangular articular disc* holds lower ends of two bones: radius and ulna. This disc isolates the inferior radioulnar joint cavity from the wrist joint.

The movements at the radioulnar joint are given in **Table 10.3**.

Table 10.3 Movements at the radioulnar joint

Movement	Prime mover/s	Accessory muscles
Supination	Supinator Biceps brachii	Forearm extensors
Pronation	Pronator teres Pronator quadrates	Forearm flexors

Wrist Joint (Radiocarpal Joint) (Figs. 10.7 and 10.8)

1. Wrist joint is a *synovial, ellipsoid* type of joint.
2. It involves the articular surface at the *lower end of the radius* and superior/proximal surface of the *scaphoid* and *lunate* (proximal row carpals) the triangular articular surface of the inferior articular disc prevents ulnar participation, hence it is also called the radiocarpal joint.
3. The joint capsule is reinforced anteriorly by the *palmar radiocarpal* and *palmar ulnocarpal ligaments*, posteriorly by the *dorsal radiocarpal ligament* and sideways by the *radial and ulnar collateral ligaments*.
4. The radiocarpal (wrist) joint permits flexion, extension, adduction, abduction and circumduction.
5. Note that the range of adduction is greater than that of abduction, owing to the lower projection of the radial styloid process.

The movements at the wrist joints are described in **Table 10.4**.

Table 10.4 Movements at the wrist joint

Movement	Prime mover/s	Accessory muscles
Flexion	Flexor carpi radialis Flexor carpi ulnaris Palmaris longus	Flexor digitorum superficialis Flexor digitorum profundus Abductor pollicis longus
Extension	Extensor carpi radialis longus Extensor carpi radialis brevis Extensor carpi ulnaris	Extensor digitorum Extensor of the thumb

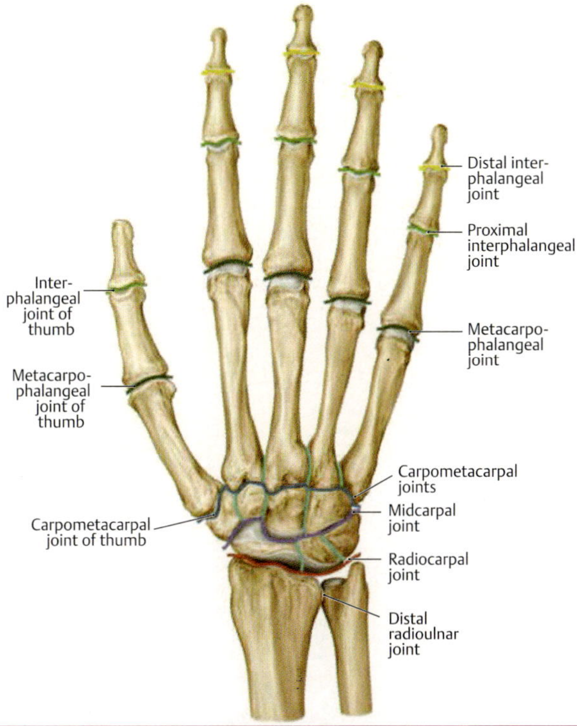

Fig. 10.7 Wrist joint and joints of the hand.

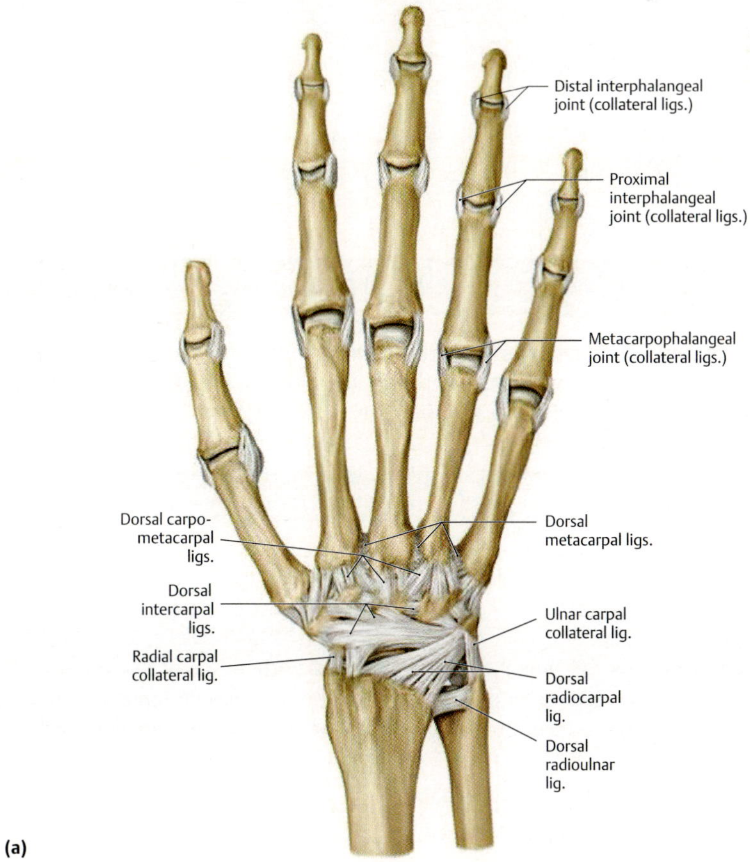

Fig. 10.8 Ligaments of the wrist joint and joints of the hand: **(a)** Posterior (dorsal) view. *(continued)*

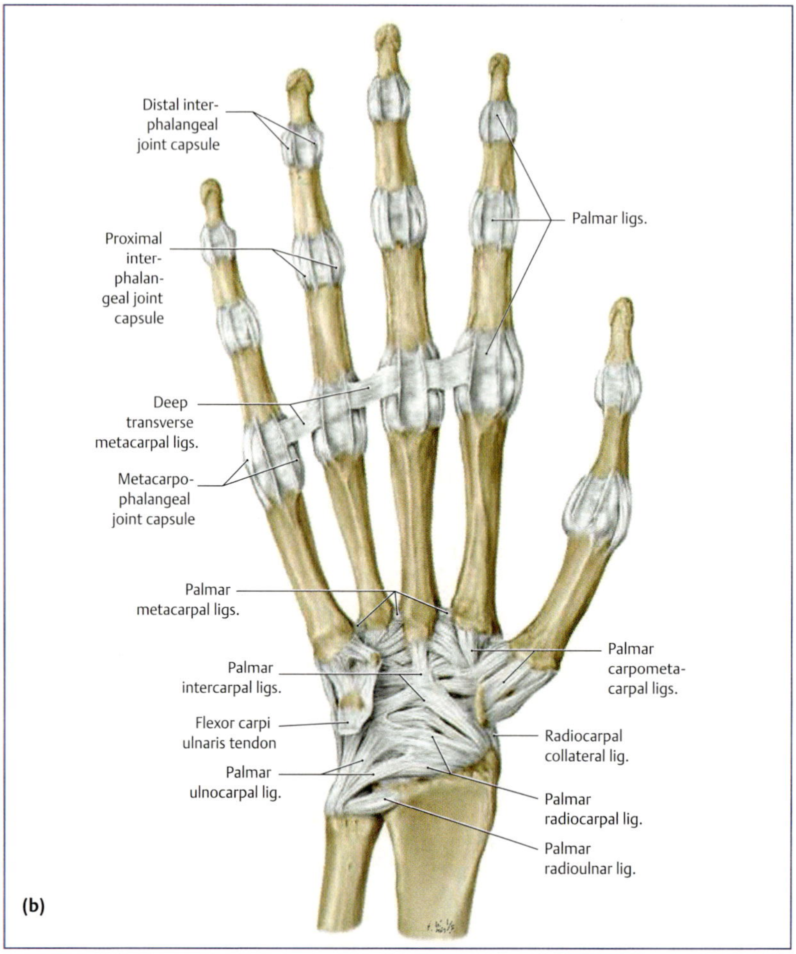

Fig. 10.8 *(continued)* Ligaments of the wrist joint and joints of the hand: **(b)** Anterior (palmar) view.

Clinical Notes

1. *Rheumatoid arthritis*: Often involves the wrist joint.
2. *Ganglion*: Back of the wrist is often the site for occurrence of the ganglion. It results from mucoid degeneration of the connective tissue of the joint capsule.

First Carpometacarpal Joint (Fig. 10.9)

1. First carpometacarpal joint is a synovial, saddle type of joint.
2. It is the only carpometacarpal joint having a separate joint cavity.
3. Articular surfaces include the *distal surface of the trapezium* and the *base of the first metacarpal* bone.
4. Since these surfaces are concavo-convex, the joint shows a wide range of movements.
5. The joint capsule is strengthened by anterior, posterior and lateral ligaments.
6. Since the thumb has undergone 90 degree of rotation, the movements of the thumb are different from those of other fingers.
   - *Flexion*: Draws the thumb in front of the palm
   - *Extension*: The reverse way, that is, the flexion and extension of the thumb occur in the plane of the palm.
   - *Adduction and abduction* occur in the plane at right angles to the plane of the palm.

Movements at the first carpometacarpal joints are given in detail in **Table 10.5**.

Table 10.5 Movements at the first carpometacarpal joints

Movement	Muscles causing movement
Flexion	Flexor pollicis longus Flexor pollicis bravis
Extension	Abductor pollicis longus Extensor pollicis longus Extensor pollicis brevis
Adduction	Adductor pollicis
Abduction	Abductor pollicis brevis Abductor pollicis longus
Opponens	Opponens pollicis Flexor pollicis brevis

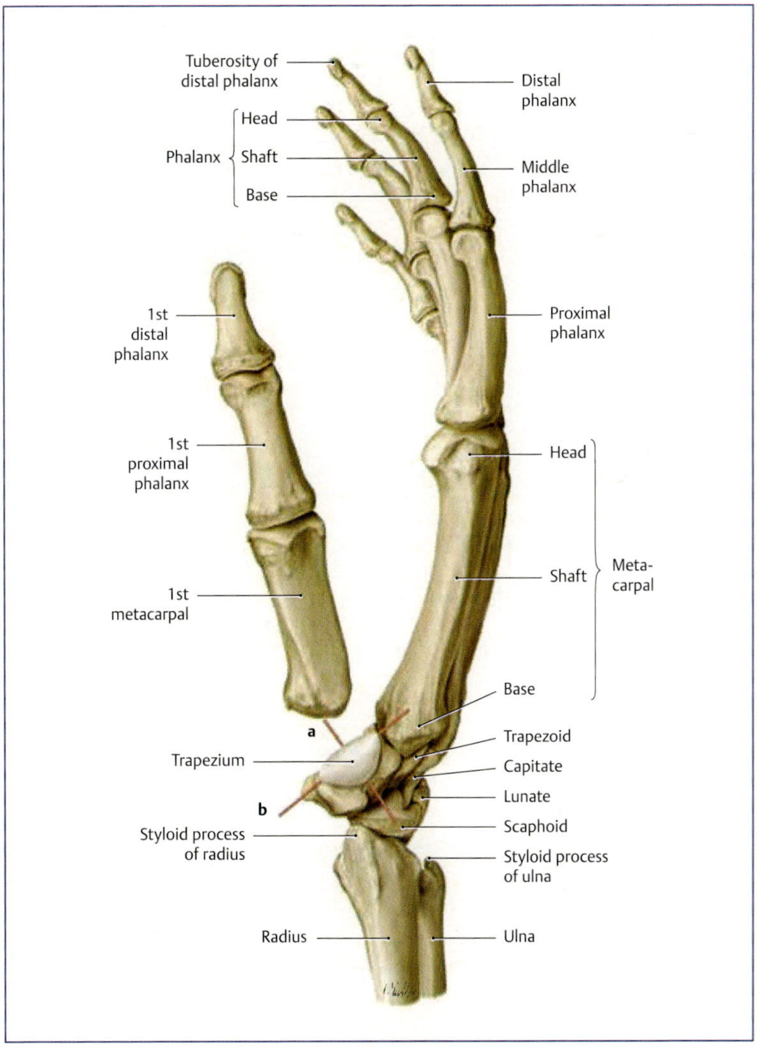

Fig. 10.9 Carpometacarpal joint of the thumb (radial view). The first metacarpal bone has been moved slightly distally to expose the articular surface of the trapezium. (**a**) Abduction/adduction and (**b**) flexion/extension.

Metacarpophalangeal Joints

Metacarpophalangeal joints are synovial, condylar type of joints. They permit flexion and extension.

Flexion is caused by the interossei and lumbricals.

Extension is caused by the extensors of the fingers.

Adduction is caused by the palmar interossei.

Abduction is caused by the dorsal interossei.

The movements at the first metacarpophalangeal joints are given in **Table 10.6**.

Table 10.6 Movements at the first metacarpophalangeal joints

Movement	Muscles causing movement
Flexion	Interossei: Palmar and dorsal Lumbricals
Extension	Extensors of the digits (extensor digitorum, extensor indicis, extensor digiti minimi, etc.)
Adduction	Palmar interossei
Abduction	Dorsal interossei

Interphalangeal Joints

1. Interphalangeal joints are synovial hinge variety of joints.
2. Only flexion and extension are permitted at these joints.
3. Flexion at the proximal interphalangeal joint is caused by the flexor digitorum superficialis and flexor digitorum profundus. In addition, profundus causes flexion at distal interphalengeal joint also.
4. Extension is caused by the interossei and lumbricals by virtue of their insertion into the extensor expansion.

Clinical Notes

Complete claw hand: It occurs due to damage to both the ulnar and median nerves, resulting in paralysis of all the lumbricals, palmar and dorsal interossei muscles. This causes claw hand with hyperextension at the metacarpophalangeal joints and flexion at the interphalangeal joints.

CHAPTER 11

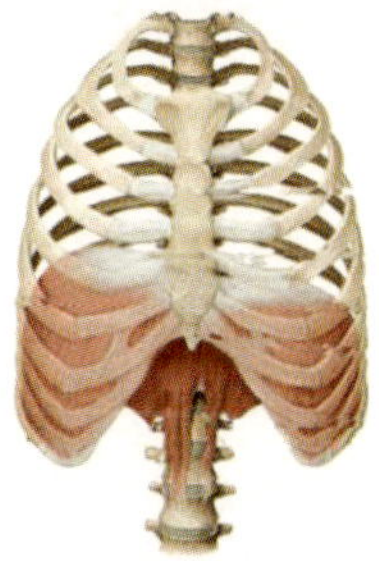

Introduction to Thorax

Learning Objectives

After reading the chapter, students should be able to understand the following:

- The location, contents, inlet and outlet of thorax.
- Importance of some surface landmarks, for example, angle of Louis, location of apex beat and palpation of trachea.

Introduction

The trunk is divided into two parts by the diaphragm. The upper part is the thorax and the lower part is the abdomen. The main function of the thorax is to house and protect the lungs and the heart. The protective function is subserved by the thoracic cage, but concomitantly it needs to be flexible to accommodate the volumetric changes involving respiration (i.e., increase in dimensions during inspiration and reduction in dimension during expiration). This is accomplished by designing the thoracic cage with alternating arrangement of the ribs and the intercostal muscles.

The thorax extends from the root of the neck to the abdomen. It contains the lungs, which are separated from each other by a median septum called the *mediastinum*. The mediastinum contains the heart and great blood vessels. Additionally, it transmits structures from the neck to the thorax and abdomen, for example, the trachea and oesophagus. It also transmits the thoracic duct in the reverse direction, that is, to the neck.

The thorax has a *superior aperture*, also called the *inlet of thorax* (**Fig. 11.1**), which is continuous with the neck. It is reniform or bean shaped. It is bounded anteriorly by the manubrium, posteriorly by the body of the first thoracic vertebra and sideways by the first ribs along with their cartilages. The plane of inlet is set obliquely being directed downwards and forwards at a 45-degree angle. The superior aperture of the thorax is sealed by the *suprapleural membrane* also called the *Sibson's fascia*. It extends as a rigid triangular fascia from the tip of the transverse process of the seventh cervical vertebra to the inner border of the first rib. It prevents puffing of lung apex into the neck during inspiration.

The *inferior aperture/outlet of the thorax* (**Fig. 11.1**) is sealed by the musculotendinous partition, the *diaphragm* which separates the thoracic cavity from the abdomen. The outlet of the thorax is bounded anteriorly by the *infrasternal angle* formed by two costal margins, posteriorly by the twelfth thoracic vertebra and on the sides by the costal margins (seventh to tenth ribs) and the floating ribs (eleventh and twelfth ribs).

The diaphragm is attached to the lower margin of the thoracic cage and bulges upwards so that the upper abdominal organs are under the cover and protection of the thoracic cage.

The diaphragm serves as a piston (**Fig. 11.2**). On contraction, the diaphragm descends, thus increasing the intrathoracic volume by increasing the vertical dimension of the thoracic cavity. This occurs during inspiration. When it relaxes, the ventral abdominal muscles push the abdominal contents and the diaphragm upwards into the thoracic cage. This occurs during expiration.

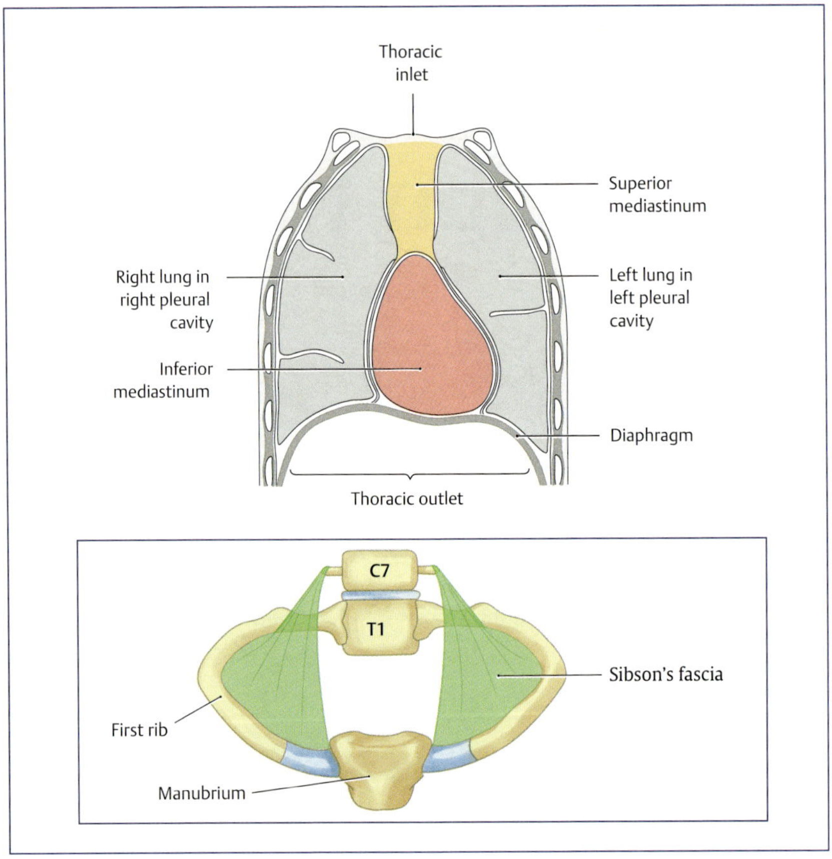

Fig. 11.1 Superior and inferior apertures of the thorax. Inset shows boundaries of superior aperture and Sibson's fascia.

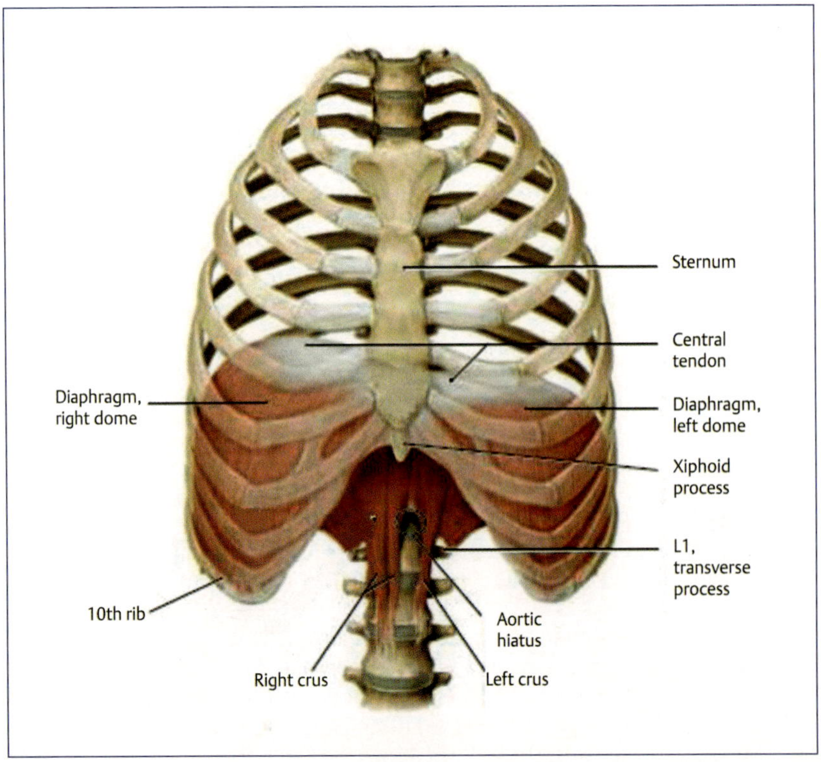

Fig. 11.2 Attachment of the diaphragm.

Surface Landmarks

The surface landmarks can be seen in **Fig. 11.3**:

1. *Jugular notch/suprasternal notch*: It is felt just above the superior border of the manubrium between the medial/sternal ends of the clavicles. It corresponds to the lower border of the second thoracic vertebra. The trachea can be palpated in this notch.
2. *Sternal angle/angle of Louis*: It presents as a transverse ridge about 5 cm below the suprasternal notch. It is at the level of the intervertebral disc between the fourth and fifth thoracic vertebrae. It marks the manubriosternal junction. The second costal cartilage joins the sternum at this junction. The ribs are counted from this level downwards tracing the finger laterally and then downwards. Sternal angle also marks the plane that separates the superior from the inferior mediastinum.
3. *Xiphisternal joint*: It lies between the two costal margins and can be felt as a short transverse ridge.
4. *Infrasternal angle*: It is formed by the two costal margins.
5. *Costal margin*: It is formed by the upturned ends of the costal cartilages of eighth to tenth ribs.
6. *Costal cartilages*: The second costal cartilage is attached to the sternal angle. The seventh costal cartilage forms the upper part of the costal margin. The linea semilunaris, that is, the lateral border of the rectus abdominis joins the costal margin at the tip of the ninth costal cartilage.
7. *Spinous processes of the thoracic vertebrae*: The first prominent spine along the back of the neck belongs to the vertebra prominens, that is, the seventh cervical vertebra. The thoracic spines can be felt in the midline below this level. The spine of T3 corresponds to the root of the spine of the scapula, and the inferior angle of the scapula lies at the level of the T7 vertebral spine.
8. *Nipple*: Its position is variable in females, but in males it usually lies at the fourth intercostal space about 10 cm away from the midsternal line.
9. *Apex beat*: It is palpable in the left fifth intercostal space about 3.5 inches away from the midsternal line.
10. *Trachea*: It can be palpated in the suprasternal notch.

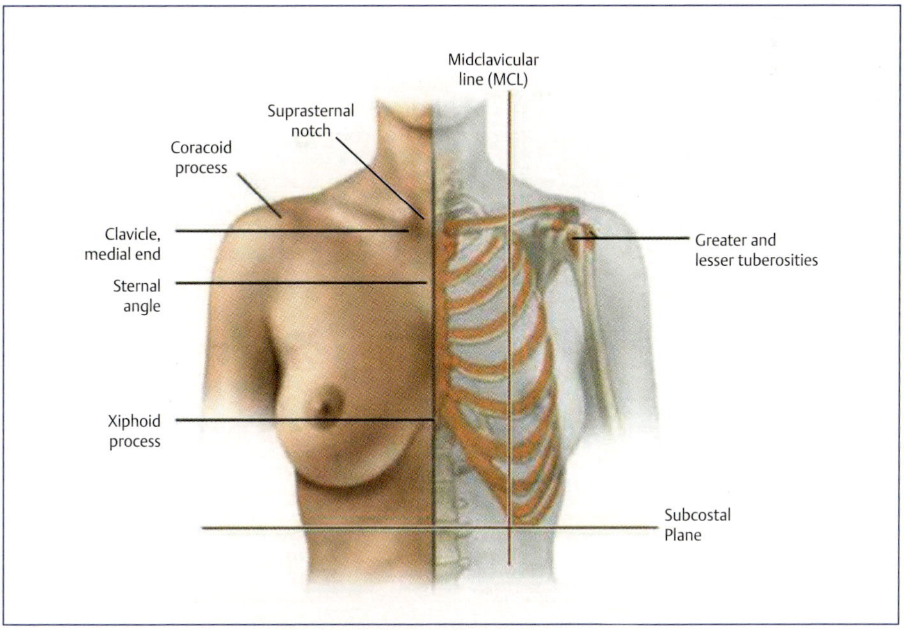

Fig. 11.3 Surface landmarks in the thoracic region.

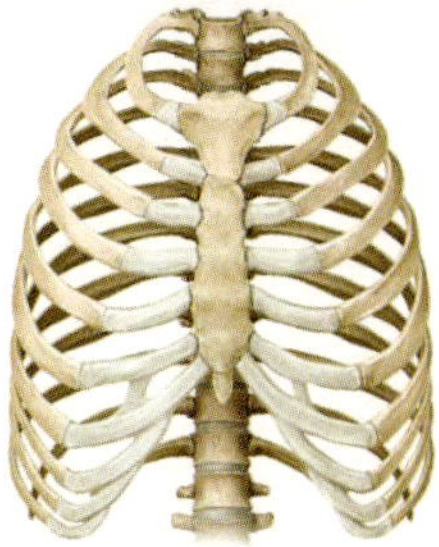

CHAPTER 12

Skeleton of the Thorax

Learning Objectives

After reading the chapter, the students should be able to do the following:

- Identify the vertebrae, the typical and atypical ones.
- Identify the ribs, the typical and atypical ones.
- Enumerate relevant relations to the bones, for example, to the sternum, first rib, etc.

Introduction

The skeleton of the thorax consists of the following bony elements (**Fig. 12.1**):

1. Twelve thoracic vertebrae
2. Twelve pairs of ribs
3. Sternum

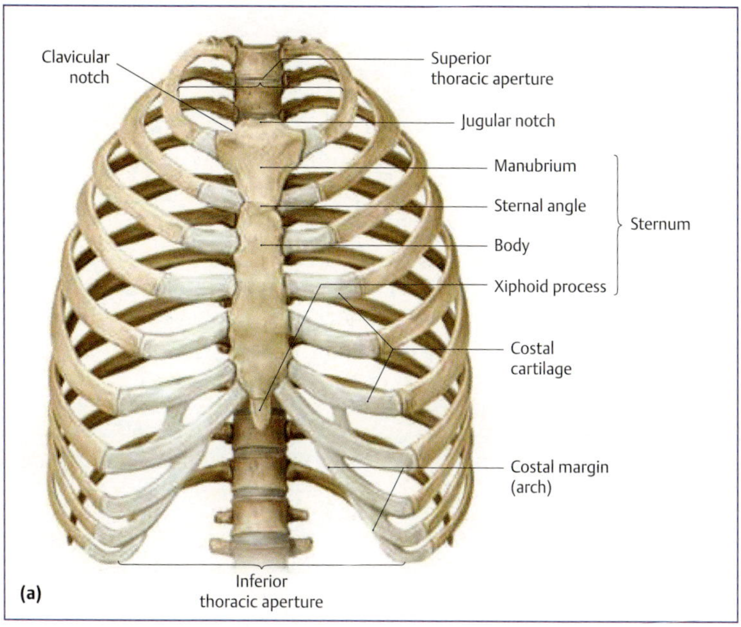

Fig. 12.1 Skeleton of thorax: **(a)** Anterior view. (*continued*)

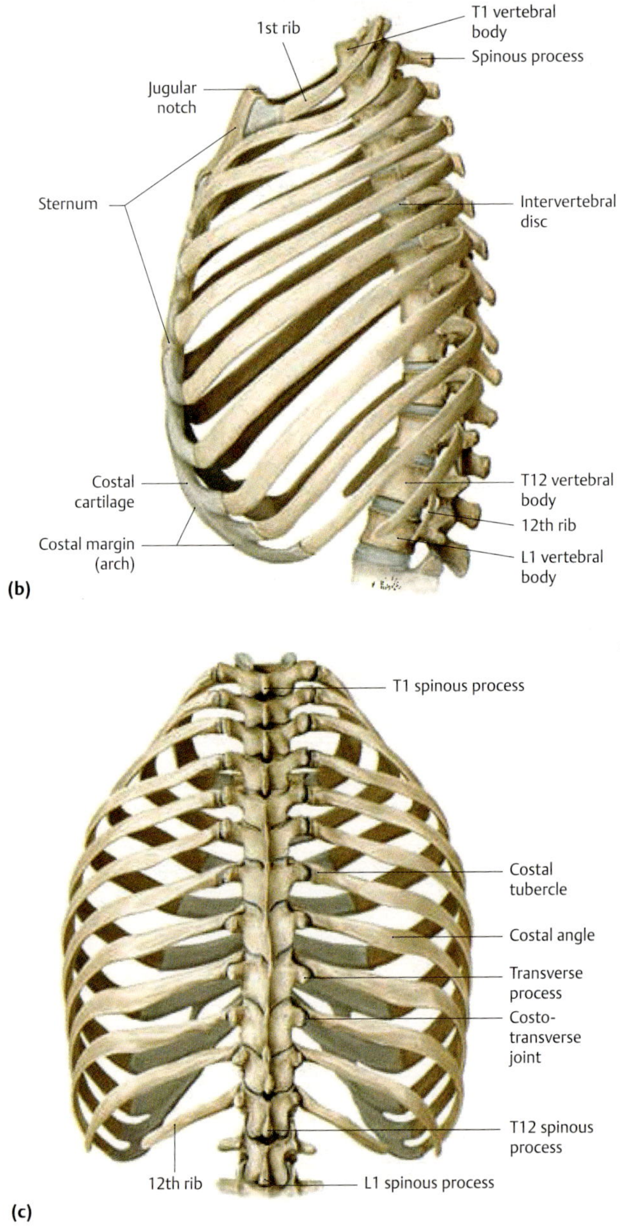

Fig. 12.1 (*continued*) Skeleton of thorax: **(b)** Left lateral view and **(c)** posterior view.

These bony elements articulate with each other to form various joints that permit a range of movements essential for respiration. In this chapter, we shall deal with the bones with their relevant general features; however, the joints have been covered in Chapter 15.

Vertebrae

The thoracic vertebrae are twelve in number (**Fig. 12.2**). Each thoracic vertebra has the following parts (**Fig. 12.3**):

1. *Body*: It lies anteriorly and is heart shaped.
2. *Pedicles*: They are two short stout bars projecting backwards and slightly laterally from the vertebral body.
3. *Laminae*: Each pedicle is continuous posteromedially with a plate of the bone, the lamina. The two laminae meet in the midline posteriorly.

4. *Vertebral arch*: It is formed by the pair of pedicles and laminae. It, along with the body of vertebra, encloses the vertebral foramen.
5. *Spinous process*: From the junction of the laminae, the spinous process passes backwards and downwards.
6. *Transverse processes*: On each side from the junction of the pedicle with the lamina, a transverse process passes laterally and slightly backwards. The spinous and transverse processes serve as a series of short levers for the movement of the vertebral column.
7. *Superior and inferior articular processes*: Projecting upwards from the junction of the pedicle and the lamina on either side, there is a superior articular process and similarly projecting downwards is an inferior articular process. Each process bears an articular facet.

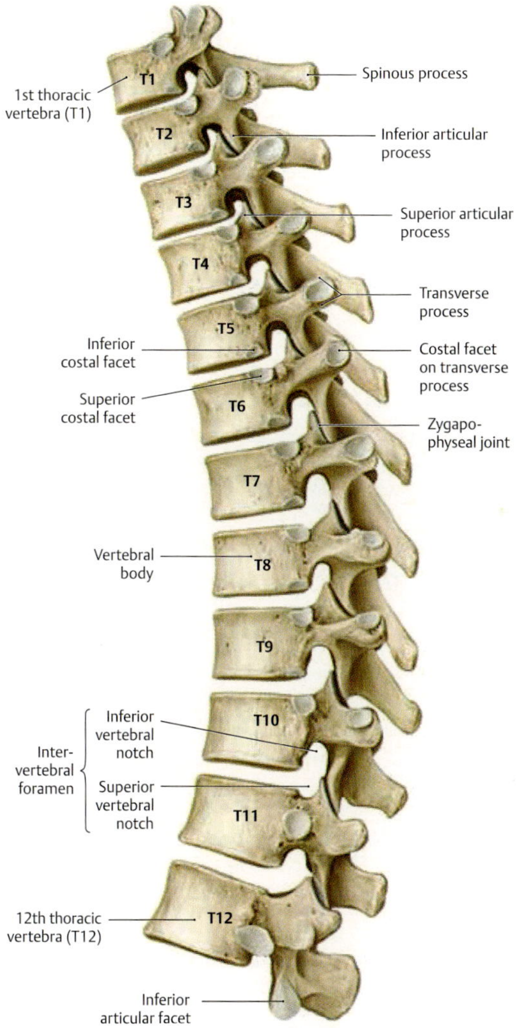

Fig. 12.2 Thoracic vertebrae (T1 to T12).

8. *Intervertebral foramen*: Each pedicle has a shallow *superior* and *a deep inferior vertebral notch*. These superior and inferior vertebral notches of the adjacent vertebrae form the intervertebral foramen. These foramina give passage to the spinal nerves arising from the spinal cord.
9. *Typical thoracic vertebrae*: The vertebral body of a typical thoracic vertebra has two *demifacets* on each side for the ribs. The *superior facet* articulates with the head of the numerically corresponding rib. The *inferior articular facet* articulates with the rib below. The transverse processes of the typical thoracic vertebra also bear a costal facet which articulates with the *articular part of the tubercle* of the corresponding rib.

10. *Atypical thoracic vertebrae*: They are the first and last two to three thoracic vertebrae. Their atypical feature being, a complete round facet for articulation with the head of the corresponding rib. The last two vertebrae, that is, the eleventh and twelfth thoracic vertebrae, do *not have costal facet on their transverse process* and do not articulate with the tubercle of the ribs. In addition, the *inferior articular process of the twelfth thoracic vertebra* has the *facet like lumbar type*, which is directed anterolaterally and is convex in nature.

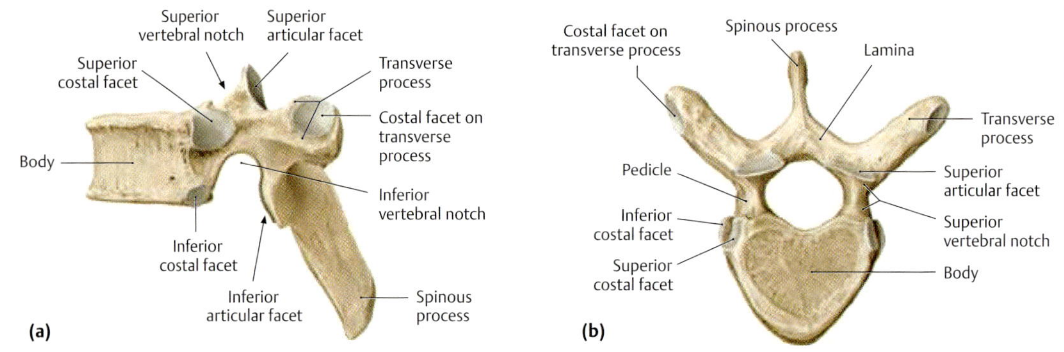

Fig. 12.3 Typical thoracic vertebra: **(a)** Lateral view and **(b)** superior view.

Ribs

1. There are twelve pairs of ribs forming a major part of the thoracic cage. The number may vary owing to the presence of the cervical or lumbar rib or absence of the twelfth rib (**Fig. 12.1**).
2. The ribs form bony arches one below the other with the intervening intercostal spaces occupied by the intercostal muscles.
3. The ribs are obliquely placed. The obliquity is maximum at the ninth rib and then decreases at the twelfth rib. The length increases up to the seventh rib and decreases till the twelfth rib.
4. *Vertebrosternal or true ribs* (**Fig. 12.4**): They articulate with the sternum at the anterior end and with the vertebrae at the posterior end, that is, the first to seventh ribs.
5. *False ribs* (**Fig. 12.4**): The remaining five ribs, that is, eighth to twelfth, are called the false ribs. Out of these, the eighth to tenth ribs have their cartilages turned upwards, joining with the higher cartilage forming the costal margin. These ribs are called the *vertebrochondral ribs.*
6. *Floating ribs*: The last two ribs, that is, the eleventh and twelfth, have their anterior ends free and are called the floating ribs or *vertebral ribs.*

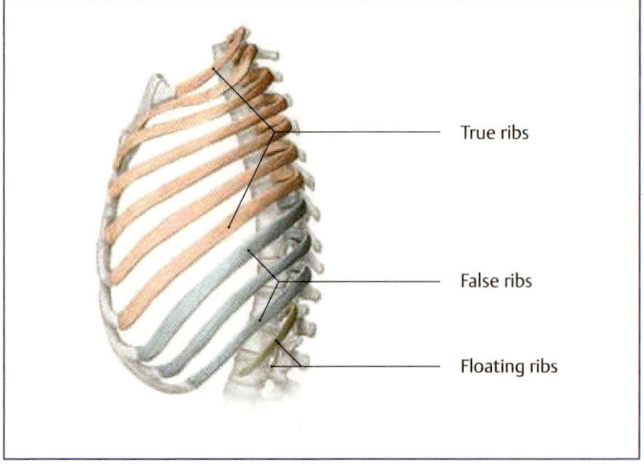

Fig. 12.4 Types of ribs.

7. *Typical ribs*: These are third to ninth ribs. Rest of the ribs, that is, the first, second, tenth, eleventh and twelfth, are called the atypical ribs. The typical rib has a *head* at the posterior end, followed

by a *neck*, a *tubercle* at the neck shaft angle, the shaft and a concave depression at the anterior end, meant for the costal cartilage (**Figs. 12.5** and **12.7**).

- *Head*: It has two facets separated by a crest. The lower larger facet articulates with the numerically corresponding vertebra, that is, the lower larger facet of the head of the fifth rib articulates with the T5 and the smaller upper facet with the T4.
- *Neck*: The neck of the rib lies in front of the transverse process of the corresponding vertebra. The neck has two surfaces, anterior and posterior, and two borders, a sharp (crest) superior and a blunt inferior border.
- *Tubercle*: It lies along the outer surface of the rib at the junction of the neck and the shaft of the rib. It has a medial *articular part* that forms the *costotransverse joint* with the transverse process of the corresponding vertebra. It also has a lateral *non-articular part* offering attachment to the *lateral costotransverse ligament*.
- *Shaft*: It is flat with outer and inner surfaces and two borders, upper and lower. The shaft is curved with the convexity outwards. It also presents an *angle*, located about 5 cm distal to the tubercle. The shaft is twisted at the angle.
- The inner surface is smooth and has a ridge which is continuous with the lower border of the neck. Below the ridge, between it and the lower border of the shaft is the *costal groove*. The costal groove contains the intercostal vessels and nerve.

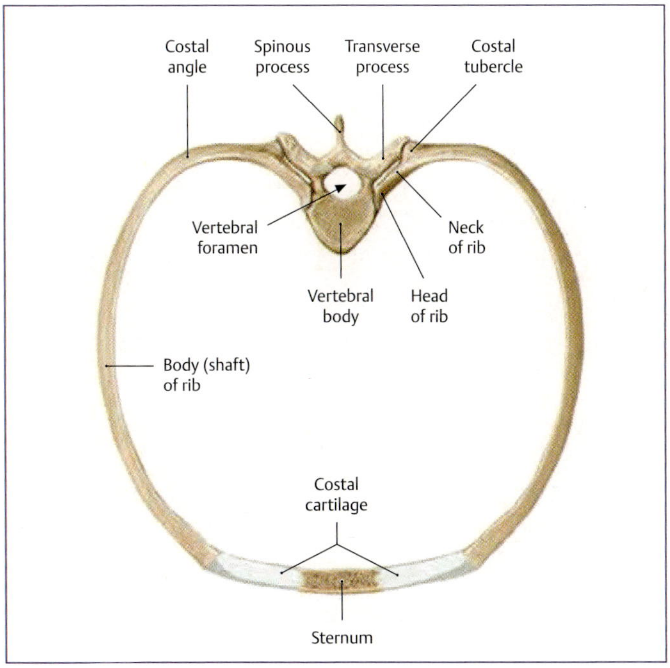

Fig. 12.5 A pair of typical ribs articulating with the vertebra posteriorly and sternum anteriorly.

Atypical Ribs

The first, second, tenth, eleventh and twelfth ribs are atypical ribs. We shall try to learn some salient features of these ribs.

First Rib (Fig. 12.6)

1. It is the shortest, broadest and the most curved rib.
2. It is not twisted like the typical ribs.
3. It is flattened from above downwards, thus presenting the superior and inferior surfaces and the inner and outer borders.
   - The superior surface is crossed by *two grooves*, an anterior for the subclavian vein and a posterior for the subclavian artery. Between these grooves, the inner border receives insertion of the

scalenus anterior muscle at the *scalene tubercle*. The inner border also gives attachment to the suprapleural membrane (Sibson's fascia). The posterior end has a small, rounded head that articulates with the first thoracic vertebra. The anterior broad end articulates with the first costal cartilage.

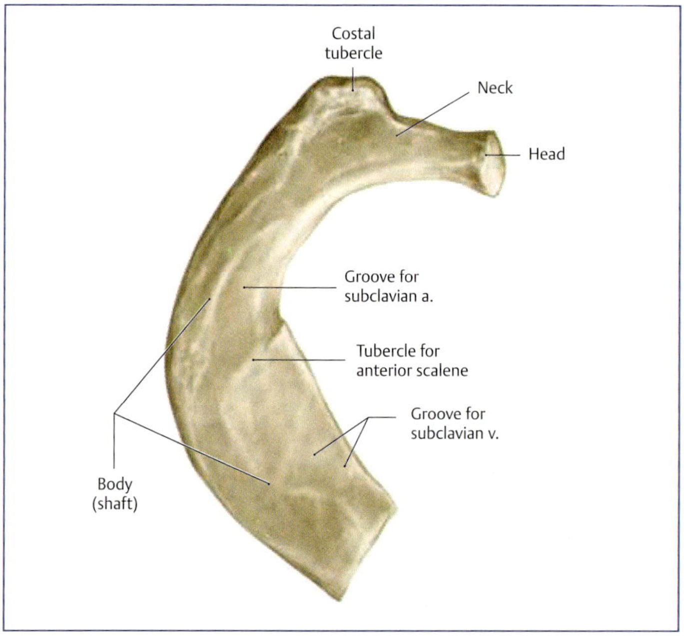

Fig. 12.6 First rib.

Second Rib (Fig. 12.7)

It has the following atypical characteristics:

1. The shaft of the second rib is not twisted.
2. Its outer surface faces upwards and the inner surface faces downwards.
3. It has a short, costal groove in the posterior part.
4. The shaft of the rib is marked by a *rough tubercle* in the middle (unique feature of the second rib) along the outer surface.

Tenth Rib

Its atypical feature is that it has only a single facet on the head for articulation with the T10 vertebra.

Eleventh (Fig. 12.7) and Twelfth Ribs

Both the ribs are short and have pointed ends without necks and tubercles. The twelfth rib may be absent.

Sternum

It is a flat bone. It forms the anterior part of the thoracic cage. It has three parts: the *manubrium, body* and *xiphoid process* (**Fig. 12.8**).

Manubrium sterni: It is the upper, thickest and broadest part of the sternum. It has two surfaces, anterior and posterior, and four borders, the superior, inferior and two lateral borders.

Its *posterior surface* is concave and forms the anterior boundary of the superior mediastinum. The *superior border* is rounded, concave and is marked by the *jugular/suprasternal/interclavicular notch* in the median portion. The lateral part of the superior border shows the *clavicular notch* which articulates with

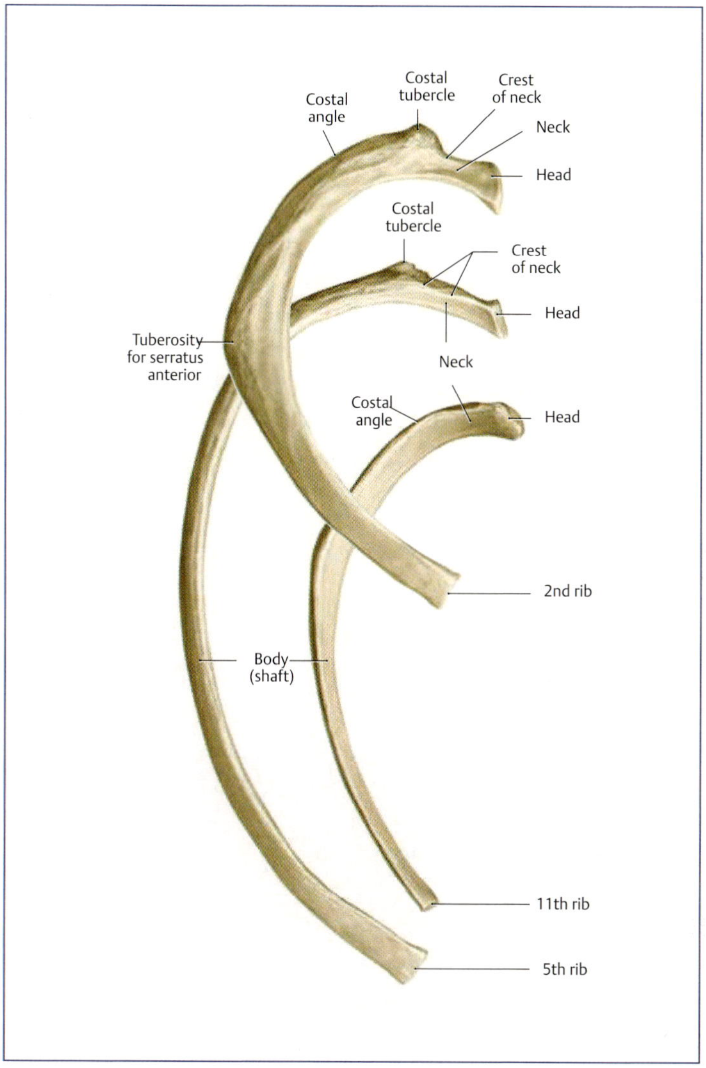

Fig. 12.7 Right ribs (superior view); 2nd, 5th and 11th.

the sternal/medial end of the clavicle at the sternoclavicular joint. The *inferior border* articulates with the body of the sternum forming the secondary cartilaginous joint. The manubrium meets the body of the sternum making the *sternal angle/angle of Louis*. The lateral border of the manubrium articulates with the first costal cartilage forming the primary cartilaginous joint. The lower part of the lateral border of the manubrium has a small demifacet for the articulation with the second costal cartilage.

Body of the sternum: It is longer, narrower and thinner as compared to the manubrium. It has an anterior and a posterior surface. The anterior surface presents three ill-defined transverse ridges indicating the lines of fusion of the four sternebrae which have eventually fused to form the body of the sternum. The *lateral borders* of the body of the sternum articulate with the third to sixth costal cartilages and part of the seventh costal cartilage. At the *upper end*, the body articulates with the manubrium forming the secondary cartilaginous joint, while at the *lower end* it articulates with the xiphisternum forming a primary cartilaginous joint.

Xiphoid process: It is the smallest and lowest portion of the sternum which is initially cartilaginous and later becomes ossified.

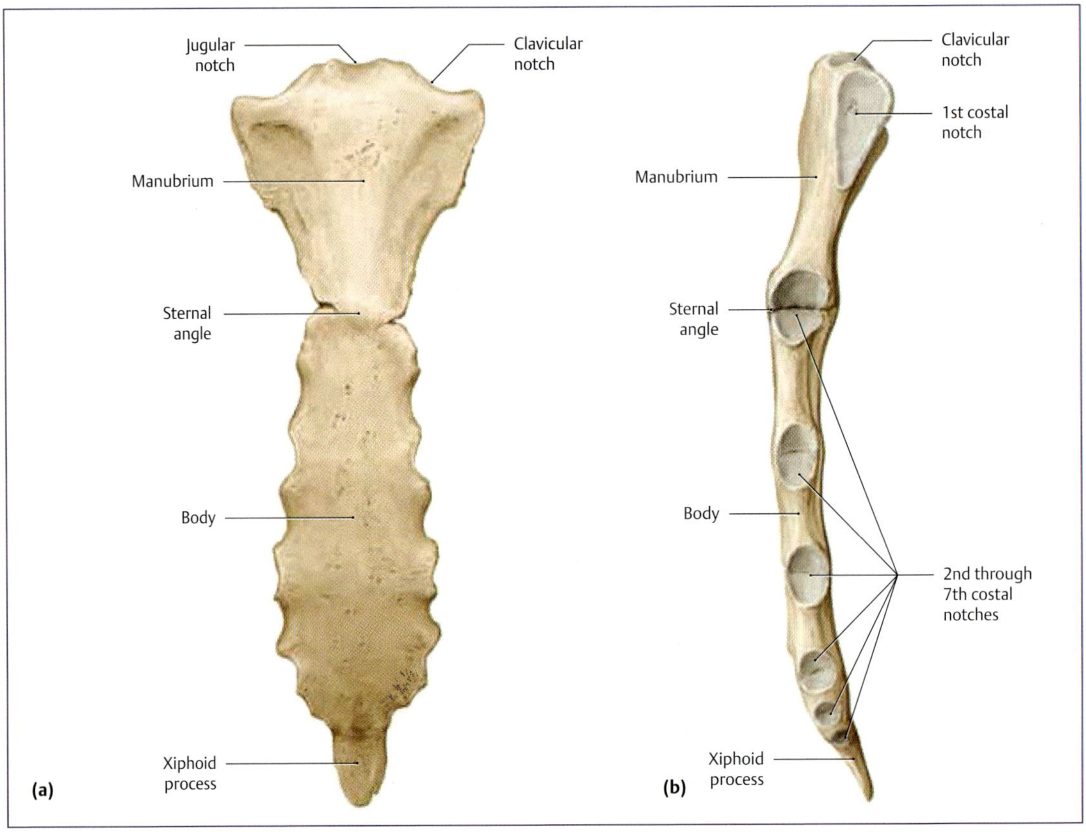

Fig. 12.8 Sternum: **(a)** Anterior view and **(b)** left lateral view.

Clinical Notes

1. *Cervical rib*: It is an anomalous rib associated with the seventh cervical vertebra. It may compress the elements of the brachial plexus and the subclavian vessels leading to neurovascular symptoms.
2. *Sternal puncture*: It is a procedure to retrieve the bone marrow from the sternum for examination.
3. *Hemivertebra*: It is a defect in the development of the vertebral body which leads to scoliosis.

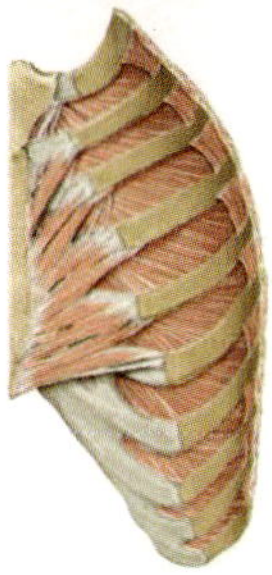

CHAPTER 13

Thoracic Wall

Learning Objectives

At the end of the dissection of the thoracic wall, you should be able to identify the following:

- Intercostal muscles.
- Intercostal nerves and their branches.
- Intercostal arteries and veins.

Introduction

The thoracic wall is overlapped by the muscles of the upper limb, muscles of the back and is encroached by the abdominal muscles. The pectoral region has already been dissected during the dissection of the superior extremity. Therefore, these overlapping muscles are removed to a great extent.

Dissection and Identification

1. Detach the serratus anterior muscle from its attachments to the ribs (upper eight ribs) and reflect it laterally.
2. Beginning at the sternal angle, palpate the ribs and intercostal spaces from the second onwards. Identify them numerically.
3. Locate the fifth intercostal space that lies between the fifth and sixth ribs.
4. Identify the external intercostal muscle (**Fig. 13.1**). It is attached to the inferior border of the fifth rib above and to the superior border of the sixth rib below (since we are dissecting the fifth intercostal space). Note the direction of its fibres. They pass obliquely towards the anterior median line. The muscle extends from the tubercle of the rib posterior to the costochondral junction anteriorly.
5. Identify the external intercostal membrane, which replaces the external intercostal muscle beyond the costochondral junction. The membrane is located between the costochondral junction and the lateral border of the sternum.
6. Pass a probe deep to the external intercostal membrane immediately lateral to the sternum. Now push the probe laterally and appreciate that it passes deep to the external intercostal muscle.
7. Using a pair of scissors, under the guiding probe, cut the external intercostal muscle from its superior attachment to the rib above. Reflect the muscle downwards (inferiorly). Your cut may be continued till you reach the midaxillary line.

https://www.winkingskull.com/dissector/V1/video.aspx?vid=233

8. Identify the internal intercostal muscle. It stretches from the floor of the costal groove of the upper rib to the inner lip of the superior border of the lower rib. The muscle depresses the upper rib. Note the direction of its fibres; they are perpendicular to the direction of the fibres of the external intercostal muscle.

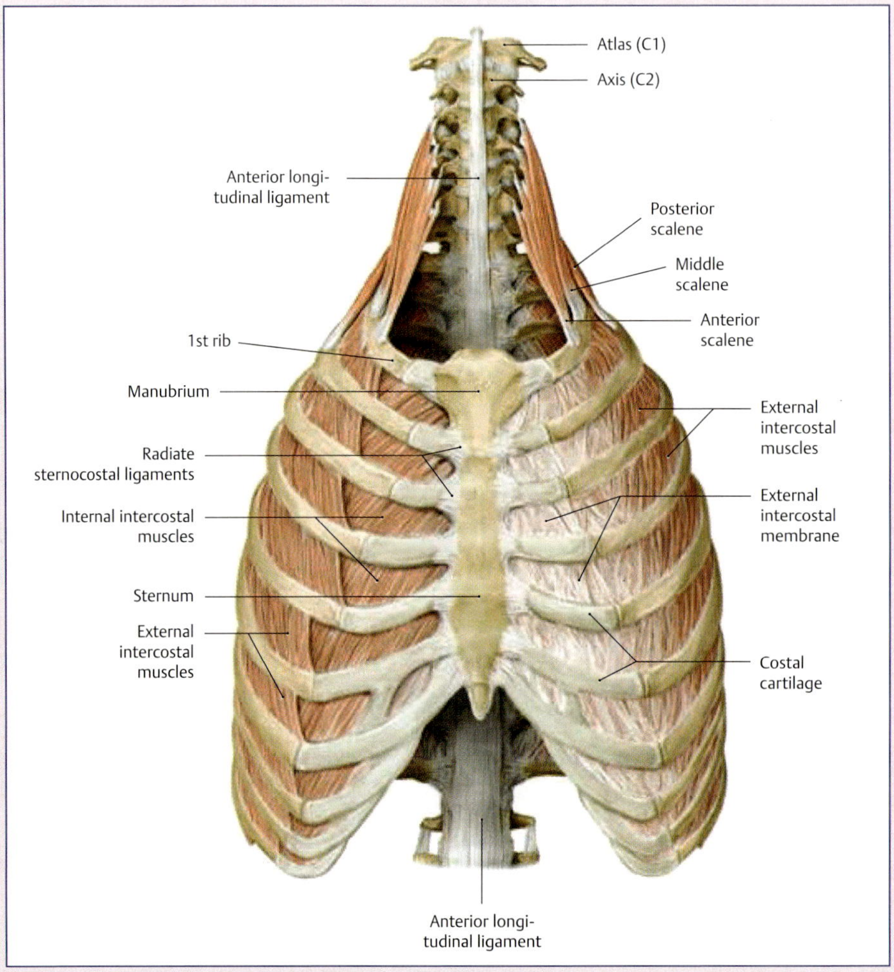

Fig. 13.1 Muscles of the thoracic wall (anterior view).

9. Starting from the lateral border of the sternum, detach the internal intercostal muscle from its lower attachment to the sixth rib. Continue it till the midaxillary line and turn the muscle upwards.
10. Now identify the fifth intercostal nerve and the corresponding posterior intercostal vessels below the fifth rib. The neurovascular plane lies between the second and third layers of muscles, that is, between the internal intercostal and innermost intercostal muscles. Note the direction of the fibres of the innermost intercostal muscle; it is like that of the internal intercostal muscle.

Opening of the thorax/removal of the anterior thoracic wall (**Fig. 13.2**):

11. Reflect the pectoralis major and serratus anterior laterally and the pectoralis minor superiorly.
12. Using a pair of scissors, cut the sternocleidomastoid near its attachment to the sternum and clavicle. Reflect it superiorly.
13. Push the infrahyoid muscles posteriorly, and using force detach them from the back of the sternum.
14. Using a saw, cut through the clavicles midway along their length.
15. At the level of the fifth intercostal space, make a transverse cut across the sternum and costal cartilages using the saw. Avoid injury to the deeper tissues.
16. With the bone cutter, cut the first to fifth ribs along the midaxillary line on both sides.

17. Cut the intercostal muscles in these spaces using a scalpel along the midaxillary line. These vertical cuts in the muscles should be aligned with the cut ribs. Make sure that the cuts are deep enough to cut the parietal layer of the pleura.

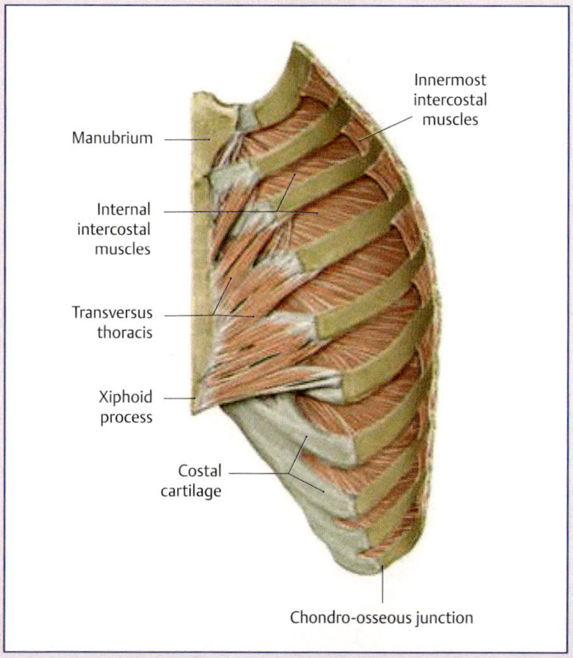

Fig. 13.2 Muscles of the thoracic wall (right half of the anterior thoracic wall removed).

18. Now cut the intercostal muscles and the parietal pleura along the upper border of the sixth rib on both sides of the thorax using a pair of scissors.
19. Now gently elevate the lower end of the sternum along with the attached portions of the cut costal cartilages and ribs.
20. Near the lower end of the sternum, identify both the *right and left internal thoracic vessels*. Cut them at the level of the fifth sternocostal joint.
21. Raise the lower end of the thoracic wall and cut the pleura with a pair of scissors where it reflects from the thoracic wall onto the mediastinum.
22. Cut the internal thoracic vessels at the level of the first rib. Remove the anterior thoracic wall along with the endothoracic fascia.
23. Identify the *transversus thoracis muscle* (**Fig. 13.2**). Trace its lower attachment to the sternum and upper attachment to the costal cartilages from the second to the sixth ribs. The subcostal muscles are shown in **Fig. 13.3**.
24. Note the internal thoracic artery and vein located between the transversus thoracis muscle and the costal cartilages. Identify the anterior intercostal branches. Note that the internal thoracic artery terminates behind the sixth or seventh costal cartilage by dividing into the superior epigastric artery and the musculophrenic artery. This division can be observed on the cadaver instead of the thoracic wall.
25. *Intercostal nerves* (**Fig. 13.4**): There are eleven intercostal nerves. The twelfth is called the *subcostal nerve*. They are ventral rami of the thoracic spinal nerves. Each intercostal nerve emerging from the intervertebral foramen below the corresponding vertebra enters the intercostal space. Here, it lies between the second (internal intercostal muscle) and the third (innermost intercostal muscle) layers of muscles, in the subcostal groove. About 1 cm lateral to the sternum, it turns forwards to continue as the *anterior cutaneous branch*.

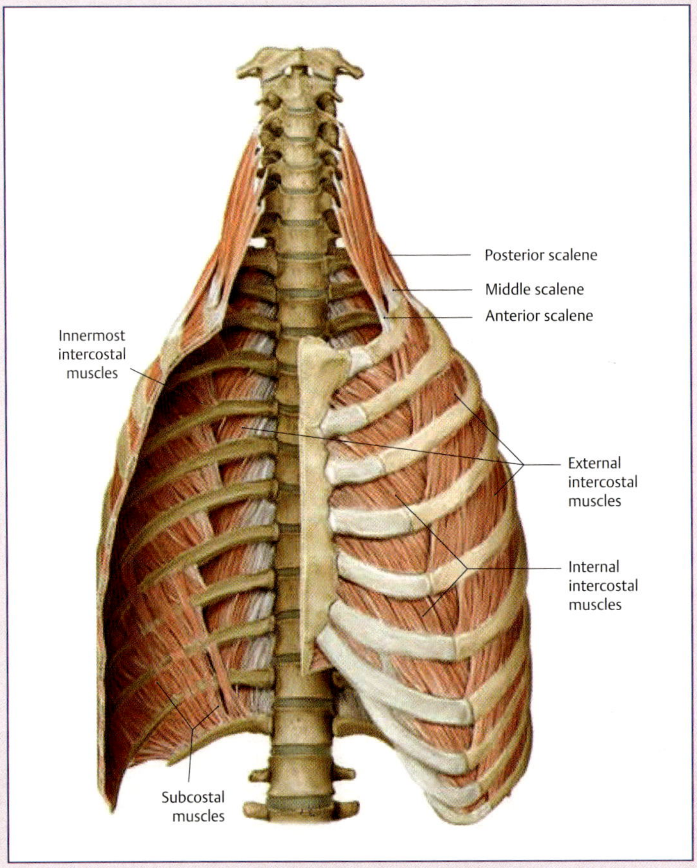

Fig. 13.3 Subcostal muscles (anterior view with thoracic cage opened to expose posterior surface of anterior wall).

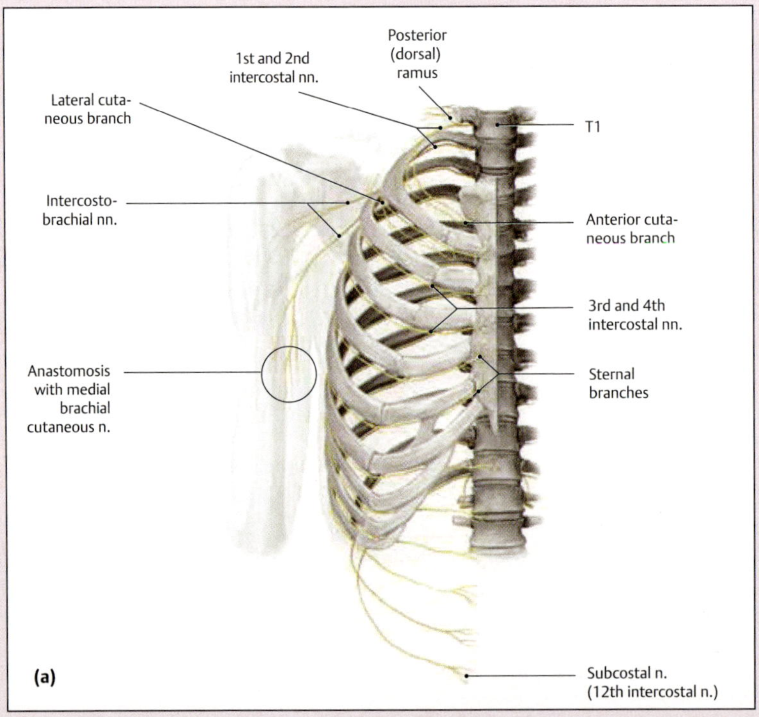

Fig. 13.4 Intercostal nerves: **(a)** Anterior view. The first rib has been removed to reveal the first and second intercostal nerves.

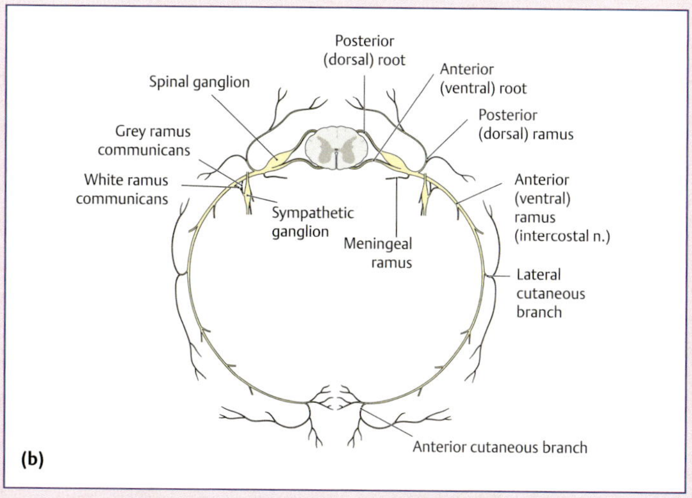

Fig. 13.4 Intercostal nerves: **(b)** A pair of typical intercostal nerves.

Branches

Each intercostal nerve is connected to the sympathetic ganglion by two branches.

1. *White ramus communicans*: Carrying the preganglionic fibres from the nerve to the ganglion.
2. *Grey ramus communicans*: Carrying the postganglionic fibres from the ganglion to the nerve.
3. *Collateral branch*: It arises near the angle of the rib. It runs along the superior border of the rib below.
4. *Lateral cutaneous branch*: It pierces the overlying muscles and divides into anterior and posterior branches.
5. *Anterior cutaneous branch*: It pierces the internal intercostal muscle, external intercostal membrane and the pectoralis major muscle and then divides into medial and lateral branches.
6. *Muscular branches*: They supply the intercostal, transversus thoracis, serratus posterior superior and inferior muscles.
7. The cutaneous innervation and dermatomes of thoracic wall are shown in **Figs. 13.5** and **13.6**, respectively.

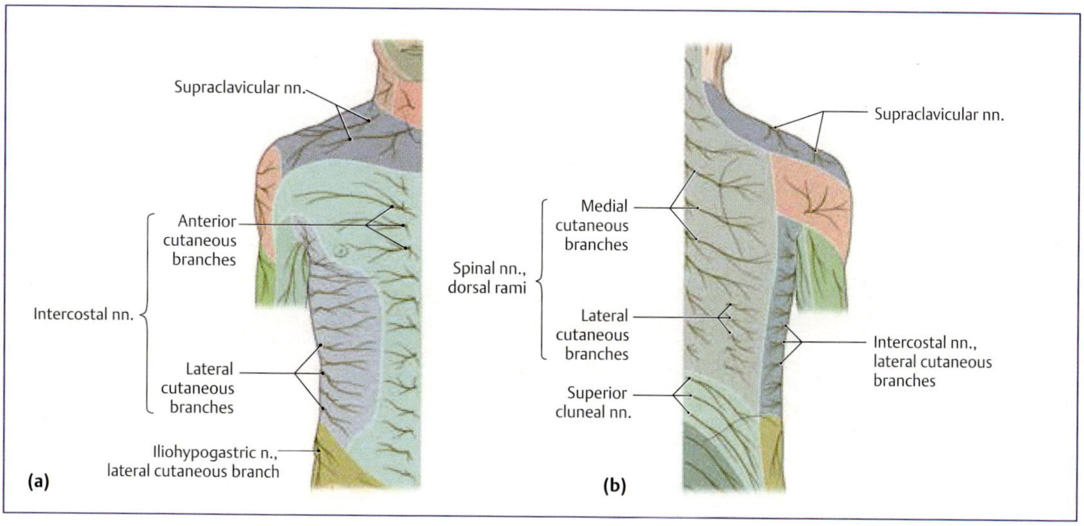

Fig. 13.5 Cutaneous innervation of the thoracic wall: **(a)** Anterior view and **(b)** posterior view.

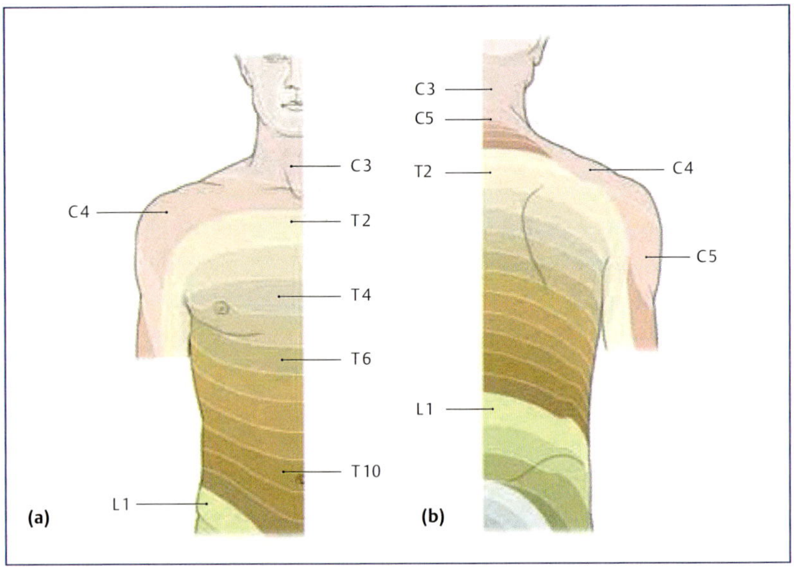

Fig. 13.6 Dermatomes of the thoracic wall (landmarks: T4 generally includes the nipple; T6 innervates the skin over the xiphoid). **(a)** Anterior view and **(b)** posterior view.

Points to Note

1. The *first intercostal nerve* has no lateral or anterior cutaneous branch. The *second* has a large lateral cutaneous branch destined to the floor of the axilla. It is called the *intercostobrachial nerve.*
2. The *seventh* nerve onwards (T7 to T11) run progressively a larger part of their course in the ventral abdominal wall, supplying the muscles and the overlying skin of the wall. The anterior cutaneous branches of the fifth to twelfth intercostal nerves pierce the rectus abdominis and its sheath to reach and supply the skin. The umbilical strip is supplied by the tenth nerve (T10).

Intercostal Vessels

Each intercostal space contains one large posterior and two smaller anterior intercostal arteries (**Figs. 13.7** and **13.8**).

1. *Posterior intercostal arteries*: They are eleven, one in each space. The first and second are derived from the superior intercostal artery, which in turn is a branch of the costocervical trunk. The third to eleventh arteries are branches of the descending thoracic aorta. The posterior intercostal artery accompanies the nerve and gives a collateral branch that passes along the superior margin of the lower rib. Both of them end up by anastomosing with the anterior intercostal arteries.
2. *Anterior intercostal arteries*: Each intercostal space has two anterior intercostal arteries.
3. In the upper six spaces, they are derived from the *internal thoracic artery*. In seventh to ninth spaces, these are derived from the *musculophrenic artery*. The corresponding *anterior intercostal veins* drain into the musculophrenic and internal thoracic veins. In the last two spaces, there are no anterior intercostal arteries. The arteries in the second, third and fourth spaces supply the mammary gland. They become enlarged during pregnancy and lactation.

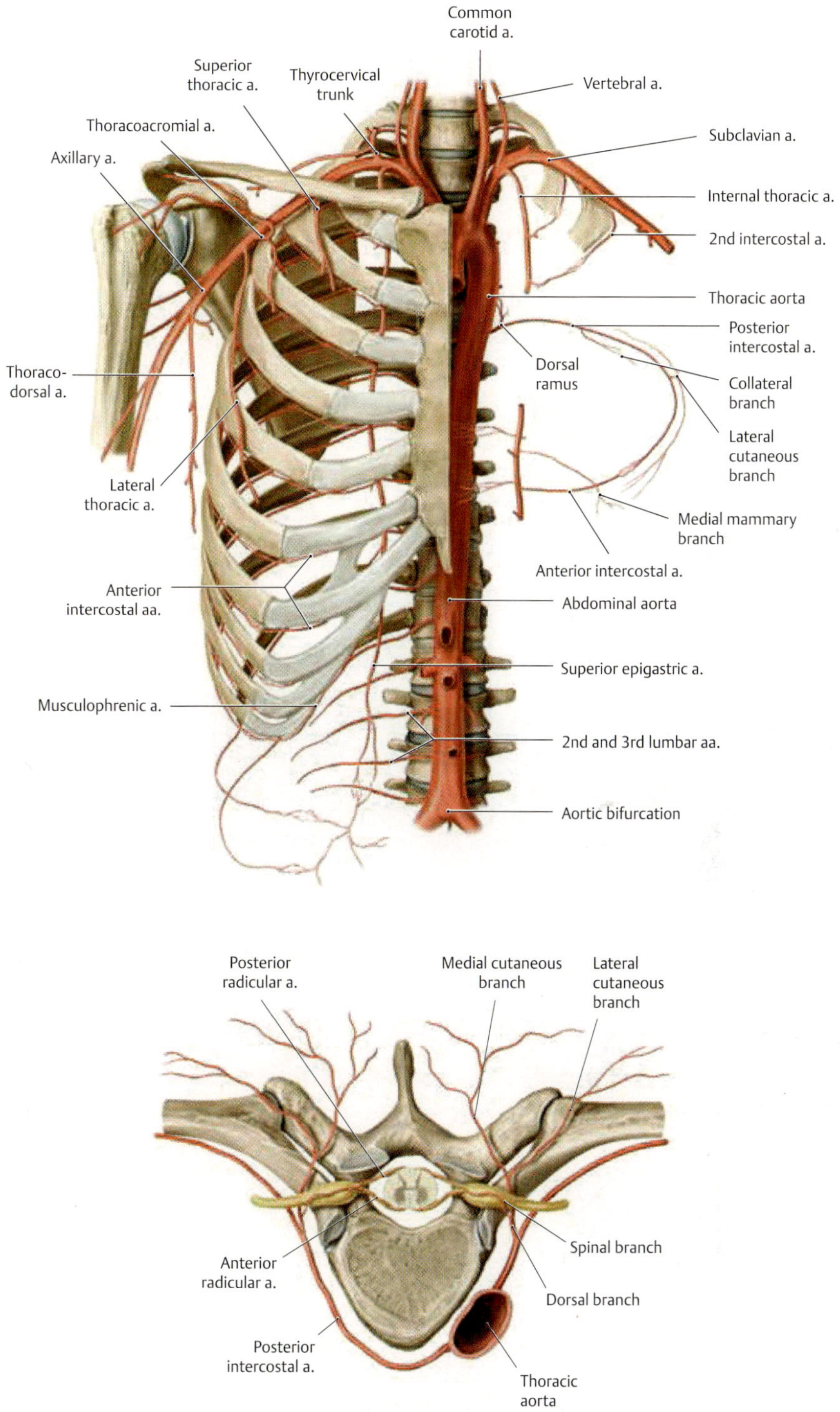

Fig. 13.7 Arteries of the thoracic wall.

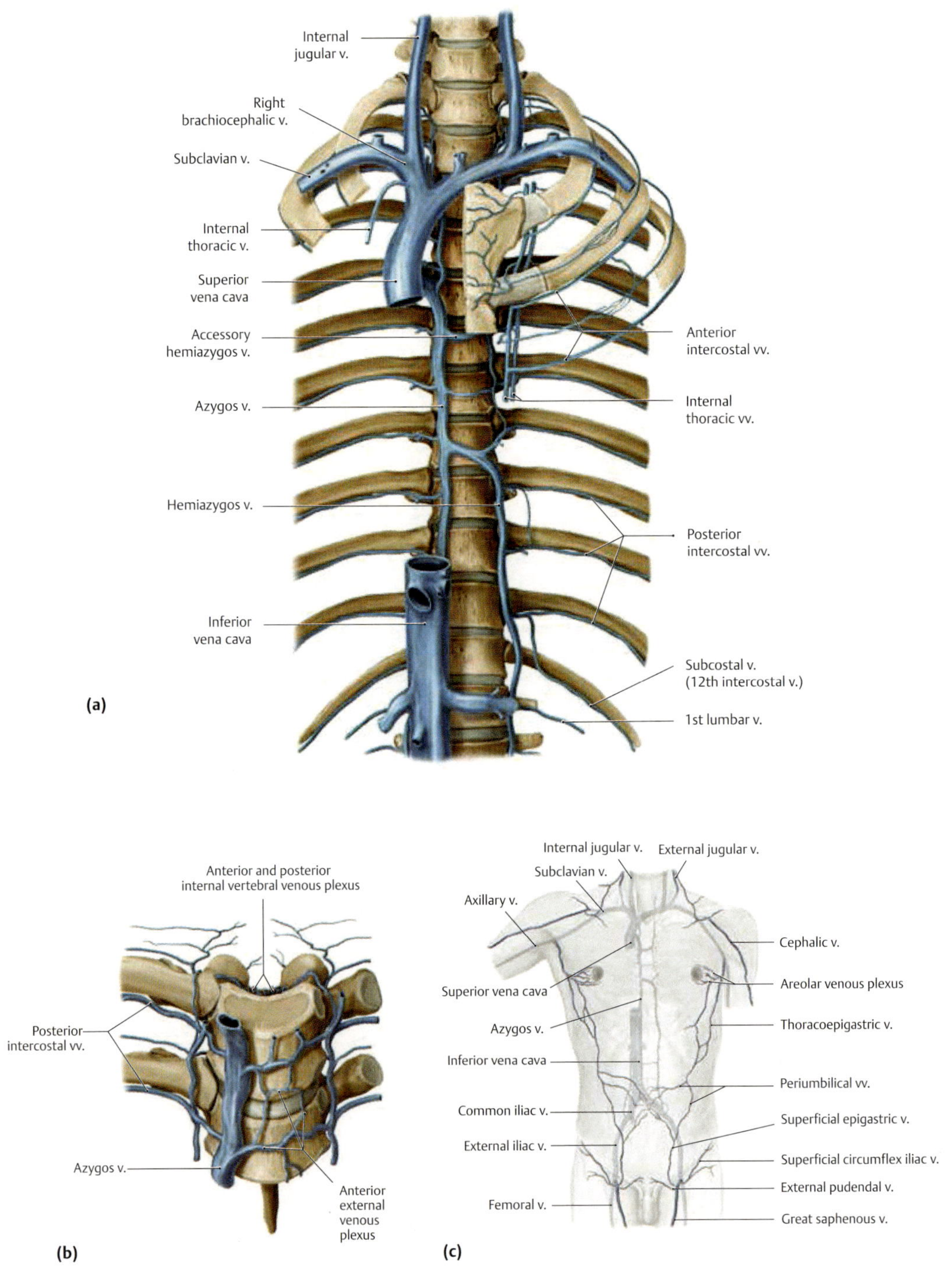

Fig. 13.8 Veins of the thoracic wall. **(a)** Anterior view with rib cage opened. **(b)** Vertebral venous plexus (anterior view). **(c)** Superficial veins (anterior view). The thoracoepigastric veins are a potential superficial collateral venous drainage route in the event of superior or inferior vena cava obstruction.

Clinical Notes

1. *Intercostal neuralgia*: Irritation of the intercostal nerve leads to referred pain in the front of the chest or abdomen.
2. A surgical approach to the thoracic contents can be sought either anteriorly or laterally. In an anterior approach, the sternum is vertically split to have an access to the heart, avoiding the major blood vessels. The sternal incision is closed subsequently by stainless steel wires. In the lateral approach, the intercostal spaces are incised to gain access to the lungs or the structures in the posterior mediastinum.

CHAPTER 14

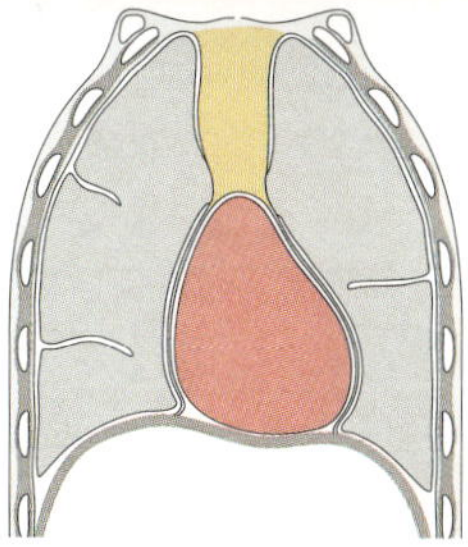

Thoracic Cavity

Learning Objectives

At the end of the dissection of the thoracic cavity, students should be able to do the following:

- Define mediastinum and tell its subdivisions.
- Define the pleura and identify its parietal and visceral layer.
- Identify the external features of lungs and tell the differences between right and left lung.
- Define bronchopulmonary segments and enumerate their number in right and left lung.
- Define pericardium and differentiate fibrous pericardium from serous pericardium.
- Identify the external features of heart and internal features of its chambers.
- Identify arch of aorta and its branches.
- Identify the extent of trachea and its relations.
- Identify the extent of curvatures and constrictions of oesophagus.
- Identify the extent of descending thoracic aorta and its branches.

Introduction

The word *mediastinum* has Latin origin and it means one that stands in the middle. The mediastinum is a bulky septum that lies between the two pleural cavities containing the lungs (refer to **Fig. 14.1a**). It extends from the root of the neck to the diaphragm vertically and from the sternum to the vertebral column anteroposteriorly.

For the sake of descriptive ease, it is subdivided into *superior* and *inferior mediastinum* by an imaginary horizontal plane passing from the sternal angle to the intervertebral disc between the T4 and T5 vertebrae (**Fig. 14.1b**).

The *inferior mediastinum* is further divided into (**Fig. 14.1b**) the following:

1. *Middle mediastinum* containing the heart and pericardium.
2. *Anterior mediastinum* lies between the heart and sternum.
3. *Posterior mediastinum* lies between the heart and vertebral column. It is pertinent to note that the anteroposterior depth of the superior aperture of the thorax is only 5 cm and that the superior mediastinum is smaller than the remaining anteroposteriorly. The posterior mediastinum extends furthest inferiorly since it passes between the diaphragm and the vertebral column up to the T12 vertebra.

Pleura

The thorax has two pleural cavities (right and left) one on either side of the mediastinum (**Fig. 14.2**). The pleural cavities are filled with the lungs. Each pleural cavity is formed by a thin serous membrane.

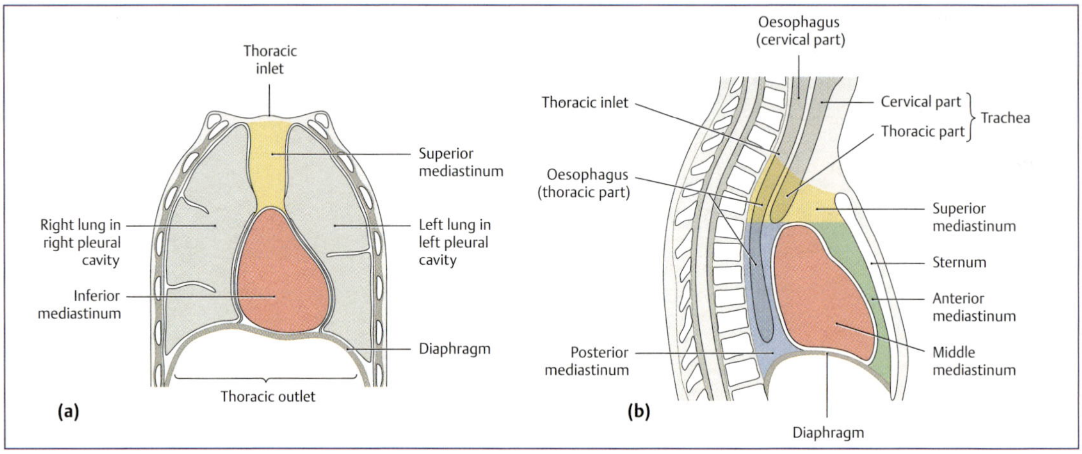

Fig. 14.1 Mediastinum. **(a)** Anterior view (coronal section). **(b)** Lateral view (midsagittal section).

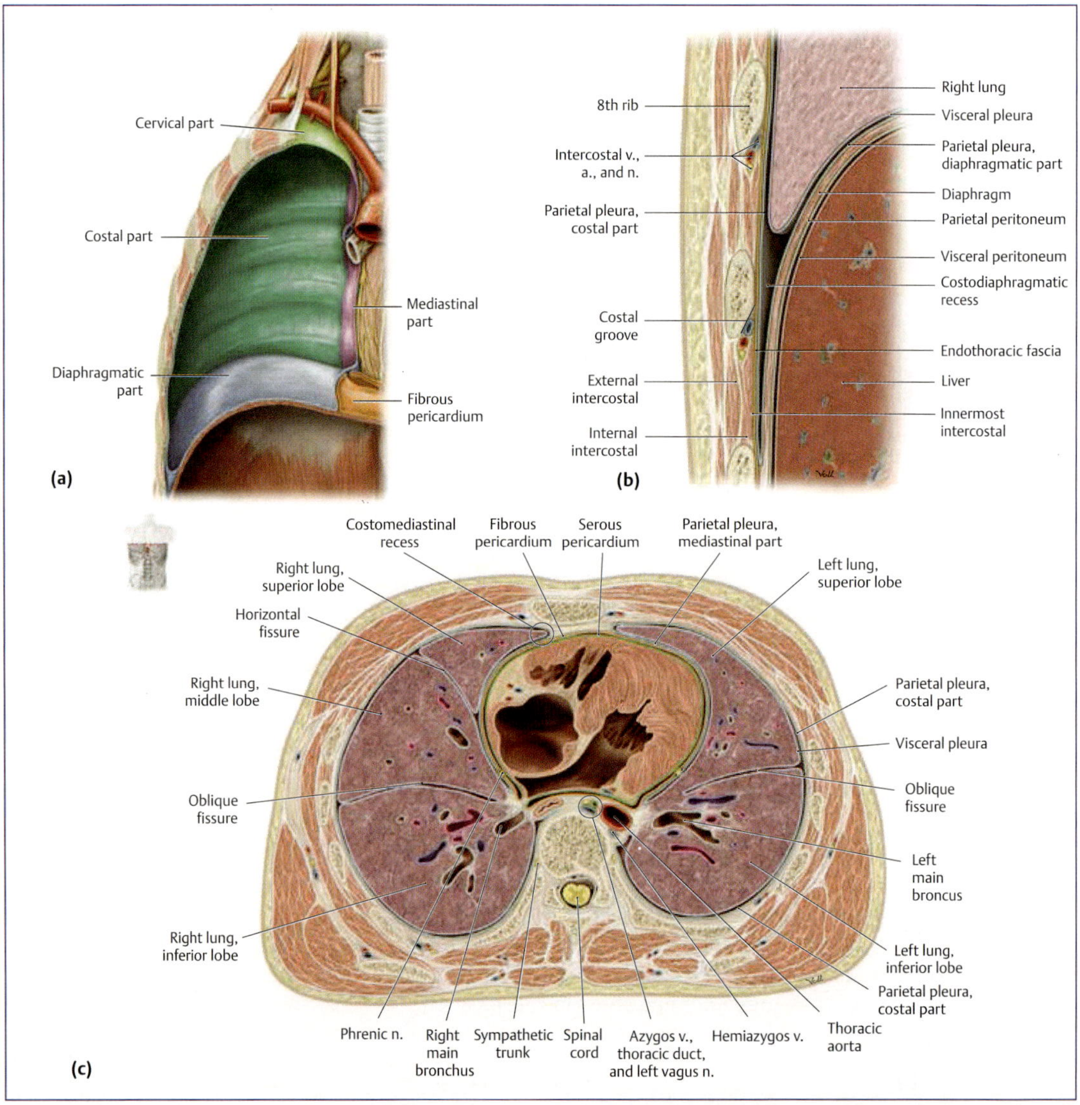

Fig. 14.2 Parietal pleura. **(a)** Parts of the parietal pleura. *Opened*: Right pleural cavity (anterior view). **(b)** Costodiaphragmatic recess, coronal section (anterior view). Reflection of the diaphragmatic pleura onto the inner thoracic wall (becoming the costal pleura) forms the costodiaphragmatic recess. **(c)** Transverse section (inferior view) showing pleural cavities and lungs.

It has two layers:

1. Parietal pleura
2. Visceral/pulmonary pleura

The *parietal pleura* is further subdivided into (**Fig. 14.3**) the following:

https://www.winkingskull.com/dissector/V1/video.aspx?vid=275

1. *Costal pleura*: It lines the inner surface of the thoracic wall.
2. *Mediastinal pleura*: It covers the mediastinum.
3. *Diaphragmatic pleura*: It covers the superior surface of the diaphragm.
4. *Cervical pleura*: It covers the apex of the lung and extends into the root of the neck. In turn, it is covered by the *suprapleural membrane/Sibson's fascia*. The cervical pleura rises about 2 inches above the first costal cartilage. The suprapleural membrane is superiorly attached to the transverse process of the seventh cervical vertebra and inferiorly along the inner border of the first rib. It contains a muscle, the *scalenus minimus*. It maintains the pleural dome against the respiratory changes, such as deep inspiration or forced expiration.

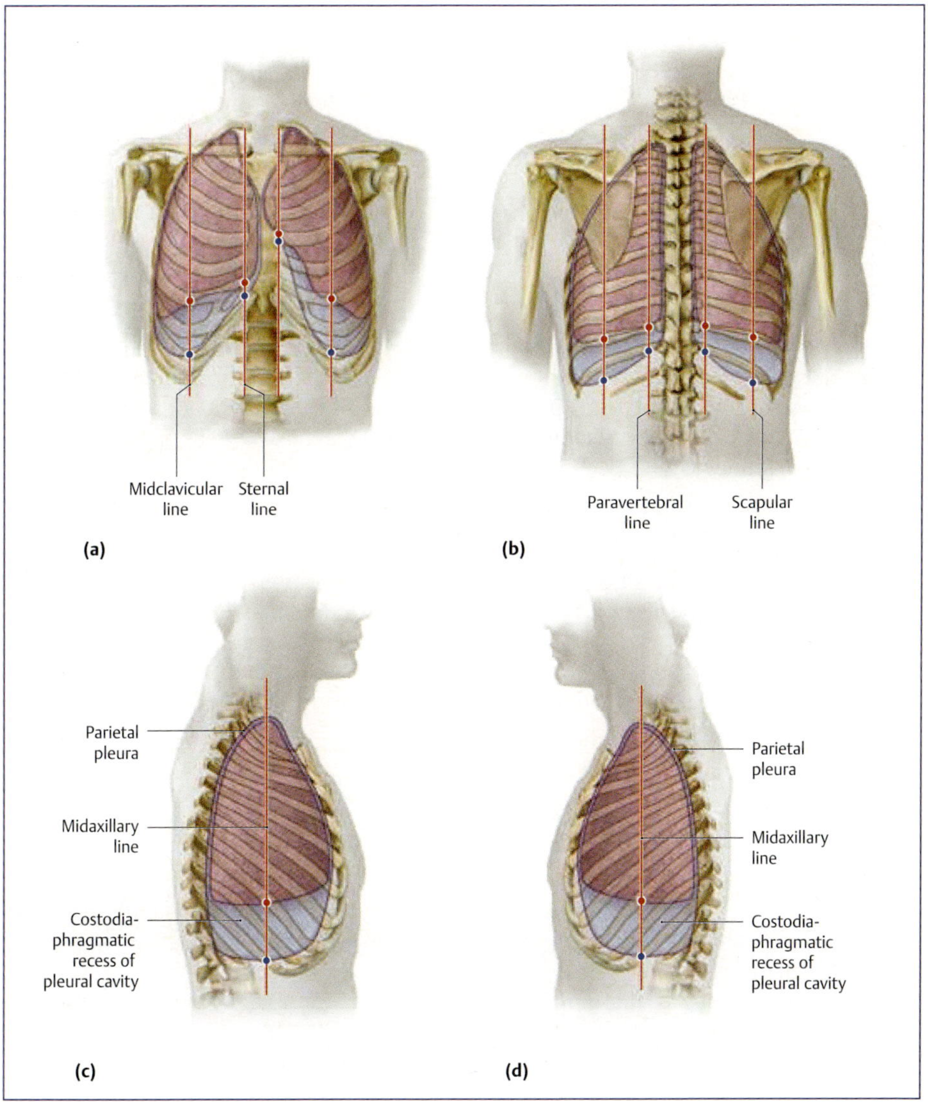

Fig. 14.3 Boundaries of the lungs and pleural cavities. **(a)** Anterior view. **(b)** Posterior view. **(c)** Right lateral view. **(d)** Left lateral view.

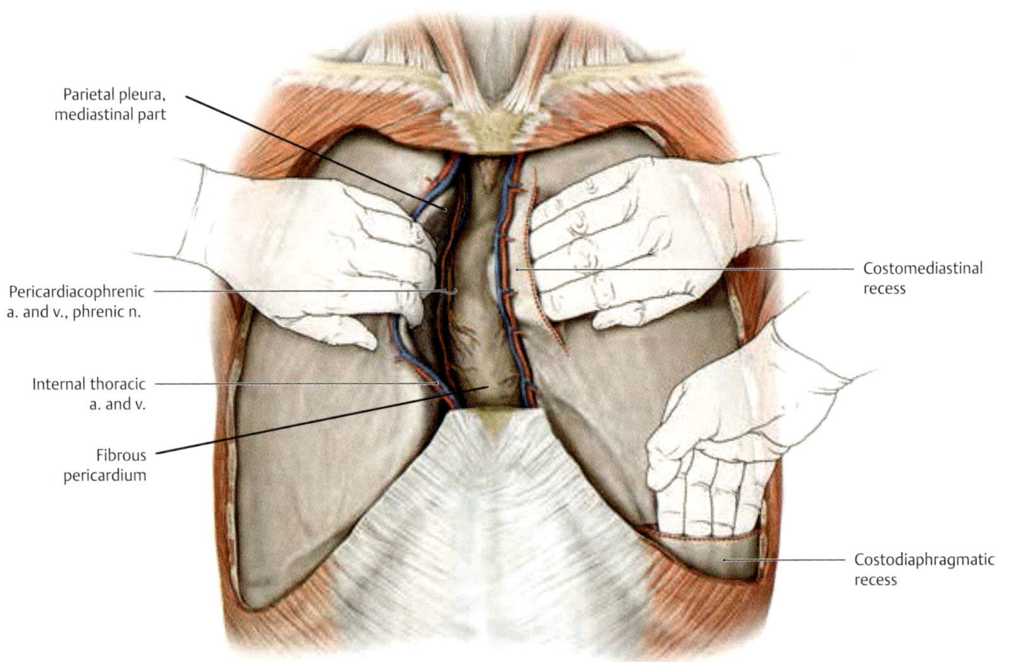

Fig. 14.4 Costomediastinal and costodiaphragmatic recesses.

The costal pleura lines the thoracic wall to which it is loosely bound by the *endothoracic fascia*. The pleura surrounding the root of the lung extends downwards beyond the root in the form of the *pulmonary ligament*. The pulmonary ligament contains loose areolar tissue and some lymphatics. Functionally, the pulmonary ligament provides dead space for expansion of the pulmonary veins during increased venous return, such as in exercise. In addition, it allows movement of the lung root during respiratory movements of the diaphragm.

Pleural recesses: These are folds of the parietal pleura serving as reserve spaces, permitting lung expansion during deep inspiration. There are two such recesses (**Fig. 14.4**):

1. *Costomediastinal recess* (**Fig. 14.4**): It lies along the anterior margin of the pleura, that is, behind the sternum and costal cartilages. It is formed by the costal and mediastinal pleura.
2. *Costodiaphragmatic recess* (**Fig. 14.4**): It lies inferiorly and follows the inferior margin of the pleura. It is formed by the costal and diaphragmatic pleura. It measures about 5 cm at the midaxillary line extending from the eighth to the tenth rib. In *pleural effusion*, it is the first to get filled, being the most dependent part.

Lines of pleural reflection: The parietal costal pleura is folded where it meets the diaphragmatic pleura (costodiaphragmatic recess) or mediastinal pleura (costomediastinal recess). These folds are called lines of pleural reflection. The cervical pleura forms a dome over the medial one-third of the clavicle about 1 inch above the bone.

The *anterior margin of the pleural reflection* extends from the sternoclavicular joint downwards to the midpoint of the sternal angle. From here on the right side, it continues vertically downwards up to the xiphisternal joint. On the left side, the line follows the same course up to the level of the fourth costal cartilage. It then follows the left sternal margin after arching outwards, descending till the sixth costal cartilage.

The *inferior margin* passes from the lower end of the anterior margin laterally and crosses the eighth rib in the midclavicular line, tenth rib in the midaxillary line and twelfth rib at the outer border of the sacrospinalis muscle on the posterior side. It then passes horizontally to the lower border of T12 vertebra, about 2 cm lateral to the spine of T12.

The *posterior margin* of pleural reflection passes vertically from 2 cm lateral to the spine of T12 vertebra to a point 2 cm lateral to the spine of C7 vertebra from where it continues as the mediastinal pleura.

Dissection and Identification

1. To explore the pleural cavities, use your hands but avoid injury from the cut ends of ribs. You can cover the cut ends of the ribs with wet cotton or paper towels.
2. Remove the fluid from the cavity by soaking it with cotton or paper towels.
3. Identify the four parts of the parietal pleura, that is, the costal, diaphragmatic, mediastinal and cervical pleura.
4. Insert your fingers in the costodiaphragmatic recess and note how the diaphragmatic pleura turns to the thoracic wall at an acute angle.
5. Placing your hand between the mediastinum and the lung, palpate the root of the lung. At the root of the lung, the mediastinal pleura is continuous with the visceral (pulmonary) pleura. Feel the *pulmonary ligament* that extends below the root of the lung.
6. All parts of the lung should slide freely against the parietal pleura. However, if there are adhesions between the visceral (pulmonary) and the parietal pleurae because of disease process, break them with fingers. Now the lung is attached to the mediastinum by the root.

Clinical Notes

1. *Pleural effusion*: Excessive accumulation of fluids in the pleural cavity is called pleural effusion. It is aspirated by a procedure called *paracentesis thoracis/pleural tap*. It is done by inserting a needle in the sixth intercostal muscle. The needle is passed in the lower part of the space to avoid injury to the intercostal nerve and vessels.
2. *Pleurisy*: It refers to the inflammation of the pleura, often accompanied by pleural effusion.
3. *Pneumothorax*: It refers to the presence of air (pneuma) in the pleural cavity and hydropneumothorax refers to the presence of fluid and air.
4. *Haemothorax*: It refers to the presence of blood in the pleural cavity.
5. *Empyema*: It refers to the presence of pus in the pleural cavity.

Dissection and Identification

Lungs in situ:

1. Observe the lung in situ (**Fig. 14.5**).
2. Each lung has three surfaces, the costal, mediastinal and diaphragmatic.
3. Identify the *oblique fissure* on both the lungs. The oblique fissure lies deep to the fifth rib laterally and anteriorly it is deep to the sixth costal cartilage.
4. Identify the *horizontal fissure* on the right lung. It lies deep to the fourth costal cartilage and the fourth rib.
5. Note that the *right lung* has two fissures, the oblique and horizontal, and has three lobes, the *superior, middle* and *inferior*. The *left lung* has only one fissure (oblique fissure) and two lobes, the *superior* and *inferior*. Note that the apex of the lung lies anterior to the neck of the first rib, above the plane of thoracic inlet.
6. Identify the *pericardium* occupying the space between the two lungs. It contains the heart.
7. Now insert your hand between the heart and the lung to palpate the *root of the lung*. The structures forming the root include the pulmonary vessels and principal bronchus.
8. Identify the *phrenic nerve* and *pericardiacophrenic vessels* that pass anterior to the root of the lung. The *vagus* nerve is posterior to the root of the lung.

Removal of the lungs:

https://www.winkingskull.com/dissector/V1/video.aspx?vid=202

1. Placing your hand between the lung and the mediastinum, retract the lung laterally to stretch the root of the lung.

2. Using a pair of scissors, transect the root of the lung midway between the lung and the mediastinum.

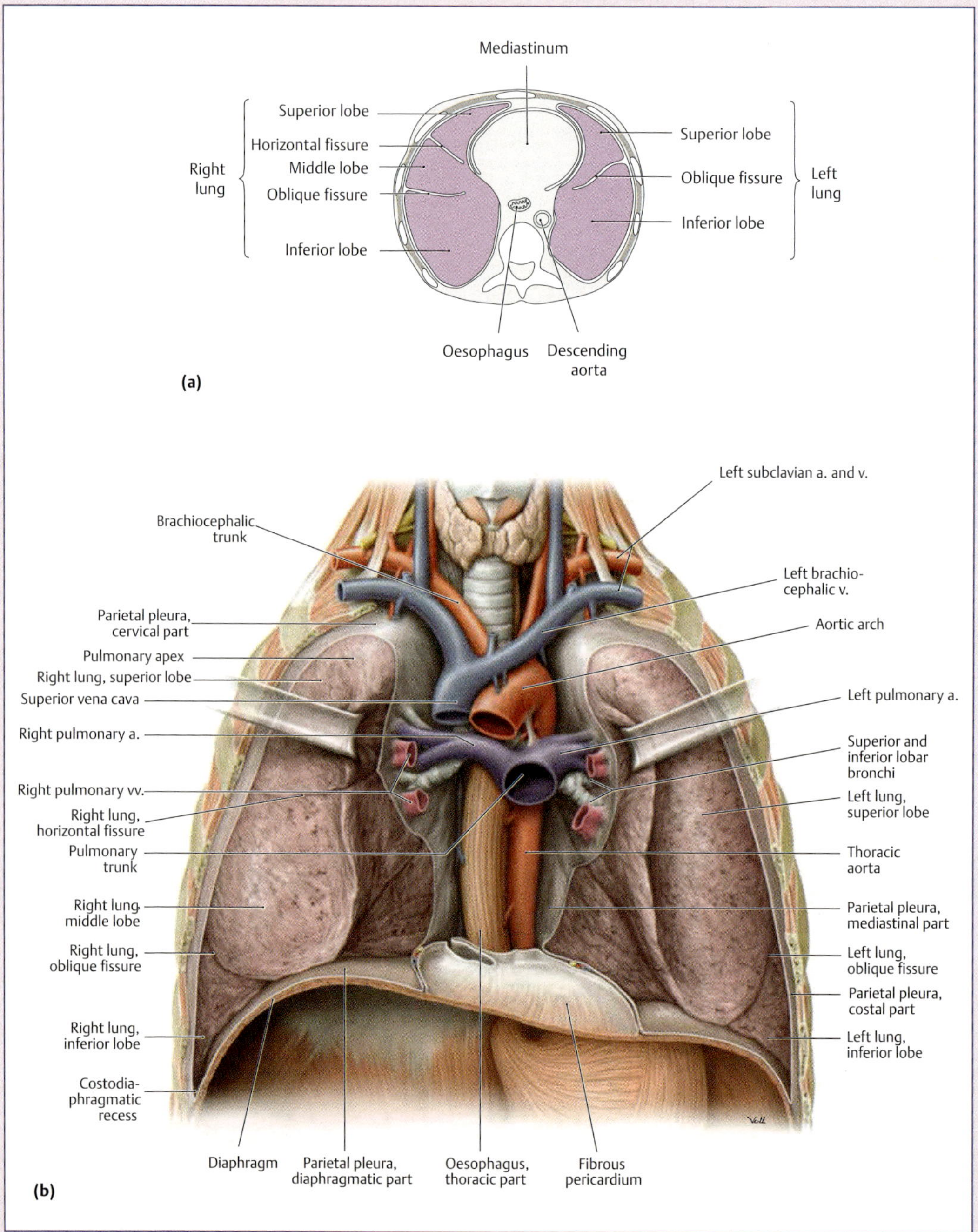

Fig. 14.5 Lungs. **(a)** Topographical relations of the lungs, transverse section, inferior view. **(b)** Anterior view with lungs retracted in situ.

3. During the removal of the lungs, preserve the phrenic nerve, pericardiacophrenic vessels and vagus nerve.
4. Remove both the lungs. Note that the right lung is shorter but bulkier than the left lung.
5. Identify the borders and surfaces of the lungs.

Lungs

The pair of lungs (**Fig. 14.6**) placed in the thoracic cavity forms the respiratory organs. They are spongy in texture. They contain air and hence are light. The right lung weighs 600 g and the left lung weighs about 550 g. In newborns/infants, they are pink in colour. In adults, due to the deposition of carbon particles inhaled, they become mottled black. Each lung is free in its pleural cavity; however, in most cadaveric specimens, the pulmonary pleura is adherent to the parietal pleura due to an old inflammation involving the pleura.

Each lung has an apex, base, three borders and two surfaces:

https://www.winkingskull.com/dissector/V1/video.aspx?vid=277

1. *Apex*: It is blunt and extends into the root of the neck about 3 to 5 cm above the anterior end of the first rib. It is crossed by the subclavian vessels (artery and vein) and is being separated from them by the pleura and suprapleural membrane (Sibson's fascia).
2. *Base*: It rests upon the diaphragm. It is semilunar in shape and concave. The right lung base is separated by the diaphragm from the right lobe of the liver, while the left one is separated from the left lobe of the liver, stomach and spleen. The sharp inferior margin of the lung separates the base from the costal surface. This margin extends into the costodiaphragmatic recess of the pleura but does not reach the lower limit of the recess except in deep inspiration. The inferior margin is blunt medially where it is related to the pericardium.
3. *Anterior border*: It is thin and extends into the costomediastinal recess of the pleura. It corresponds to the anterior line of the pleural reflection on the right side. On the left side, the anterior margin shows a wide *cardiac notch* below the level of the fourth costal cartilage. Below this notch, it

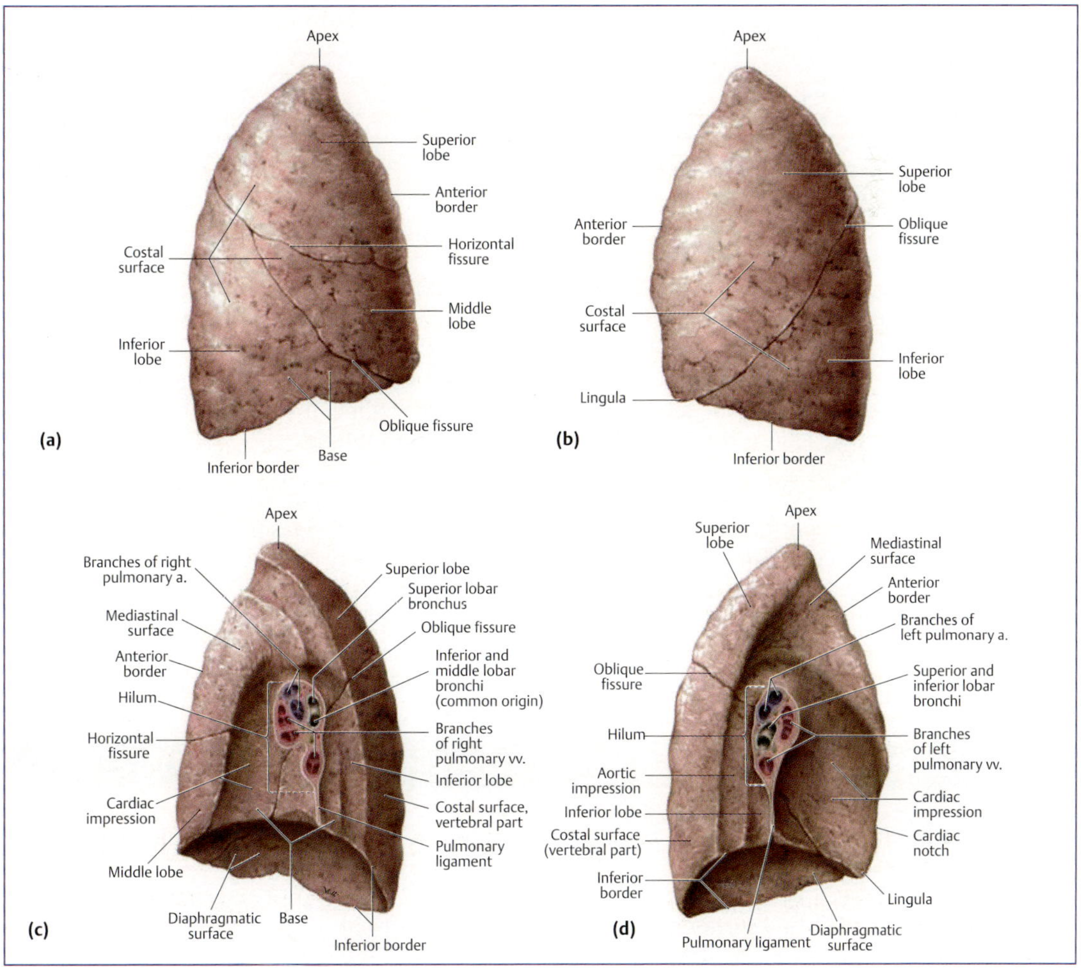

Fig. 14.6 Gross anatomy of the lungs. **(a)** Right lung (lateral view). **(b)** Left lung (lateral view). **(c)** Right lung (medial view). **(d)** Left lung (medial view).

extends medially to form the lingula. In the region of the cardiac notch, the pericardium is not covered by the lung.

4. *Posterior border*: It is thick and rounded and lies in paravertebral gutters. It extends from the level of the spine of C7 vertebra to the T10 spine.
5. *Inferior border*: It is thin and separates the base from the costal and mediastinal surfaces.
6. *Medial surface*: It is related to the vertebral column and mediastinum. It is indented by the heart and great blood vessels, more so on the left side.
7. *Hilum of the lung*: It is an area of the mediastinal surface placed nearly in the centre, through which various structures either enter or leave the lung.
8. *Root of the lung*: All the structures that enter or leave the lung constitute the root of the lung. It is formed by bronchus/bronchi, a pulmonary artery, two pulmonary veins, bronchial vessels along with the pulmonary plexus of nerves, lymphatics and some amount of connective tissue. The pleura extends below the hilum as the pulmonary ligament. The large structures at the hilum of the lung can be identified. The *bronchus* can be recognized by a firm hyaline cartilage in its wall. The cartilage helps to maintain patency of the bronchial lumen. The cartilage is found along the wall of the bronchial tree as it ramifies into finer channels from primary, secondary, tertiary and so on. It is missing in the bronchioles, that is, when the calibre of the bronchial element is less than 1 mm. There are *spiral bundles of smooth muscles and elastic tissue* between the cartilages and the lining ciliated columnar epithelium of the intrapulmonary bronchi. This allows elongation of the bronchi during expansion of the lung in inspiration and shortening in expiration. The muscle, however, may cause severe reduction in the luminal size of the bronchi in some cases, for example asthma. The parasympathetic nerves cause contraction and the sympathetic nerves cause relaxation of the bronchial musculature. Therefore, the sympathomimetic drugs are used to treat bronchial asthmatic attacks.

The single pulmonary artery can be identified by this thicker wall against two pulmonary veins at the hilum of the lung.

Fissures and Lobes

1. *Right lung*: It has two fissures, an oblique fissure and a horizontal fissure. It has three lobes, the superior, middle and inferior lobes.
   - *Oblique fissure*: It passes through the entire thickness of the lung except the hilum. It passes obliquely downwards and forwards crossing the posterior border about 6 to 6.5 cm below the apex of the lung and the inferior border about 5 cm away from the median plane. Owing to its obliquity, the inferior lobe is most posterior and the superior (and middle) lobe is more anterior.
   - *Horizontal fissure*: The right lung has an additional horizontal fissure passing from the anterior border to the oblique fissure. It lies at the level of the fourth costal cartilage and by running horizontally meets the oblique fissure in the midaxillary line. It separates the superior lobe from the middle lobe. It corresponds to the lingula of the left lung.

   https://www.winkingskull.com/dissector/V1/video.aspx?vid=279

2. *Left lung*: It has only one fissure and two lobes. The oblique fissure divides the left lung into superior and inferior lobes. Projection of cardia (heart) more onto the left side produces the so-called *cardiac notch* along the left lung. Just below this notch, the part of the left lung is called the *lingula*. It corresponds to the middle lobe of the right lung. Lungs may show variations in the number of lobes. The right lung may have only two lobes (*superior* and *inferior*) with only an oblique fissure, and the horizontal fissure may be missing. Alternatively, there may be an additional lobe, for example the *azygos lobe*.

Dissection and Identification

Mediastinal surface of the lungs and hilum:

1. Observe the hilum of the lung. The arrangement of the structures in the hilum is a bit different on the two sides (**Fig. 14.6c,d**).
   Hilum of the right lung: It shows the following structures from above downwards:

   https://www.winkingskull.com/dissector/V1/video.aspx?vid=281

   - Eparterial bronchus

- Pulmonary artery
- Hyparterial bronchus
- Inferior pulmonary veins

Hilum of the left lung: The structures from above downwards are:

https://www.winkingskull.com/dissector/V1/video.aspx?vid=280

- Pulmonary artery
- Bronchus
- Inferior pulmonary veins

2. Some of the structures related to the mediastinal surface of the lung produce contact impressions.
3. Identify the following on the mediastinal surface of the left lung:

   https://www.winkingskull.com/dissector/V1/video.aspx?vid=282

   - *Cardiac impression*: It is related to the left ventricle, left auricle, infundibulum and adjacent part of the right ventricle.
   - *Aortic arch impression*: Arch of the aorta.
   - *Thoracic aorta impression*: Caused by the descending thoracic aorta.
4. In addition, the mediastinal surface of the left lung is related to the phrenic nerve, pericardiacophrenic vessels, anterior and posterior pulmonary plexus and vagus nerve.
5. Identify the following impressions on the mediastinal surface of the right lung.
   - *Cardiac impression*: Caused by the right atrium and auricle.
   - *Superior vena caval impression*: Related to the superior vena cava.
   - *Impression of the azygos vein*: It arches over the hilum of the right lung.
   - *Oesophageal impression*: In addition to these impressions, the mediastinal surface of the right lung is related to the lower part of the brachiocephalic vein, inferior vena cava, trachea, right vagus and right phrenic nerves, the anterior and posterior pulmonary plexuses and pericardiacophrenic vessels.
6. Examine the main bronchus at the hilum; follow it in the lung by blunt dissection.
7. Identify the division of the main bronchus into eparterial and hyparterial bronchus and their subsequent division into the *superior, middle* and *inferior lobar bronchi.* Note that the superior lobar branches pass above the pulmonary artery.
8. In the left lung, identify the *superior* and *inferior lobar bronchi.*
9. Using blunt dissection, trace the lobar bronchus for about 3 to 4 cm into the lung tissue and observe that it divides into *segmental bronchi.* Each segmental bronchus/tertiary bronchus ventilates a *bronchopulmonary segment.* There are 10 such bronchopulmonary segments in each lung.
10. Identify the *bronchial artery.* It courses along the surface of the principal (main) bronchus.

    https://www.winkingskull.com/dissector/V1/video.aspx?vid=89

11. Note that the hilum of the lung contains lymph nodes, lymphatics and autonomic nerves. The sympathetic nerves are derived from the right and left sympathetic trunks, while the parasympathetic component comes from the vagi. Together they form anterior and posterior pulmonary plexuses.

Blood Vessels

The branches of the *pulmonary artery* carry deoxygenated blood to the lungs. Each branch follows the bronchus to each lobe and subsequent segmental (tertiary) bronchus. The terminal capillaries reach the walls of the respiratory bronchioles and the alveoli for gaseous exchange (**Fig. 14.7**).

After this, the oxygenated blood is drained by the lobular tributaries to be finally delivered through the *pulmonary veins* to the left atrium of the heart. The veins are intersegmental. The *right superior pulmonary vein* drains the superior and middle lobes, while the *left superior pulmonary vein* drains the superior lobe of the left lung. The *inferior pulmonary veins* on both sides drain the corresponding inferior lobes. The blood supply to the lungs, that is the bronchial tree and to the pulmonary parenchyma, is given by the *bronchial arteries.* On the *right side,* there is one bronchial artery which is derived from the third posterior intercostal artery or from the left bronchial artery.

On the *left side,* there are two bronchial arteries which are branches of the descending thoracic aorta. Venous blood from the lung tissue is carried on both sides (right and left) by *two bronchial veins.* The

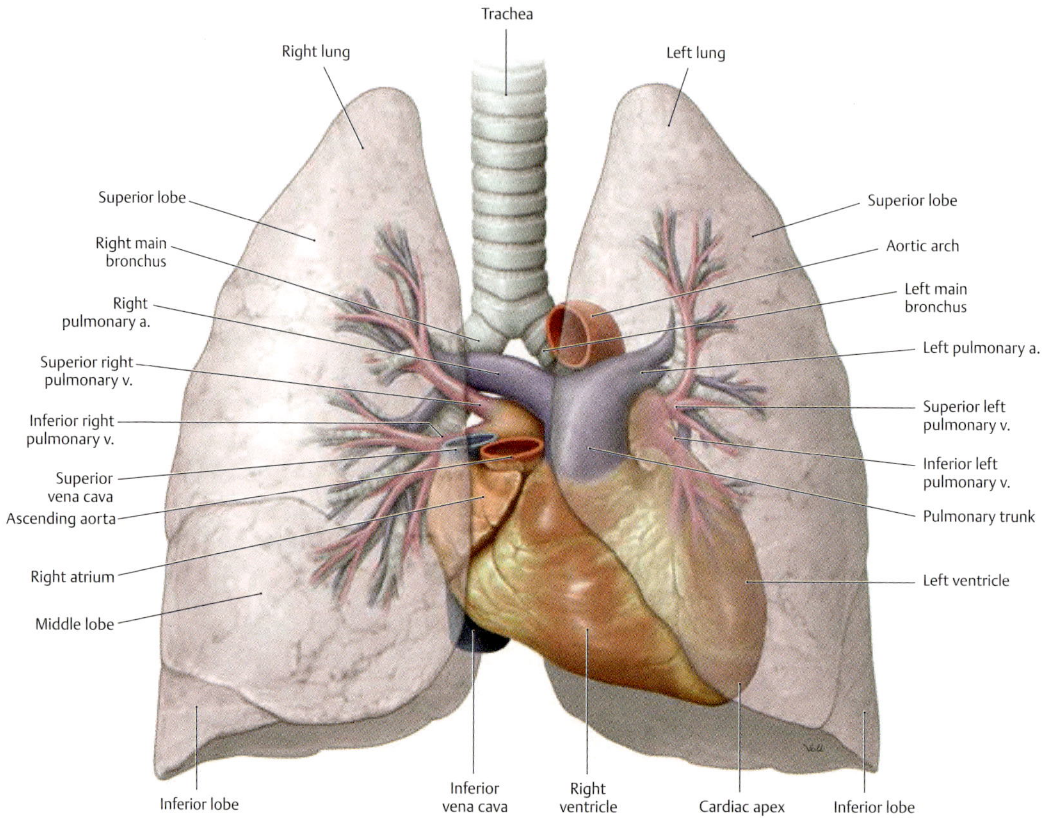

Fig. 14.7 Distribution of the pulmonary arteries and veins (anterior view).

right bronchial veins drain into the azygos vein, while the left bronchial veins drain either into the left superior intercostal vein or into the hemiazygos vein.

Lymphatics and the Lymph Nodes

There are two sets of lymphatic vessels, superficial and deep. The *superficial plexus* of lymph vessels is placed deep to the pleura and drains the peripheral part of the pulmonary parenchyma. These vessels pass around the borders and reach the hilum and drain into the *bronchopulmonary nodes*. The deep set of lymphatic vessels drain the bronchial tree and deeper tissue and terminate into the bronchopulmonary nodes at the hilum. The bronchopulmonary nodes lie laterally along the principal bronchus. The most medial lymph nodes reach the tracheal bifurcation. These are the *tracheobronchial nodes*. They drain through the *bronchomediastinal trunk* into the brachiocephalic vein of the corresponding side or through the thoracic duct on the left side.

Bronchopulmonary Segments

Each bronchopulmonary segment forms well-defined sector of the pulmonary parenchyma, is ventilated by the tertiary/segmental bronchus and has its own artery while the veins are intersegmental in position. Each segment is pyramidal in shape with its apex directed towards the hilum of the lung and the base to the periphery (**Figs. 14.8** and **14.9**).

The intersegmental planes are formed by the connective tissue which is continuous on the surface with the pulmonary pleura. During segmental resection (conservative surgery), the surgeons explore these planes following the pulmonary vein which lies in these planes.

In the right lung, the segments are as follows:

I. Apical
II. Posterior } Superior lobe
III. Anterior

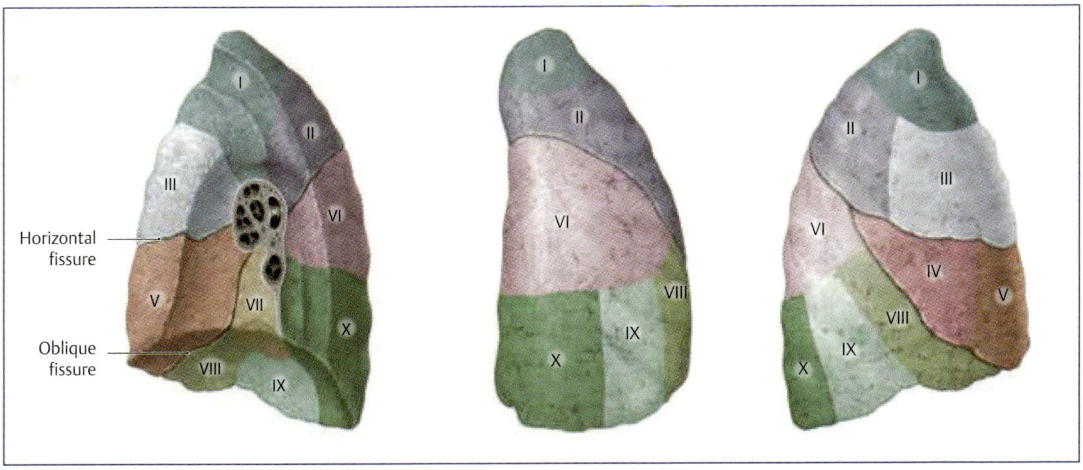

Fig. 14.8 Right lung: bronchopulmonary segments.

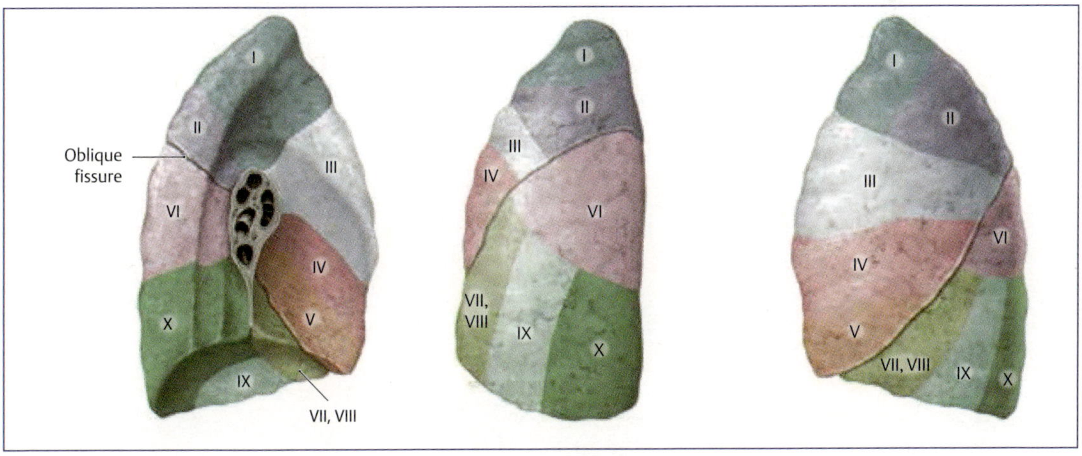

Fig. 14.9 Left lung: bronchopulmonary segments.

IV. Lateral } Middle lobe
V. Medial

VI. Superior
VII. Medial basal
VIII. Anterior basal } Inferior/lower lobe
IX. Lateral basal
X. Posterior basal

In the left lung, the segments are as follows:

I. Apical } or Apicoposterior
II. Posterior } Superior lobe
III. Anterior
IV. Superior lingular
V. Inferior lingular
VI. Superior
VII. Anterior basal
VIII. Medial basal
IX. Lateral basal
X. Posterior basal

In the left lung, the number of segments may be reduced to nine if there exists an apicoposterior segment in the superior lobe.

Clinical Notes

1. The purulent lesions (pus-forming lesions) are restricted to the segment involved.
2. Tuberculosis or bronchogenic carcinoma can involve adjacent segments crossing the segmental barrier.
3. Knowledge of the bronchopulmonary segments helps in segmental resection, that is, performing conservative surgical procedures.
4. Postural drainage can be done in case of lung abscess or bronchiectasis by giving a particular position to the patient.
5. Interpretation of bronchogram can be done if we have the knowledge of the bronchopulmonary segments.
6. In performing bronchoscopy, the knowledge of bronchopulmonary segments is essential.

Mediastinum

Observe the structures under the mediastinal pleura. The mediastinal pleura is in contact with the following structures from the anterior to the posterior side (**Fig. 14.10**). *On the right side*, they are the pericardium, root of the right lung and oesophagus.

Note that the right *brachiocephalic vein* descends down to the first costal cartilage and further it leads to the *superior vena cava passing* down towards the heart (right atrium), creating a sort of ridge. The *inferior*

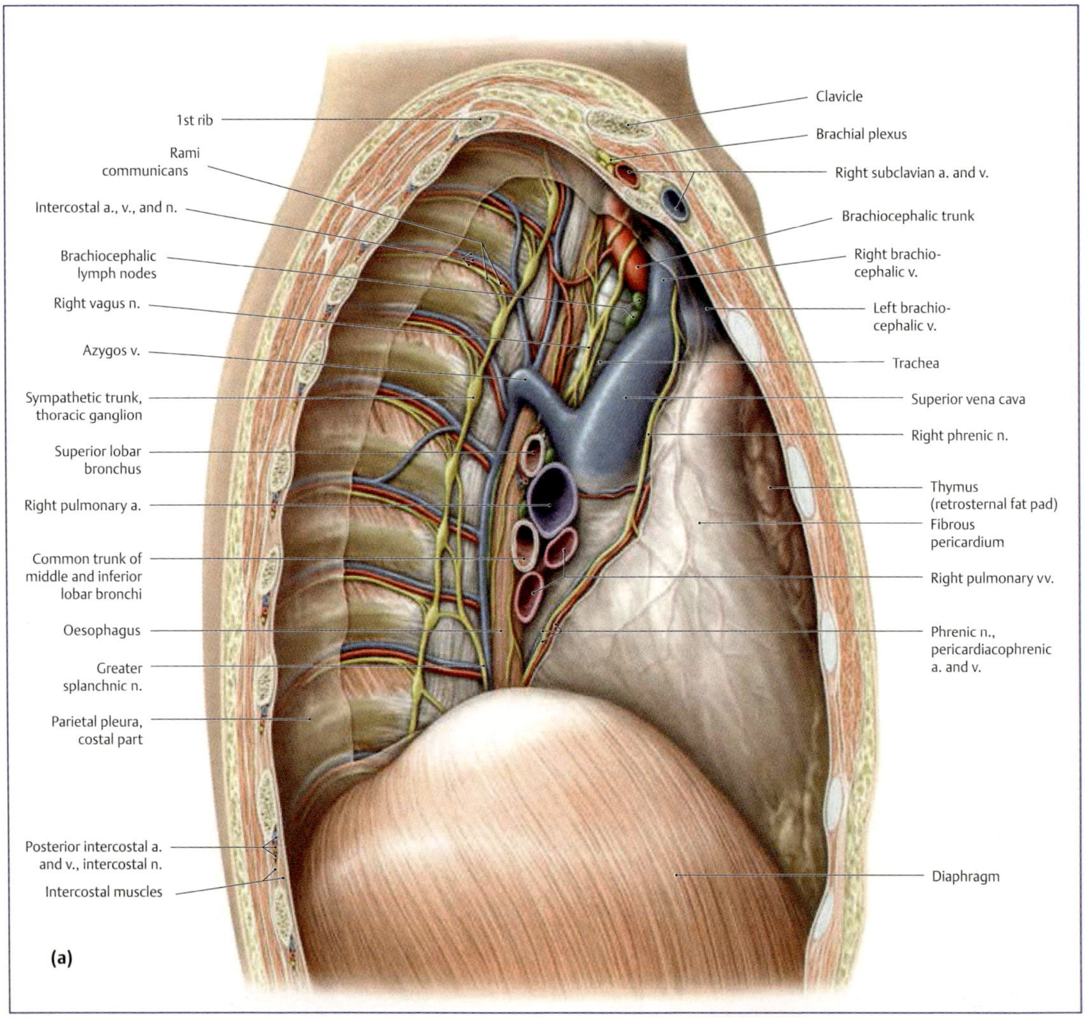

Fig. 14.10 Structures related to the mediastinal surfaces of the lungs. **(a)** Right lateral view, parasagittal section. Note the many structures passing between the superior and inferior (middle and posterior) mediastinum.

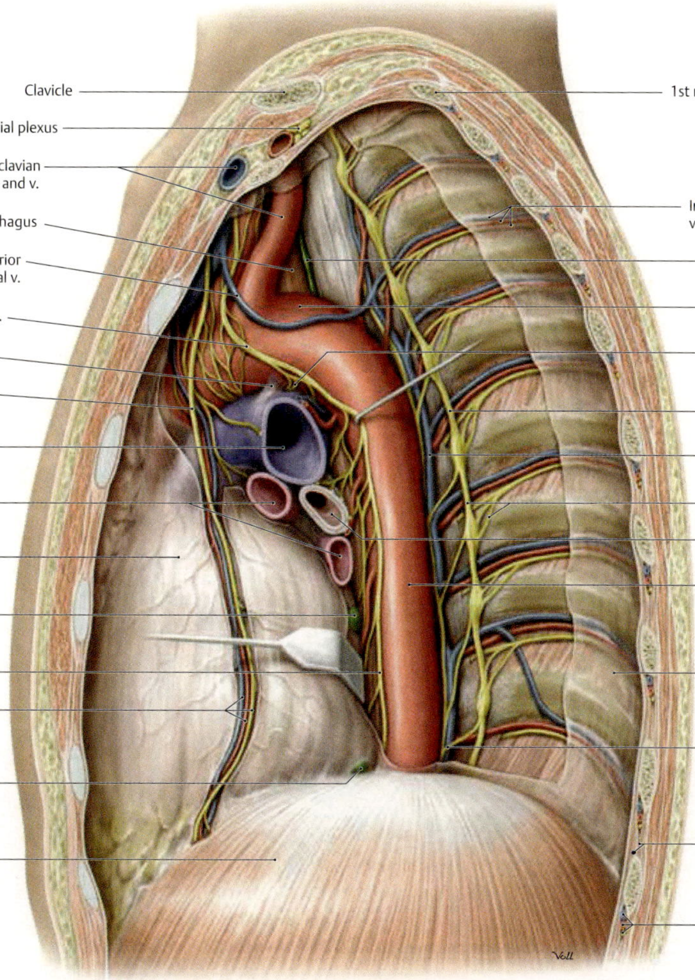

Fig. 14.10 Structures related to the mediastinal surfaces of the lungs. **(b)** Left lateral view, parasagittal section. *Removed*: Left lung and parietal pleura. *Revealed:* Posterior mediastinal structures.

vena cava similarly forms a short ridge ascending from the diaphragm to the posteroinferior aspect of the cardiac bulge. The *phrenic nerve* and accompanying pericardiacophrenic vessels form a vertical ridge passing on the surface of the pericardium. They pass about 1.5 cm anterior to the root of the lung. Note the *azygos vein* arching over the root of the lung to enter the superior vena cava. Above this level, the *trachea* and *oesophagus* can be seen or palpated posterior to the phrenic nerve and superior vena cava.

Observe the *right vagus nerve* descending across the trachea passing behind the root of the lung. It accompanies the oesophagus. Posterior to the oesophagus, note the thoracic vertebrae with the posterior intercostal vessels and the azygos vein. Observe the *sympathetic trunk* on the heads of the upper ribs and on the sides of the vertebral bodies at the lower level. Note the roots of the *greater splanchnic nerve* passing anteroinferiorly from the lower part of the trunk. *On the left side*, observe the bulge of the heart within the pericardium with the root of the lung posterosuperior to it. They are separated from the vertebral column by the *descending thoracic aorta*. The *oesophagus* can be seen superior to the arch of aorta. Just above the diaphragm, it lies between the pericardium and the aorta. Observe the *arch of the aorta* curving over the root of the left lung. The left common carotid and left subclavian arteries pass superiorly from the convexity of the arch of the aorta anterior to the oesophagus.

The *phrenic* and *vagus* nerves descend between these arteries on the lateral aspect of the arch of the aorta. The vagus nerve passes posterior to the lung root. The phrenic nerve with the accompanying vessels passes vertically over the pericardium.

The thoracic duct may be observed along the oesophagus superior to the aortic arch.

The sympathetic chain and greater splanchnic nerve are present in a similar manner as on the right side; however, they are partly concealed by the aorta (**Fig. 14.10a,b**).

Dissection and Identification

1. Make a longitudinal cut through the pleura parallel to the phrenic nerve on each side of it.
2. Strip the posterior flap backwards to the intercostal spaces. Avoid injury to the underlying structures.
3. Strip the anterior flap forward to reveal the pericardium and superior vena cava on the right side and the arch of the aorta on the left side.
4. Remove the fat and connective tissue from the *sympathetic trunk* and its anterior branches.
5. Observe that superiorly these branches pass to the pulmonary plexus and inferiorly to the splanchnic nerves.
6. In at least two ganglia, identify the *rami communicans* which pass back to the corresponding intercostal nerves.
7. Follow the *posterior intercostal vessels* on the vertebral column and in the posterior parts of the intercostal spaces.
8. Trace them in the first two spaces on each side to the neck of the first rib. On the right side, the remaining veins join the *azygos vein*. On the left side, they terminate into the *left superior intercostal* and *hemiazygos veins.*
9. The left superior intercostal vein can be followed passing obliquely across the arch of the aorta to the left brachiocephalic vein.
10. Identify the vagus nerve on each side and trace it to the posterior side of the root of the lung. Note its branches to the pulmonary plexus at the root of the lung.
11. On the right side, identify and trace the trachea and oesophagus down to the root of the lung and the superior and inferior vena cava reaching to the pericardium.
12. On the left side, find the *superior cervical cardiac branch of the left sympathetic trunk* and the *inferior cervical cardiac branch of the left vagus* on the arch of the aorta between the vagus and phrenic nerves. Inferiorly, they pass under the concavity of the aortic arch.
13. Identify and follow the left subclavian artery and the oesophagus superior to the aortic arch. Avoid injury to the thoracic duct that lies immediately to the left of the oesophagus and the recurrent laryngeal nerve coursing anterolateral to the oesophagus.

Autonomic Nervous System

Autonomic nervous system has two components: parasympathetic and sympathetic.

Parasympathetic component: The *parasympathetic component* supplies the eye, gut tube, heart and the respiratory and urogenital systems. Its preganglionic fibres are derived from the cranial nerves and S2–4 spinal nerves (craniosacral outflow). The parasympathetic innervation to the thorax comes from two *vagus nerves*. They innervate the heart, lungs, trachea and oesophagus.

Sympathetic component: The *sympathetic* component derives its preganglionic fibres, that is, the white rami communicans from the thoracic (T1–T12) and upper lumbar nerves. The sympathetic postganglionic fibres supply the same thoracic structures, that is, the heart, lung, trachea and oesophagus. In addition, they supply the blood vessels and involuntary structures of the body wall, for example, the erector pilorum muscle and sweat glands. The postganglionic fibres in the sympathetic system follow the blood vessels to reach their destination, that is, the target organ/structure.

The sympathetic part comprises two elements:

1. *Sympathetic trunks*
2. *Sympathetic plexuses*

Sympathetic trunks: They extend from the upper cervical region to the coccyx. There are two sympathetic trunks, one each on either side of the front of the vertebral column. From the ganglia, the *postganglionic fibres* pass to the cranial and spinal nerves in the form of *grey rami communicans*. Some of these postganglionic fibres pass through the visceral branches. These are called the *splanchnic nerves*. They reach the sympathetic plexuses.

Sympathetic plexuses: They are formed by a network of fine nerve fibres with the scattered ganglia. They are associated with the arteries that supply the visceral organs. The main plexuses in the thorax are the *cardiac and pulmonary plexuses*. They also carry parasympathetic fibres.

The sympathetic trunk in the thorax consists of 11 or 12 ganglia connected by longitudinal fascicles of the pre- and postganglionic fibres. There are ganglion cells scattered along these bundles. The first thoracic ganglion is often fused with the inferior cervical ganglion to form the *stellate/cervicothoracic ganglion* that lies on the neck of the first rib.

The sympathetic system in the thorax shows the following branches:

1. *White and grey rami communicans*. Each ganglion receives the *white ramus* (preganglionic fibres) from the intercostal nerve and reciprocally sends the *grey ramus* (postganglionic fibres) to the nerve to be distributed to the target organ.
2. The visceral branches include:
   - *Aortic* and *oesophageal* branches which are derived from the upper five thoracic ganglia and also from the greater splanchnic nerve.
   - *Cardiac* and *pulmonary branches* which are derived from the third and fourth ganglia. They pass anteroinferiorly along the vertebral bodies to reach the corresponding plexuses.
   - *Greater splanchnic nerve* is formed by the branches of the fifth to ninth ganglia. The greater splanchnic nerve issues branches to the aorta and oesophagus. It presents a small splanchnic ganglion along its course just before its penetration of the crus of the diaphragm to enter the abdomen.
   - *Lesser splanchnic nerve* is derived from the branches of the tenth and eleventh thoracic ganglia.
   - *Lowest splanchnic nerve* is formed by the branch from the last thoracic ganglia. The lesser and the lowest splanchnic nerves enter the abdomen together piercing the crus of the diaphragm.

Azygos Vein

It is formed in the abdomen by the union of the lumbar azygos, right subcostal and right ascending lumbar veins. It enters the thorax through the aortic orifice of the diaphragm lying immediately to the right of the aorta and the thoracic duct. It then runs upwards initially posterior to the diaphragm and then to the oesophagus on the anterior surface of the vertebral bodies. At the fourth thoracic vertebra, it arches anteriorly above the root of the right lung and terminates by joining the posterior aspect of the superior vena cava. At times, part of the lung, called the *azygos lobe* surrounded by the pleura, extends upwards between the arch of azygos vein and the structures medial to it (oesophagus, trachea and right vagus nerve). It can be detected radiographically.

The tributaries of the azygos vein are (a) *right superior intercostal vein* which is formed by the union of the second and third posterior intercostal veins, (b) *fourth* to *seventh right posterior intercostal veins*, (c) *hemiazygos vein*, (d) *accessory hemiazygos vein*, (e) *right bronchial vein* and (f) *oesophageal, mediastinal and pericardial veins*.

The oesophageal tributaries communicate with the gastric vein near the oesophageal orifice of the diaphragm. This communicates the portal and systemic veins. The azygos vein also forms a channel of anastomosis the superior and inferior vena cava.

Phrenic Nerves

Phrenic nerves are the only motor nerves to supply the diaphragm. They innervate the diaphragm and the structures derived from the septum transversum, that is, the diaphragm, pericardium, mediastinal and diaphragmatic pleura, liver, gall bladder and inferior vena cava. They are derived from the ventral rami of C3, C4, C5; hence the referred pain from the involvement of these structures is felt at the shoulder, for example, acute cholecystitis.

Course: The phrenic nerve derived from C3, C4, C5 descends into the thorax posterolateral to the internal jugular vein and is accompanied by the pericardiacophrenic artery, a branch from the internal thoracic artery. It then passes over the mediastinum and supplies the mediastinal pleura. At the root of the lung, it is present anteriorly.

The *left phrenic nerve* passes over the left surface of the arch of the aorta between the left common carotid and left subclavian arteries. It then lies on the pericardium and supplies the pericardium over the left auricle and left ventricle.

The *right phrenic nerve* passes posterolateral to the right brachiocephalic vein and the superior vena cava. It passes over the pericardium covering the right atrium and inferior vena cava to reach the diaphragm.

Both the phrenic nerves pierce the diaphragm and supply the diaphragm along its inferior surface to which they are attached.

Anterior Mediastinum

It lies between sternum anteriorly and the pericardium and pleura posteriorly. It contains the lower part of the *thymus*. In addition, there is some loose fatty tissue between the sternum and the costomediastinal recess of the pleura.

Thymus: It is a primary lymphoid organ comprising a bilobed mass. It develops as a bilateral structure derived from the ventral elongate portion of the third pharyngeal pouch. It then descends from the neck to the thorax along with the inferior parathyroid glands with which it may retain a fibrous connection. In foetal life and in newborn, the thymus is large. It grows till puberty; however, it then regresses in size. In cadavers, it is reduced to two strips of fibro-fatty tissue with the lymphoid element. Functionally, it is concerned with the development of the immune response. It produces T lymphocytes, essential elements of the immune system of the body.

Middle Mediastinum

The middle mediastinum contains the pericardium, heart and the roots of the great blood vessels that enter or leave the heart.

Posterior Mediastinum

The posterior mediastinum contains thoracic aorta, thoracic duct, oesophagus and azygous venous system. The contents of anterior, middle and posterior mediastinum are shown in **Fig. 14.11**.

Pericardium

It is a sac that encloses the heart and is pierced by the great blood vessels, that is, the aorta, pulmonary trunk, superior and inferior vena cava and four pulmonary veins. It consists of the outer fibrous pericardium and the inner serous pericardium.

Fibrous Pericardium

It is a conical sac of fibrous tissue with its apex at the level of the sternal angle and has a broad base blended imperceptibly with the central tendon of the diaphragm. In some lower mammals, it is separated from the diaphragm by the *infracardiac bursa*. The fibrous pericardium is connected anteriorly to the two ends of the body of the sternum by the *superior* and *inferior sternopericardial ligaments*. Posterior to it are the principal bronchi, oesophagus and the descending thoracic aorta. Laterally, it is related to the mediastinal pleura, lungs, phrenic nerve and the pericardiacophrenic vessels (**Figs. 14.11a** and **14.12**).

Serous Pericardium

It forms a double-layered thin serous sac around the heart. It has an outer *parietal layer* that lines the fibrous pericardium and an inner *visceral layer* (the epicardium) covering the heart. These parietal and visceral layers of the pericardium are derived from the *somatopleuric* and *splanchnopleuric layers* of the intra-embryonic coelom (lateral plate mesoderm), respectively. Between these layers is the potential space called the pericardial cavity, containing a thin film of serous fluid that lubricates the surfaces allowing smooth movement of the heart during systole and diastole.

Sinuses of the Serous Pericardium

The visceral layer of the pericardium encloses the roots of the great blood vessels in the form of two tubes, an *arterial* and a *venous tube*. The arterial tube encloses the aorta and pulmonary trunk. The venous tube encloses the superior and inferior venae cavae and the four pulmonary veins. The passage between these two tubes is the *transverse pericardial sinus*. It is developed when the dorsal mesocardium degenerates and disappears. The transverse sinus is bounded anteriorly by the aorta and pulmonary trunk and posteriorly by the superior vena cava and the left atrium (**Fig. 14.13**). The *oblique pericardial sinus* is bounded anteriorly by the left atrium and posteriorly by the parietal pericardium.

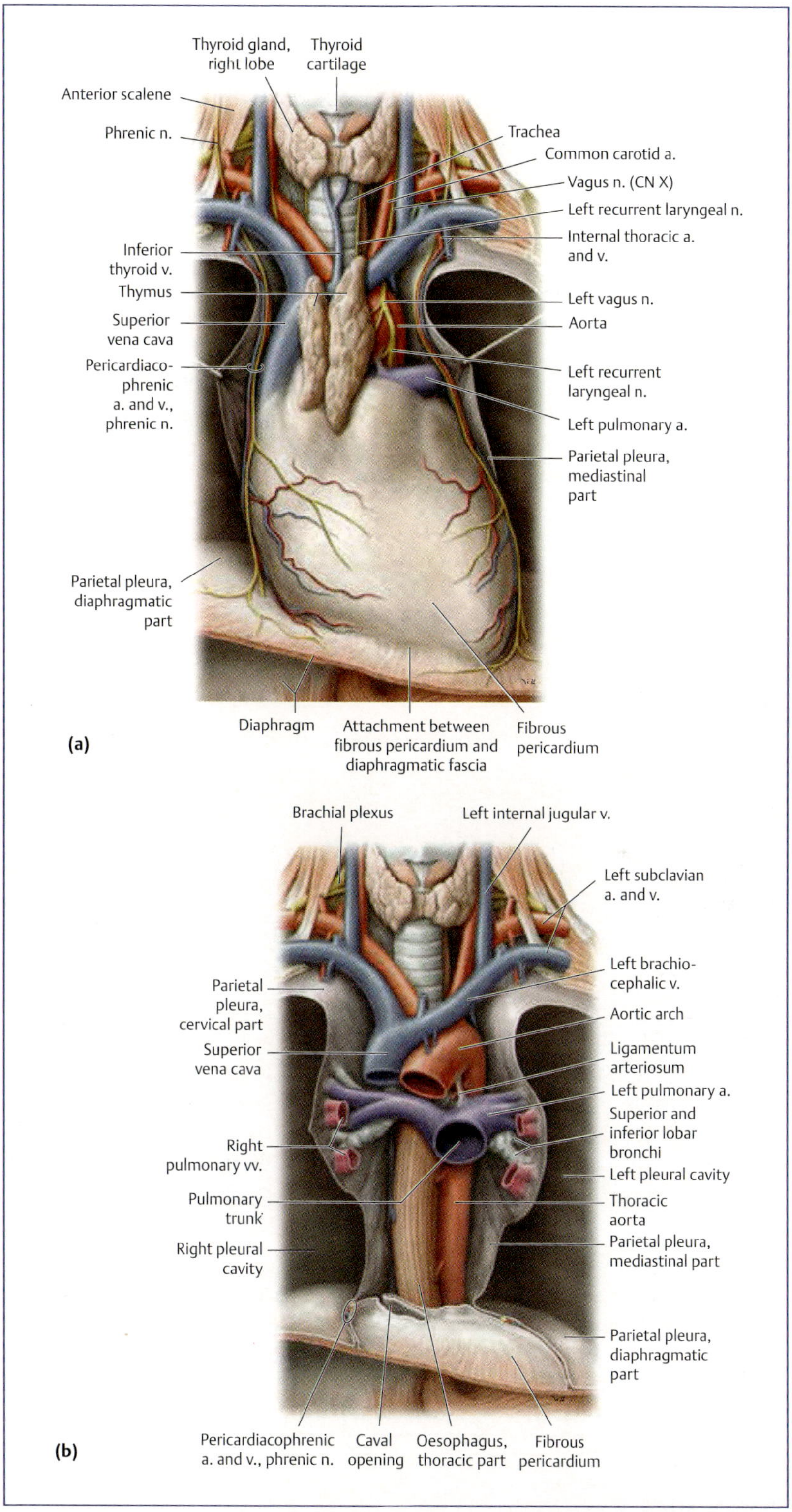

Fig. 14.11 Contents of the mediastinum. **(a)** Anterior view with thymus, heart and pericardium in place. **(b)** Anterior view with heart, pericardium and thymus removed. (*continued*)

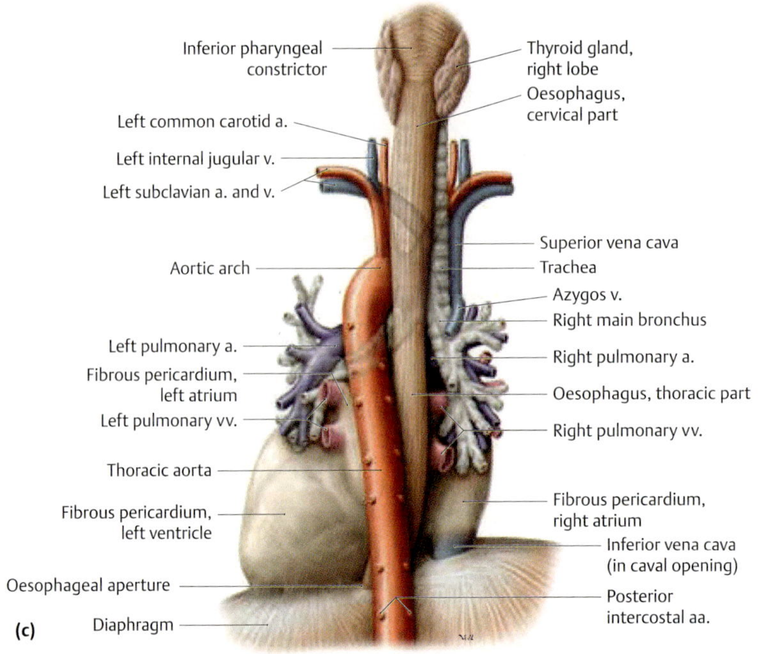

Fig. 14.11 (*continued*) Contents of the mediastinum. **(c)** Posterior view.

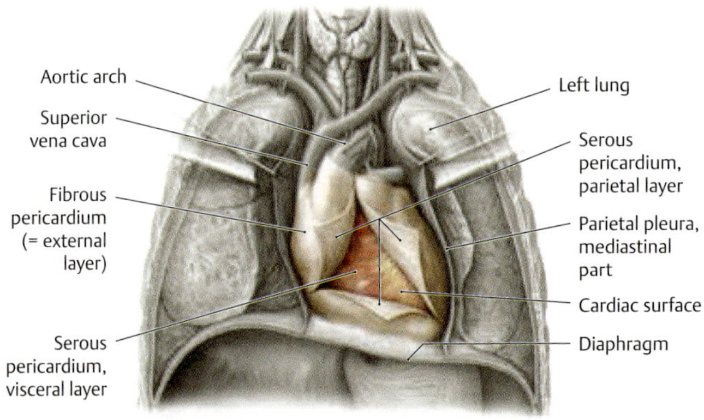

Fig. 14.12 Anterior view of the opened thorax with the thymus removed and flaps of the anterior pericardium reflected to reveal the heart.

Blood and Nerve Supply of the Pericardium

The blood supply to the pericardium is derived from the branches of the following:

1. Internal thoracic artery
2. Musculophrenic artery
3. Descending thoracic aorta

These branches supply the fibrous and parietal layers of the pericardium.

The nerve supply of the fibrous and parietal pericardium is by the phrenic nerve and it carries pain sensation. The epicardium (visceral layer) is supplied by the autonomic nerves.

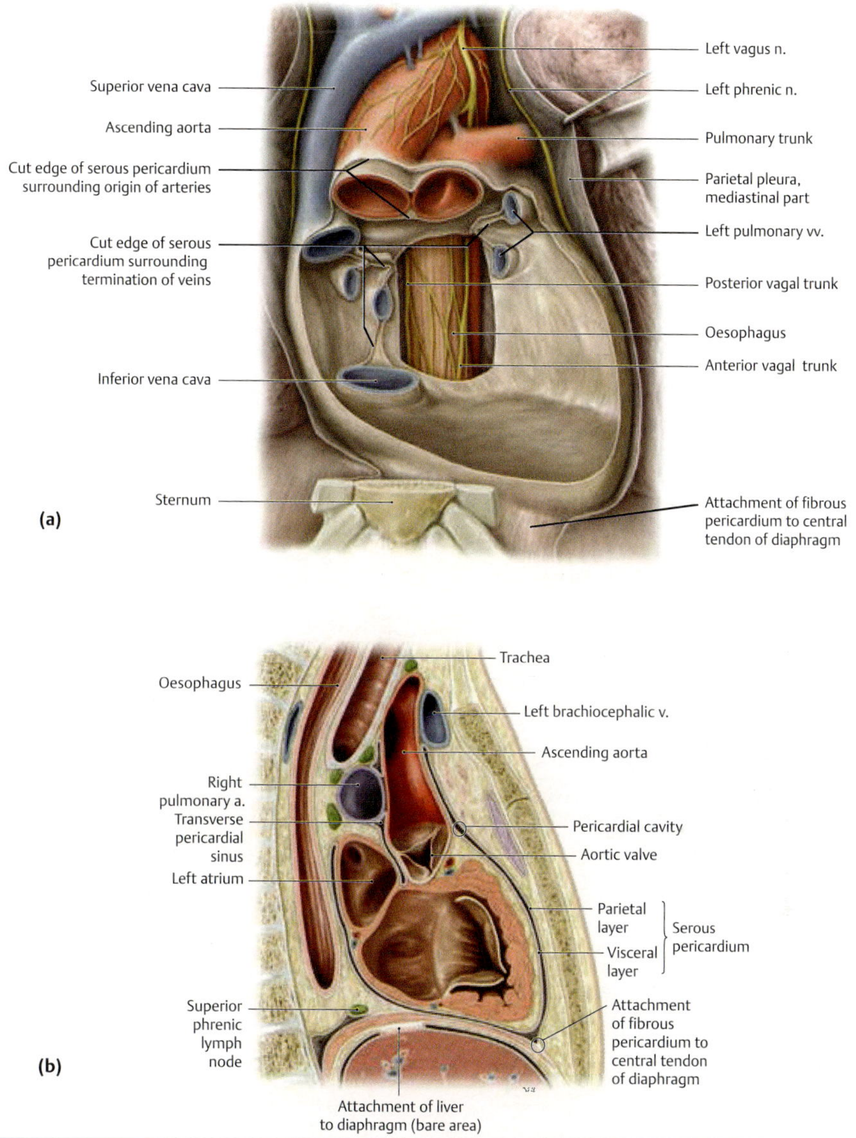

Fig. 14.13 Sinuses of serous pericardium. **(a)** Anterior view with serous pericardium cut open. **(b)** Sagittal section showing pericardium, pericardial cavity and transverse pericardial sinus.

Dissection and Identification

To open the pericardium, transect it as shown in **Fig. 14.14**. Initially, elevate the pericardium with the help of forceps and then use a pair of scissors to give cuts. Make a vertical cut from the diaphragm to the ascending aorta. Then give two transverse cuts at the upper and lower limits of the pericardium.

1. Identify the superior vena cava, ascending aorta, arch of the aorta and pulmonary trunk.
2. Using your finger, gently open the gap between the arch of the aorta and the pulmonary trunk to identify the *ligamentum arteriosum*. It connects the left pulmonary artery to the arch of the aorta (and is derived from the distal part of the left sixth aortic arch artery).

   https://www.winkingskull.com/dissector/V1/video.aspx?vid=285
3. Using a probe, clean the *left vagus* as it crosses the left side of the aortic arch. Now try to find and trace the *left recurrent laryngeal nerve* coursing under the concavity of the aortic arch posterior to the ligamentum arteriosum.

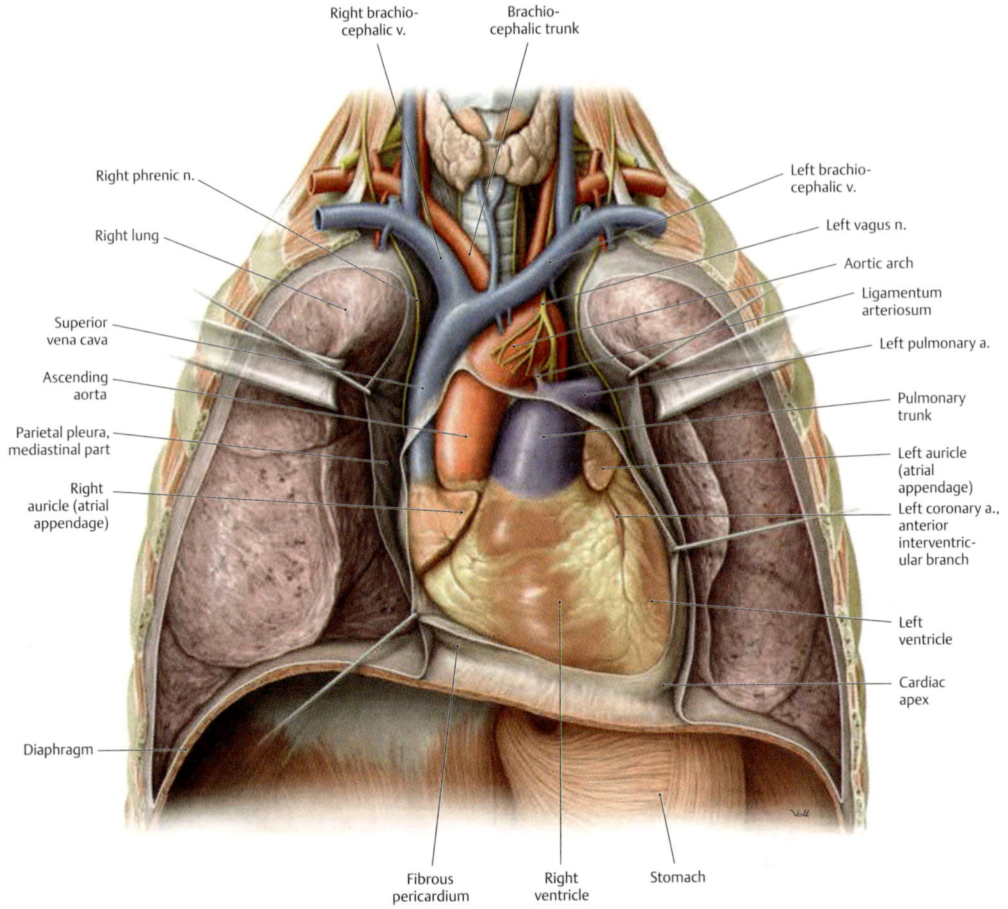

Fig. 14.14 Anterior view of the opened thorax with thymus and anterior pericardium removed to reveal the heart.

4. Now identify the chambers of the heart seen from the anterior aspect. These are the *right atrium*, the *right ventricle* and the *left ventricle*. Note that the right ventricle forms most of the anterior/*sternocostal surface* of the heart.
5. Define/identify the borders of the heart (**Fig. 14.15**).
   - *The right border*: It is formed by the right atrium.
   - *The left border*: It is formed by the left ventricle.
   - *The inferior border*: It is formed by the right ventricle plus a small part by the left ventricle.
   - *The superior border*: It is formed by both atria, the right and left, along with the auricles.

Note that these borders are also evident on the radiograph of the chest except the superior border which is not seen clearly.

6. *Apex of the heart*: It is formed by the left ventricle (apex beat) and can be felt in a living being in the fifth intercostal space about 9 cm from the midline.
7. *Base of the heart*: Identify the base of the heart which is formed by the left atrium and the small part of the right atrium.
8. Note that the inner surface of the pericardium is lined by a smooth and shiny parietal layer of the serous pericardium.
9. Note that the parietal layer of serous pericardium is reflected over the heart as a visceral layer and this line of reflection is placed at the roots of the great blood vessels.
10. *Pericardial cavity*: The potential space between the parietal and visceral layers of the serous pericardium is the pericardial cavity. It contains a thin film of serous fluid lubricating the apposed surfaces permitting free movement of the cardia within the pericardium.

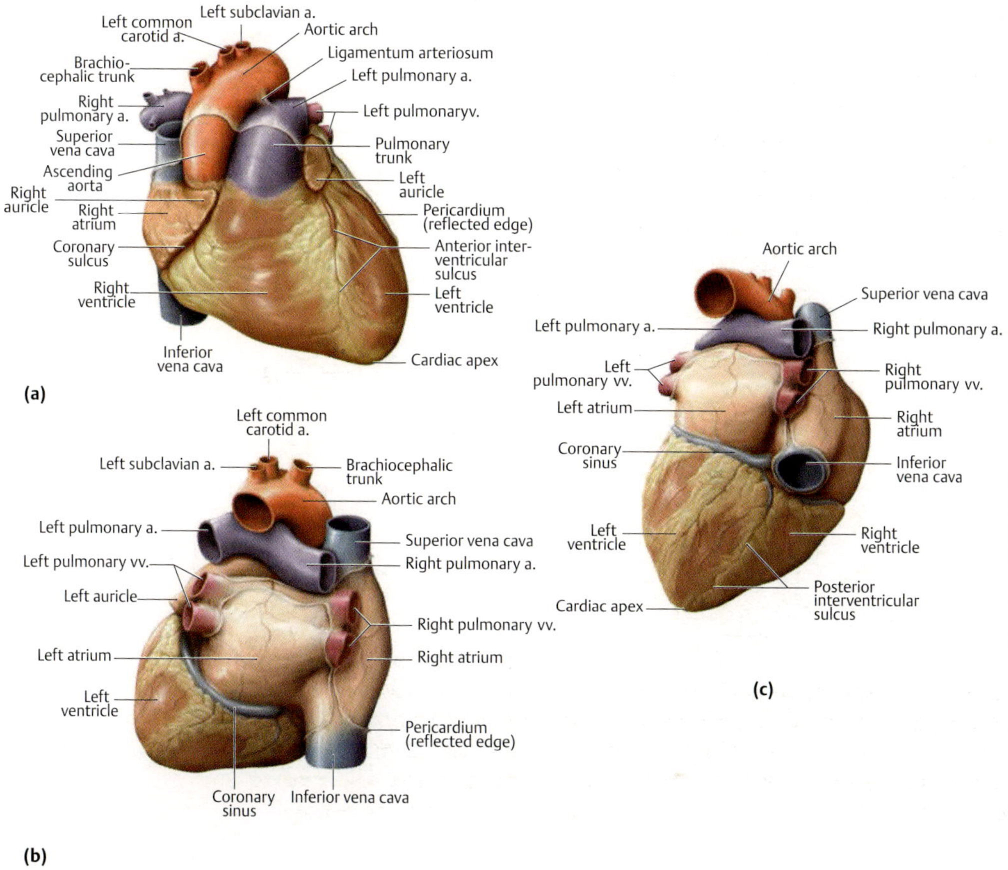

Fig. 14.15 External features of the heart. **(a)** Anterior (sternocostal) surface. **(b)** Posterior surface (base). **(c)** Inferior (diaphragmatic) surface.

11. Identify the *oblique pericardial sinus* as follows. Place your right hand with the fingers lying posterior to the heart. Lifting the heart gently, push your fingers superiorly till they are obstructed by the reflection of the serous pericardium. Now your fingertips are in the oblique pericardial sinus.

https://www.winkingskull.com/dissector/V1/video.aspx?vid=204

12. *The transverse pericardial sinus* can be identified in the following manner. Put your right index finger behind the pulmonary trunk and ascending aorta. Push the finger from the left to the right until the fingertip emerges between the superior vena cava and the arch of the aorta. Now your finger is in the transverse pericardial sinus.

https://www.winkingskull.com/dissector/V1/video.aspx?vid=203

Clinical Notes

1. *Pericardial effusion*: Collection of fluid in the pericardial cavity. It can be drained through the fifth or sixth intercostal space or in the angle between the xiphoid process and the left costal margin with the needle being directed upwards, backwards and to the left.

2. *Pericarditis*: Inflammation involving the pericardium. The pain is due to the involvement of parietal pericardium, whereas in angina pectoris it is from myocardium.
3. *Hemopericardium*: Bleeding into the pericardial cavity. It may be caused by penetrating wounds.
4. *Cardiac tamponade*: Compression of the heart due to accumulation of fluid in the pericardial cavity.

Surface Anatomy of the Heart

Superior border: It extends from a point on the lower border of the left second costal cartilage (about 1.25 cm from the sternal margin) to a point on the upper border of the third right costal cartilage (about 1.25 cm from the sternal margin) (**Fig. 14.16**).

Inferior border: It is marked by a line joining a point at the lower border of the sixth costal cartilage 2 cm from the sternal margin to a point at the apex, that is, in the fifth intercostal space 9 cm away from the midline.

Right border: It is marked by a line slightly convex to the right and joining the right ends of the superior and inferior borders.

Left border: It is marked by a line fairly convex to the left and joining the left ends of the superior and inferior borders. The area of the thoracic wall overlying the heart is called the *precordium*.

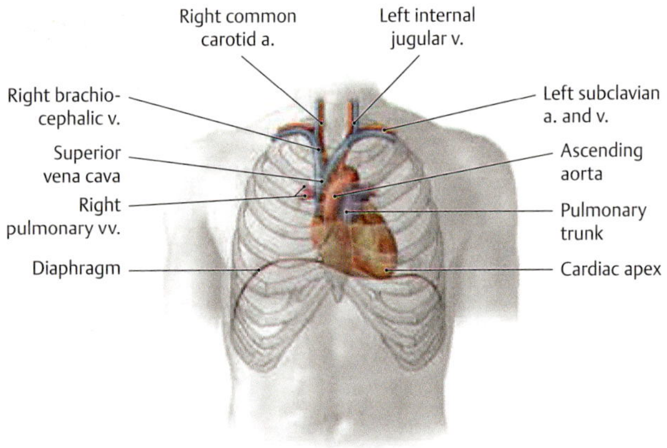

Fig. 14.16 Projection of the heart and great vessels onto chest (anterior view).

Dissection and Identification

Removal of the heart:

https://www.winkingskull.com/dissector/V1/video.aspx?vid=91

1. To detach the heart from the great blood vessels, the lines of the serous pericardial reflection are followed.
2. Place a probe in the transverse sinus of the pericardium.
3. With a pair of scissors, cut the *ascending aorta* and *pulmonary trunk* anterior to the probe, about 1.5 cm above their emergence from the heart.
4. Cut the *superior vena cava* with a pair of scissors about 1 cm above its junction with the right atrium.
5. Lift the heart by its apex and superiorly cut the inferior vena cava close to the diaphragm.
6. Lift the heart by its apex and cut the four *pulmonary veins* where they form the boundary of the oblique pericardial sinus.
7. At this stage, the heart is retained in a position only by the reflections of the serous pericardium from the posterior surface to the inner surface of the pericardial sac. Cut through these reflections to release the heart.
8. Referring to the illustration, identify the openings of all the great blood vessels.

External features of the heart:

https://www.winkingskull.com/dissector/V1/video.aspx?vid=286

https://www.winkingskull.com/dissector/V1/video.aspx?vid=287

1. Identify the following structures on the external surface of the heart (**Figs. 14.15**):
   - *Coronary sulcus*: It runs around the heart and separates the atria from the ventricles.
   - *Anterior interventricular sulcus*: It runs along the sternocostal surface of the heart between two ventricles and lodges the anterior interventricular branch of the left coronary artery.
   - *Posterior interventricular sulcus*: It runs between two ventricles on the diaphragmatic surface of the heart and lodges the posterior interventricular branch of the right coronary artery. Note that the interventricular sulci indicate the location of the interventricular septum and they join the coronary sulcus (atrioventricular sulcus) at right angles.
2. *Surfaces of the heart*:
   - *Anterior/sternocostal surface*: It is mainly formed by the right ventricle and a small part of the left ventricle and atria.
   - *Inferior/diaphragmatic surface* (**Fig. 14.15**): It is mainly formed by the left ventricle and a small part of the right ventricle.
   - *Left surface*: It is formed by the left ventricle and is related to the cardiac impression of the left lung.
   - *Right surface*: It is formed by the right atrium and is related to the right lung.
   - *Base of the heart*: It is the posterior or vertebral surface and is formed by the atria, mainly the left atrium. It is separated from the diaphragmatic surface by the posterior part of the *coronary sulcus*. This contains parts of both the right and left coronary arteries and the *coronary sinus*.
3. Note that the coronary sulcus and interventricular sulci mark the boundaries of the four chambers of the heart.
4. Now identify the four chambers starting from the right atrium, right ventricle, left ventricle and left atrium.
5. Examine the heart from the superior side to view and identify the following:
   - Aorta and aortic valve
   - Pulmonary trunk and pulmonary valve
   - Superior vena cava
6. Now view the diaphragmatic surface of the heart and identify the following:
   - Orifice of the inferior vena cava.
   - Posterior interventricular sulcus.
   - Note that the cardiac veins and coronary arteries with their branches are located in the coronary (atrioventricular) and interventricular sulci and that the veins are superficial to the arteries.

Cardiac veins:

1. Note that the vessels of the heart are located between the epicardium (visceral pericardium) and the muscle (myocardium) of the heart (**Fig. 14.17**).
2. The cardiac veins are superficial to the coronary arteries; hence, they can be viewed and dissected first.
3. The fat accompanying these veins and arteries is to be removed from the coronary and interventricular sulci using blunt dissection.
4. Identify the *coronary sinus* on the diaphragmatic surface. It is the dilated portion of the venous draining system of the heart located in the coronary sulcus. It is about 2 to 2.5 cm long and opens into the right atrium by an orifice located to the left of the inferior vena caval opening. We shall view this when we study the interior of the right atrium at a later stage.
5. Using blunt dissection, clean the surface of the coronary sinus.
6. Trace the coronary sinus superiorly in the coronary sulcus to the point where it receives the *great cardiac vein*.
7. Using blunt dissection, follow the great cardiac vein on the sternocostal surface of the heart as it courses from the apex of the heart and then along the anterior interventricular sulcus upwards to the coronary sinus.

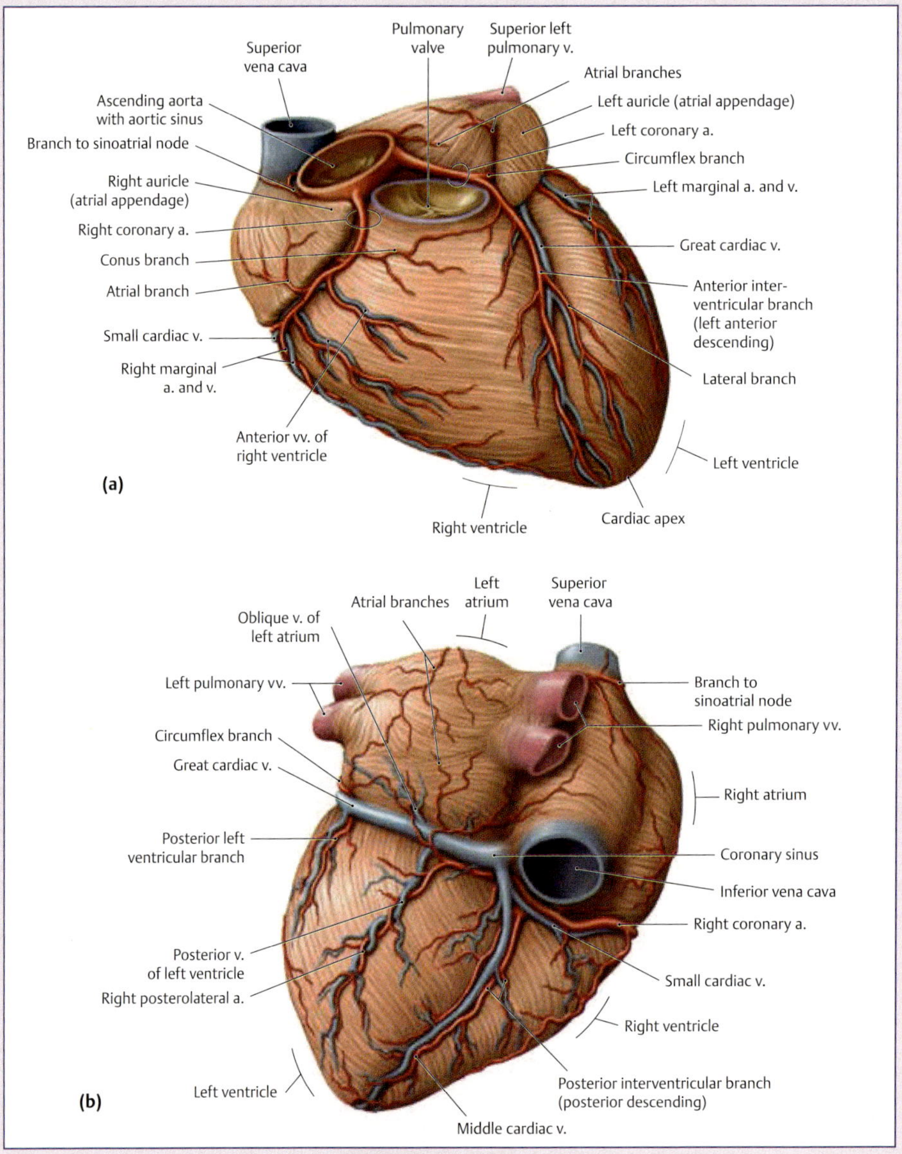

Fig. 14.17 Coronary arteries and cardiac veins. **(a)** Anterior view. **(b)** Posteroinferior view. *Note:* the right and left coronary arteries typically anastomose posteriorly at the left atrium and ventricle.

8. *Middle cardiac vein*: Identify the middle cardiac vein in the posterior interventricular sulcus. Trace it up to the coronary sinus.
9. *Small cardiac vein*: Identify the small cardiac vein near the inferior end of the coronary sinus. Using blunt dissection, dissect and follow it to the anterior surface (sternocostal surface) where it courses along the inferior border of the heart.
10. *Anterior cardiac veins*: They bridge the atrioventricular sulcus between the right atrium and the ventricle. They directly open into the right atrium along its anterior wall. On their way, they pass superficial to the right coronary artery.
11. *Posterior vein of the left ventricle*: It runs on the diaphragmatic surface of the left ventricle and drains into the middle of the coronary sinus.
12. *Oblique vein of the left atrium (vein of Marshall)*: It is a small vein running on the posterior surface of the left atrium. It terminates by joining the left end of the coronary sinus. It develops from the left common cardinal vein (Duct of Cuvier).
13. *Right marginal vein*: It accompanies the marginal branch of the right coronary artery. It drains into the small cardiac vein or directly into the right atrium.

14. *Venae cordis minimae (Thebesian veins)*: These are small veins present in all four chambers of the heart and they directly open into the cavity. They are more in number on the right side than on the left.

Coronary arteries:
To begin with, observe the aortic valve in the lumen of the ascending aorta. Identify the three semilunar cusps of the aortic valve, one anterior and two posterior cusps. The wall of the aorta shows outpocketing against each cusp. These are called the aortic sinuses (of Valsalva). Thus, there are three aortic sinuses, one anterior and two posterior (**Fig. 14.18**).

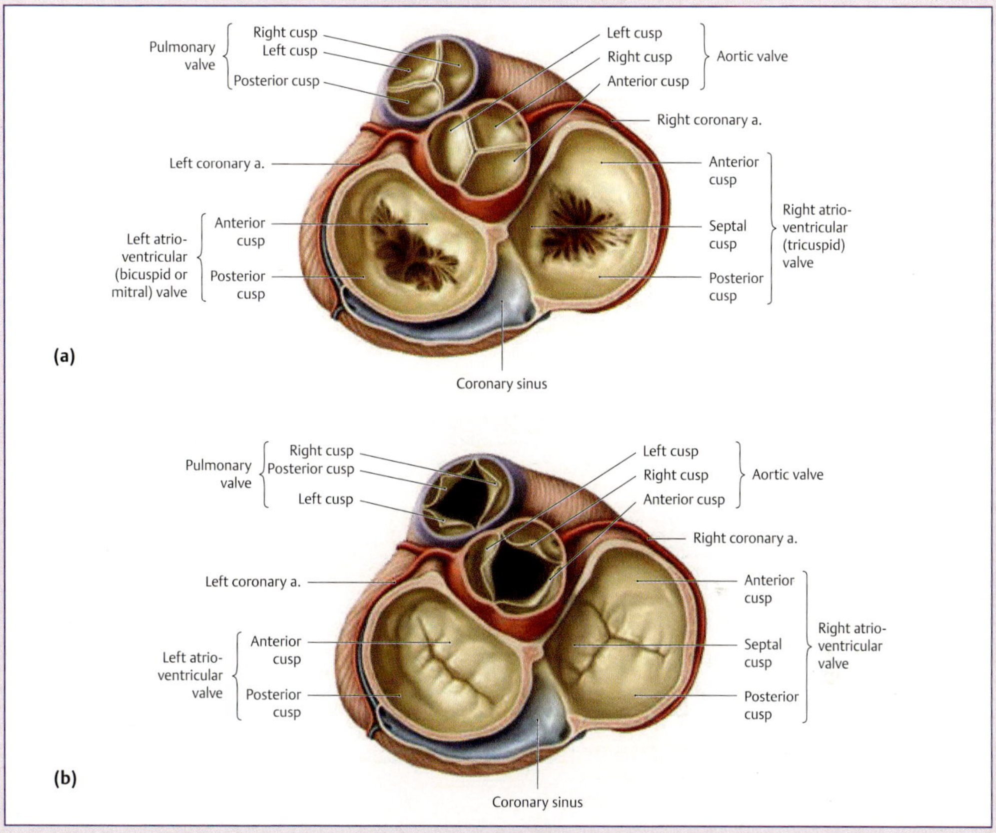

Fig. 14.18 Cardiac valves (plane of cardiac valves, superior view). *Removed*: Atria and great arteries. **(a)** Ventricular diastole (relaxation of the ventricles). *Closed*: Semilunar valves. *Open*: Atrioventricular valves. **(b)** Ventricular systole (contraction of the ventricles). *Closed*: Atrioventricular valves. *Open:* Semilunar valves.

Right coronary artery: It arises from the *anterior aortic sinus*. Identify its opening in the sinus. Insert the tip of the probe into the opening, and on the surface of the heart, palpate the tip of the probe in the place between the right auricle and the ascending aorta. This is the beginning of the right coronary artery.

https://www.winkingskull.com/dissector/V1/video.aspx?vid=92

https://www.winkingskull.com/dissector/V1/video.aspx?vid=288

1. Using blunt dissection, clean the right coronary artery and identify its anterior *right atrial branch*. It arises close to the origin of the right coronary artery. It ascends along the anterior wall of the right atrium towards the superior vena cava. It gives off the *sinoatrial nodal branch* that supplies the sinoatrial node (pacemaker) of the heart.
2. Follow the right coronary artery further along the coronary sulcus. Close to the inferior border of the heart, it gives rise to its *right marginal branch*. The branch accompanies the small cardiac vein and follows the inferior border of the heart.
3. To explore the further course of the right coronary artery, trace it along the coronary sulcus to the diaphragmatic surface of the heart. On reaching the posterior interventricular sulcus, it issues a branch, the *posterior interventricular branch*. It runs down along the interventricular

sulcus to the apex of the heart. The posterior interventricular branch of the right coronary artery is accompanied by the middle cardiac vein.

4. *Artery to the atrioventricular node*: It is a branch of the right coronary artery. It arises from the right coronary artery at the junction of the posterior interventricular sulcus with the coronary sulcus. This is also referred to as the *crux of the heart*.

Left coronary artery: It arises from the left posterior aortic sinus, locate the opening of the left coronary artery. Insert the tip of the probe in the opening. On the surface of the heart, palpate the tip of the probe between the left auricle and the pulmonary trunk. This is the beginning of the left coronary artery.

https://www.winkingskull.com/dissector/V1/video.aspx?vid=205

https://www.winkingskull.com/dissector/V1/video.aspx?vid=289

1. Using blunt dissection, clean the left coronary artery. After its short course, it divides into an *anterior interventricular branch* and the *circumflex branch*.
2. Follow the *anterior interventricular branch* along the anterior interventricular sulcus down to the apex of the heart. It is often called the *left anterior descending* (LAD) artery by the clinicians. It is accompanied by the great cardiac vein.
3. Trace the *circumflex branch* of the left coronary artery in the coronary sulcus around the left border. This circumflex branch gives numerous unnamed branches that supply the posterior wall of the left ventricle. In the coronary sulcus, the circumflex branch accompanies the coronary sinus.

Areas of Distribution and Branches of the Coronary Arteries

The right coronary artery has the following branches (**Fig. 14.19**):

1. Major branches: (a) Marginal and (b) posterior interventricular
2. Small branches: (a) Nodal (to SA node), (b) right atrial and (c) infundibular

Areas of distribution:

1. Right atrium
2. Greater part of the right ventricle (except the part close to the anterior interventricular sulcus)
3. Small part of the left ventricle close to the posterior interventricular groove
4. Posterior part of the interventricular septum
5. The entire conducting system of the heart except the left branch of the AV bundle

The left coronary artery has the following branches:

1. Major branches: (a) Anterior interventricular and (b) circumflex
2. Small branches: (a) Left atrial and (b) pulmonary

Areas of distribution:

1. Left atrium
2. Greater part of the left ventricle (except the part close to the posterior interventricular sulcus)
3. Small part of the right ventricle close to the anterior interventricular sulcus
4. Anterior part of the interventricular septum
5. Left branch of the AV bundle

Clinical Notes

1. Thrombosis of the coronary artery leads to myocardial infarction which may prove fatal.
2. An incomplete obstruction can lead to *angina pectoris*. In this, the patient experiences pain in the precordial region and radiating down along the medial side of the left arm and forearm.
3. *Coronary angiography*: To evaluate the extent of patency/blockage involving coronary arteries and their branches, radio-opaque dye is injected and the coronaries are visualized.
4. *Coronary angioplasty*: Stent is inserted at the site of blockage along the coronary artery or its major branch to reinstate the flow of blood.

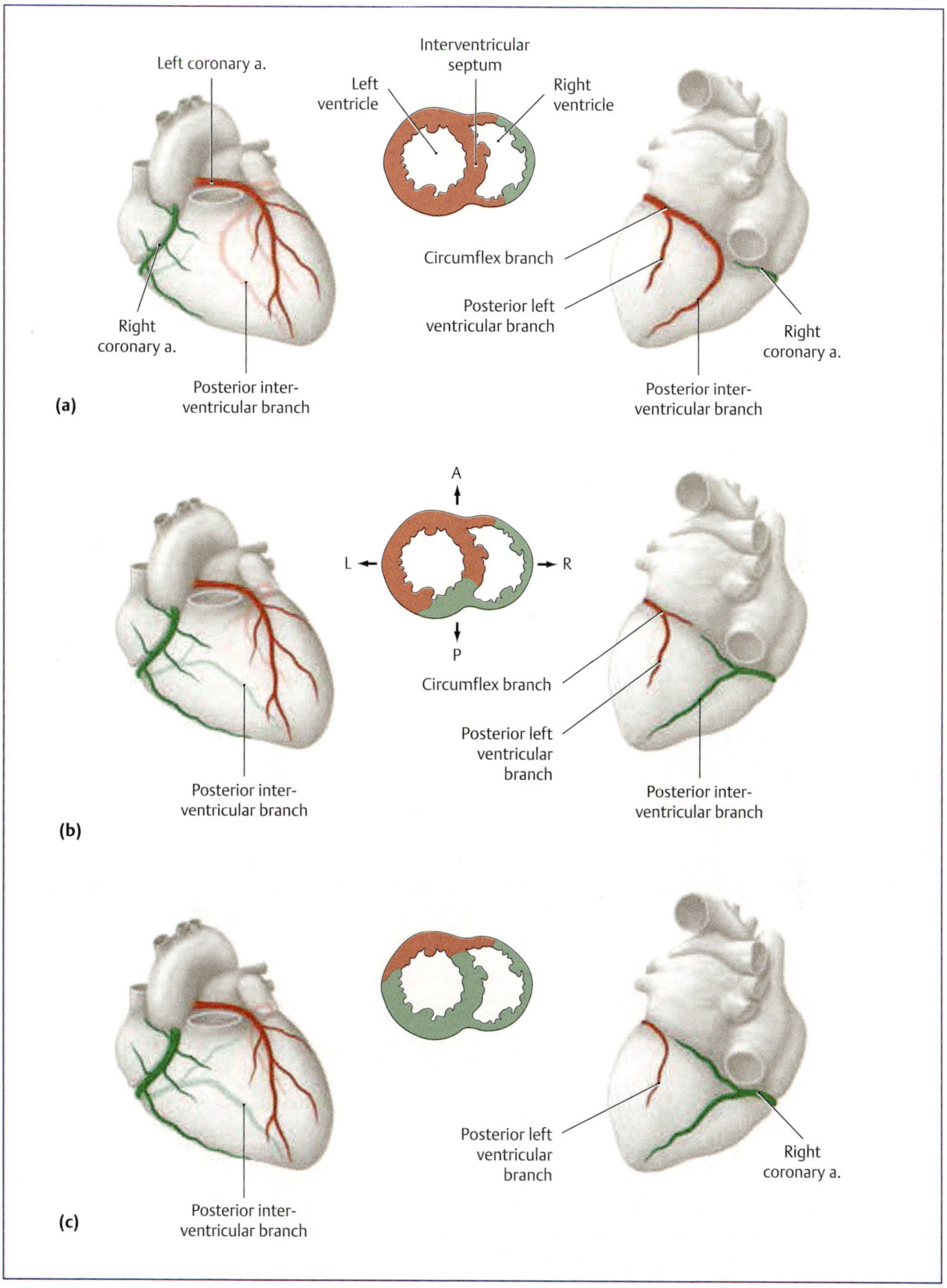

Fig. 14.19 Distribution of the coronary arteries. **(a)** Left coronary dominance (15–17%). **(b)** Balanced distribution, right coronary artery dominance (67–70%). **(c)** Right coronary dominance (~15%).

Lymphatics of the Heart

The lymphatics of the heart follow the coronary arteries. They form two trunks. The right trunk drains into the brachiocephalic nodes, while the left one ends into the tracheobronchial nodes located at the bifurcation of the trachea.

Nerves of the Heart

Both components of the autonomic nervous system contribute to the heart. The sympathetic fibres come from the cervical and upper thoracic ganglia of the sympathetic chain. The parasympathetic fibres are carried by the vagus and they are cardioinhibitory, while the sympathetic fibres are cardioacceleratory, that is, vagal stimulation causes bradycardia (slowing the heart rate) and sympathetic stimulation causes tachycardia (increase in heart rate).

Both the sympathetic and parasympathetic nerves form the superficial and deep cardiac plexuses (**Fig. 14.20**). The *superficial cardiac plexus* is located below the arch of the aorta in front of the right pulmonary artery. It is formed by the:

1. Superior cervical cardiac branch of the left sympathetic chain.
2. The inferior cervical cardiac branch of the left vagus.

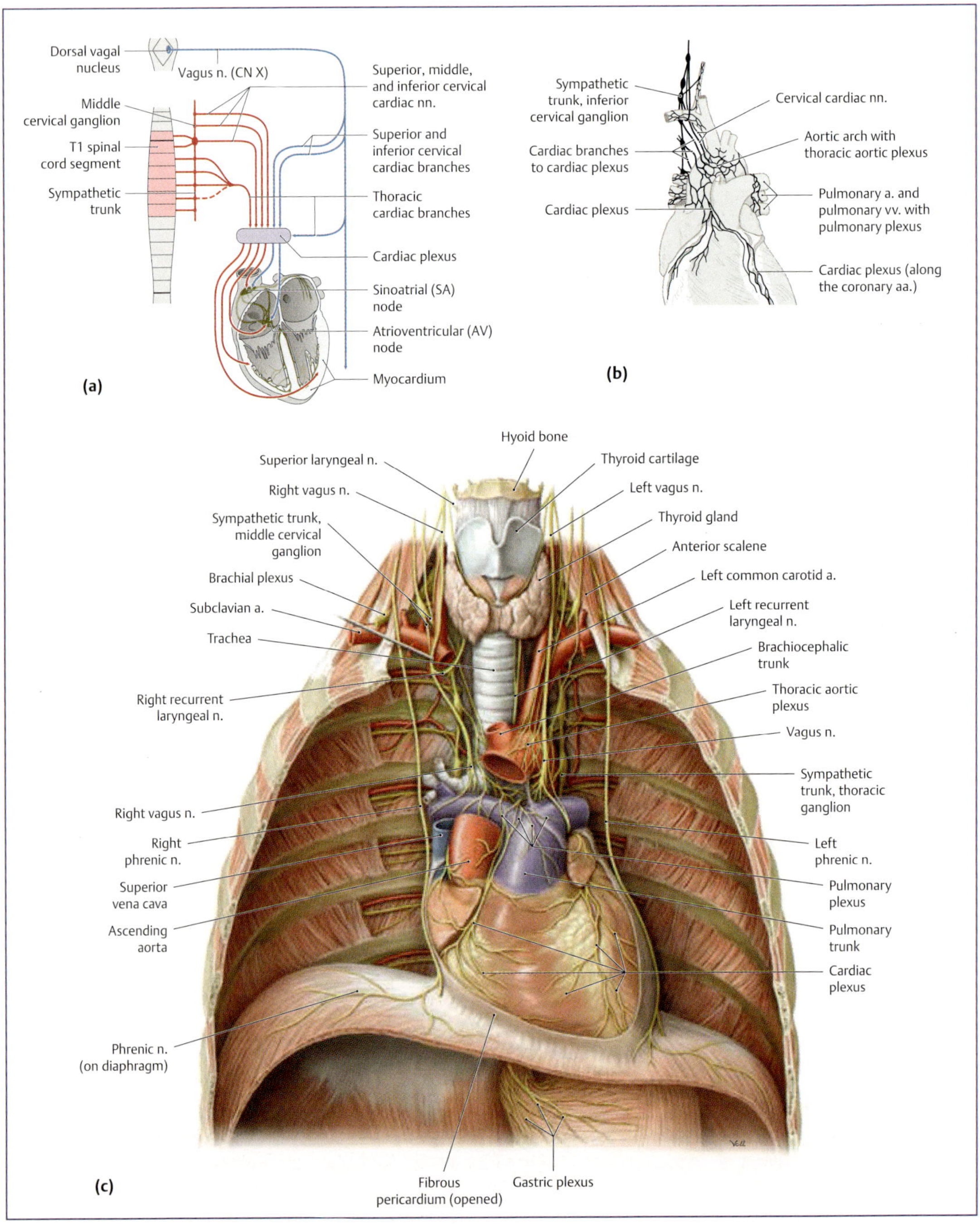

Fig. 14.20 Nerves of the heart. **(a)** Schematic. **(b)** Autonomic plexus of the heart, right lateral view. Note the continuity between the cardiac, aortic and pulmonary plexuses. **(c)** Autonomic nerves of the heart. Anterior view of opened thorax.

The *deep cardiac plexus* is located in front of the tracheal bifurcation, behind the arch of the aorta. It is formed by the:

1. Cardiac branches from the cervical and upper thoracic ganglia of the sympathetic trunk.
2. Cardiac branches of the vagus and recurrent laryngeal nerves.

Branches of these cardiac plexuses follow the coronary arteries to reach the myocardium.

Internal Features of the Atria and Ventricles

To observe and study the internal features of the four chambers of the heart (**Fig. 14.21**), the incisions are made as per the illustration.

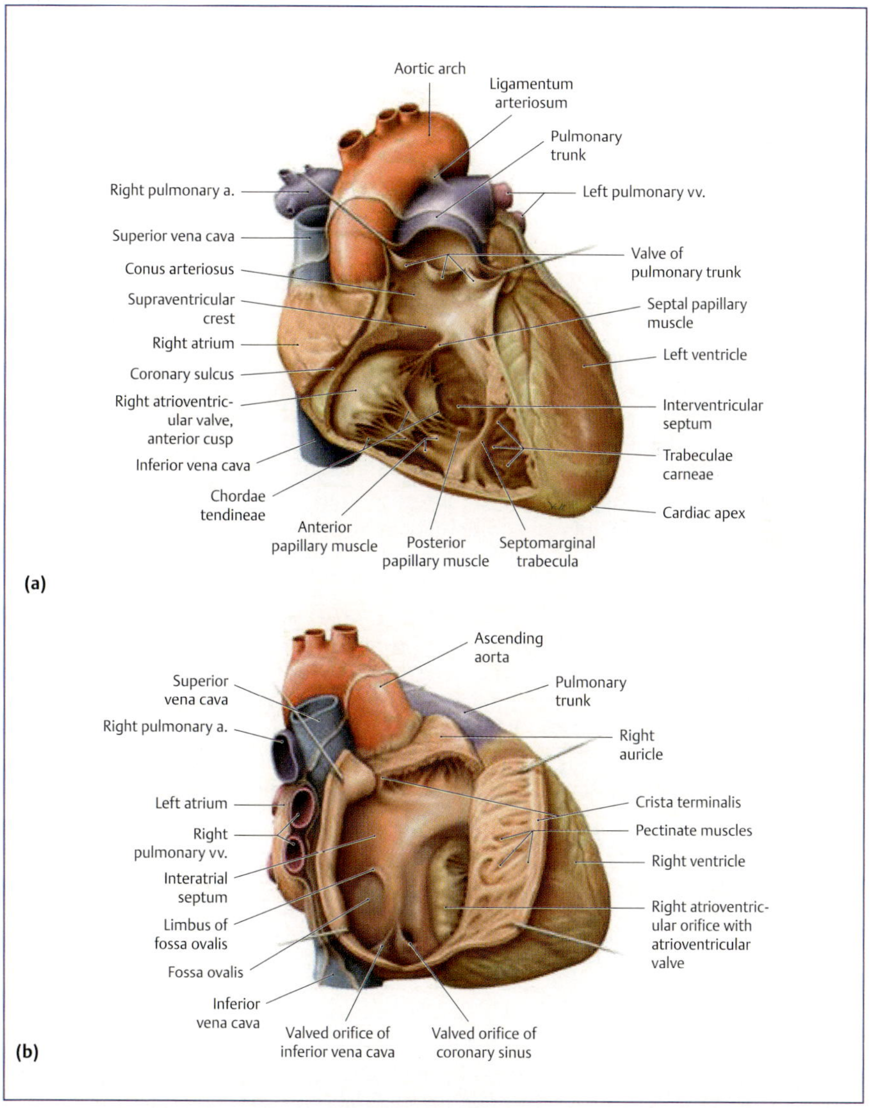

Fig. 14.21 Chambers of the heart. **(a)** Right ventricle, anterior view. Note the supraventricular crest, which marks the adult boundary between the embryonic ventricle and the bulbus cordis (now conus arteriosus). **(b)** Right atrium (right lateral view). (*continued*)

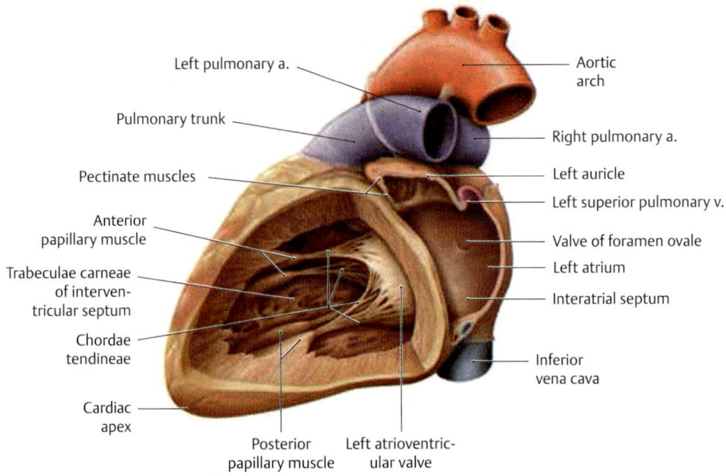

Fig. 14.21 (*continued*) Chambers of the heart. **(c)** Left atrium and ventricle (left lateral view). Note the irregular trabeculae carneae characteristic of the ventricular wall.

Dissection and Identification

To study the interior of the right atrium:

https://www.winkingskull.com/dissector/V1/video.aspx?vid=93

1. Use a pair of scissors to make a cut at the tip of the right auricle. Inserting one blade of the scissors through this opening, carry the cut horizontally to the right.
2. Now turn the scissors to cut through the anterior wall of the right atrium in the downward direction till you reach just superior to the inferior vena cava.
3. Turn the scissors to continue this cut horizontally to the left, stopping little short of the coronary sulcus.
4. Turn the flap of the atrial wall towards the left to open the right atrium. Remove the clotted blood and rinse the chamber with water taking the heart to the sink. Observe along the interior of the right atrium following:

   https://www.winkingskull.com/dissector/V1/video.aspx?vid=291

   - *Crista terminalis*: It is a vertical ridge.
   - *Musculi pectinati*: It consists of muscular ridges running horizontally.
   - Opening of the superior vena cava.
   - Opening and valve of the inferior vena cava.
   - Opening and valve of the coronary sinus.
   - Fossa ovalis and limbus fossa ovalis.

Right Atrium

The interior of the right atrium shows two distinct parts separated by the *crista terminalis*: (a) The posterior smooth part called the *sinus venarum* receives the superior vena cava, inferior vena cava and coronary sinus. This part develops from the *right horn of the sinus venosus* (the sinus venosus is placed at the venous end of the developing heart tube). (b) The anterior part shows parallel muscular ridges called the *musculi pectinati* (pectin = comb). They extend into the auricle. This part develops from the right portion of the primitive atrium.

Crista terminalis: It is a vertical ridge extending from a point just anterior to the superior vena caval opening to the ridge at the inferior vena caval orifice, that is, the valve of the inferior vena cava (Eustachian valve). This ridge is continuous on the left side with a small flap at the opening of the coronary sinus. This small flap is the *valve of the coronary sinus*; both the valves are derived/developed from the *right sinus* (sinoatrial) *valve* of the sinoatrial orifice between the sinus venosus and the primitive atrium.

Further, this ridge continues superiorly with the *limbus fossa ovalis* bordering the *fossa ovalis*. The posteromedial wall of the right atrium is formed by the *interatrial septum*. The fossa ovalis is a depression seen along this wall and marks the site of the foramen ovale. The *foramen ovale* is a valvular foramen present in prenatal life. It is between the septum secundum and the caudal limb of the septum primum. It closes after birth. It directs better oxygenated blood (including placental blood) coming from the inferior vena cava (across this foramen ovale) from right atrium to the left atrium during prenatal life. Foramen ovale permits flow from the right to the left atrium because the right atrium receives blood from the superior vena cava, inferior vena cava and coronary sinus, that is, blood from almost the entire body of the foetus. Therefore, pressure within the right atrium is more as compared to the left atrium, which receives scanty amount of blood from the non-functional lungs. At birth, the lungs start functioning (prenatally they are non-functional). So, more blood is diverted to the pulmonary beds for oxygenation at birth. More of it now returns to the left atrium, so the pressure within the left atrium increases. Once it equalizes with the pressure in the right atrium, the valvular foramen ovale closes. Initially, it is the functional closure that occurs at birth. However, subsequently fibrosis occurs between the septum primum and secundum ensuring the anatomical closure that occurs in about a week's time.

Note that the opening of the inferior vena cava into the right atrium faces the fossa ovalis (site of the foramen ovale) to which the valve of the inferior vena cava directs the blood without mixing it with less oxygenated blood coming along the superior vena cava.

Intervenous tubercle: An elevation between the two venae caval orifices in the right atrium prevents admixture of less oxygenated blood of the superior vena cava and better oxygenated blood coming through the inferior vena cava. The intervenous tubercle is well developed in quadrupeds and not so much in human beings.

Dissection and Identification

1. To determine the level of the pulmonary valve, insert a finger in the pulmonary trunk. Using a pair of scissors, make a short horizontal cut through the anterior wall of the right ventricle, immediately below the level of the pulmonary valve.

   https://www.winkingskull.com/dissector/V1/video.aspx?vid=94

2. Now insert one blade of the scissors at the right end of this cut and extend it downwards parallel to but 1 cm away from the coronary sulcus. During this, avoid damage to the cusps of the tricuspid valve at the atrioventricular orifice.
3. Insert your finger through this opening in the ventricular wall and feel the *interventricular septum*.
4. From the left end of the earlier upper horizontal cut, make a cut towards the inferior border of the heart 2 cm to the right of the anterior interventricular sulcus.
5. Turn the cut flap of the ventricular wall downwards.
6. Remove the blood clots in the cavity and rinse the chamber with water. Take care not to damage the *chordae tendineae*.
7. In the interior of the right ventricle, identify the *right atrioventricular orifice* and the *tricuspid valve*. Identify the three cusps of the tricuspid valve, namely the *anterior* (ventral), *posterior* (dorsal) and *septal cusps*.

   https://www.winkingskull.com/dissector/V1/video.aspx?vid=292

8. Observe the *chordae tendineae*. These are thin strands stretching from the summit of the papillary muscles to the ventricular surface of the cusps of the tricuspid valve.
9. Identify the three *papillary muscles*, the anterior (ventral), posterior (dorsal) and *septal*.
10. Observe the *trabeculae carneae* along the inner surface of the ventricular wall.
11. Trace the *septomarginal trabecula* from the lower part of the interventricular septum to the base of the ventral papillary muscle.
12. Identify the *infundibulum* (conus arteriosus), the opening of the *pulmonary trunk* and the *pulmonary valve*.
13. Identify the *three semilunar cusps* of the pulmonary valve. These are two anterior (right and left) and one posterior cusps.

Right Ventricle

The cavity of the right ventricle is roughly triangular in shape when viewed from the anterior side (**Fig. 14.21a**). It receives blood from the right atrium through the *right atrioventricular orifice* which is guarded by the tricuspid valve. The blood leaves the right ventricle through the *pulmonary orifice* guarded by the pulmonary valve. The anterosuperior part of the ventricular cavity is smooth and is called the infundibulum. It develops from the bulbus cordis. The remaining part of the interior of the ventricle shows irregular muscular ridges called the *trabeculae carneae.* The *supraventricular crest* separates the rough (trabeculae carneae) and smooth (infundibulum) parts of the right ventricle. In addition to these ridges, there are three papillary muscles. They are conical with their bases attached to the ventricular wall and the apices being connected by thin tendinous strands called the chordae tendineae to the ventricular face of the cusps of the tricuspid valve. The three papillary muscles are named after the ventricular wall to which their bases are attached. These are the anterior/ventral and septal papillary muscles. The dorsal/posterior papillary muscle is attached to the inferior wall. From the base of the ventral papillary muscle to the lower part of the interventricular septum, there is a *moderator band* or *septomarginal trabecula*. It conveys the right branch of the atrioventricular (AV) bundle (bundle of His), a part of the conducting system of the heart, to the right ventricular wall.

When the papillary muscles contract, they draw the margins of the adjacent cusps closer and prevent them from being forced into the atrium when the intraventricular pressure increases during ventricular contraction. Concurrently, it allows complete filling of the atrium during ventricular contraction. The *moderator band* or *septomarginal trabecula* is in fact one of the trabeculae carneae from the interventricular septum to the base of the anterior papillary muscle.

Right Atrioventricular Orifice and Tricuspid Valve

The right atrioventricular orifice is about 2.5 cm in diameter and is surrounded by a fibrous ring. The ring gives attachment to the cusps of the atrioventricular valve and the atrial as well as ventricular muscles.

The tricuspid/right atrioventricular valve has three cusps: The *anterior/ventral cusp* separates the atrioventricular foramen from the infundibulum. The *posterior/dorsal cusp* is along the inferior wall of the right ventricle. The septal cusp is along the interventricular septum. The atrial surfaces of the cusps are smooth. The chordae tendineae are attached to the margins and the ventricular surfaces of the cusps.

Pulmonary Orifice and the Pulmonary Valve

The pulmonary orifice is located at the apex of the infundibulum. It is surrounded by a thin fibrous ring and gives attachment to the valvules of the pulmonary valve.

Pulmonary Valve

It has three semilunar cusps/valvules. Each valvule is concave on its arterial surface and is formed by a thin fibrous tissue covered by endothelium. It has a thickened free margin with a small *nodule* in the middle of the free margin and a thin smooth margin with the *lunules* on each side of the nodule. The valve is closed during ventricular diastole and the cusps bulge towards the ventricular cavity. Opposite each cusp, the wall of the pulmonary trunk is dilated to form a sinus.

Pulmonary Trunk

It begins at the level of the pulmonary valve. It is anterior and to the left of the ascending aorta. It is posterior to the sternal end of the third left costal cartilage. It is about 5 cm long and 2 cm wide. It ends in the concavity of the aortic arch (behind the second left costal cartilage) by dividing into the right and left pulmonary arteries. With the ascending aorta, the pulmonary trunk lies in a single serous pericardial tube (both being developed from a single source, the truncus arteriosus).

Dissection and Identification

Left ventricle:

Observe the aorta from above and identify the aortic valve. Identify its three semilunar cusps, an anterior and two posterior (the right non-coronary and the left one).

1. Insert one blade of the scissors between the anterior and left posterior cusps.

2. Cut through the anterior wall of the ascending aorta between these cusps.

   https://www.winkingskull.com/dissector/V1/video.aspx?vid=207
3. Continue this cut downwards towards the apex of the heart. Let this cut be parallel to and about 2 cm to the left of the anterior interventricular sulcus. Note that this will cut across the anterior interventricular branch of the left coronary artery as well as the great cardiac vein accompanying it.
4. Open the left ventricle and aorta, remove the blood clots and rinse the chamber with water.
5. Identify the *left atrioventricular orifice* and the *bicuspid/mitral valve* guarding the orifice. Identify the *two cusps*, the *anterior* and *posterior papillary muscles* with the chordae tendineae associated with them.

   https://www.winkingskull.com/dissector/V1/video.aspx?vid=294
6. Observe the interior of the left ventricle studded with the *trabeculae carneae*, the muscular ridges.
7. Palpate the muscular part of the *interventricular septum* by putting the right thumb in the right ventricle and the index finger in the left ventricle. Feel the thickness of the *muscular part of the interventricular septum.*
8. Now move your thumb and index finger upwards to palpate the *thin membranous part of the interventricular septum* located just below the attachment of the anterior cusp of the aortic valve.

In the ascending aorta, identify the openings of the right and left coronary arteries arising from the aortic sinuses.

Left Ventricle (Fig. 14.21c)

The cavity of the left ventricle is circular in cross section and shows much thicker wall since it has to propel blood against greater resistance (systolic pressure 120 mm Hg) as against the right ventricle that encounters low vascular resistance (pulmonary systolic pressure being 25–30 mm Hg). The *trabeculae carneae* in the left ventricle are finer and more in number than the right ventricle. There are two large anterior and posterior *papillary muscles*. The anterior papillary muscle is attached to the left wall and the posterior muscle is attached to the inferior wall.

Each papillary muscle has *chordae tendineae* connecting it to both the cusps of the bicuspid valve. The *aortic vestibule* has a smooth wall and it leads to the aorta. It develops from the bulbus cordis.

The left atrioventricular orifice is surrounded by a fibrous ring and is guarded by the mitral/bicuspid valve. There are two cusps, a large anterior cusp that lies between the mitral and aortic orifices and a small posterior cusp.

Aortic Orifice and the Aortic Valve

The aortic orifice is located in the right posterosuperior part of the left ventricle. It is surrounded by a fibrous ring. The ring has attachment of valves/cusps of the aortic valve. The aortic valve has three semilunar cusps like the pulmonary valve. These cusps are an anterior and two posterior, that is, the left posterior and right posterior. The wall of the aorta shows a bulge at these cusps. They are called the *aortic sinuses*. The right coronary artery arises from the *anterior aortic sinus* and the left coronary artery arises from the *left posterior aortic sinus*. In addition to this, the aorta shows a swelling of its right border called the *bulb of the aorta*. It is due to the thrust of the blood ejected from the left ventricle. The bulb of the aorta is usually the site of an abnormal dilatation called the *aneurysm*.

Fibrous Skeleton of the Heart

It consists of the fibrous rings surrounding the two atrioventricular orifices and the two major arterial orifices, that is, the aorta and pulmonary trunk. The fibrous rings around the AV orifices form a shape like number '8'. Substantial amount of fibrous tissue is placed between the aortic ring in front and at the atrioventricular rings behind. The tissue between the aortic ring and the right AV ring is called the *trigonum fibrosum dextrum*. In some mammals, for example, in sheep, it may have a small bone called the *os cordis*. The fibrous tissue between the aortic ring and the left AV ring is called the *trigonum fibrosum sinistrum*. Yet another fibrous band called the *tendon of the infundibulum* lies between the infundibulum of the right ventricle and the aortic ring.

Conducting System of the Heart

It consists of specialized myocardial cells meant for initiation and subsequent conduction of the cardiac impulse (**Fig. 14.22**). These fibres are finer as compared to the other myocardial fibres. The conducting system has the following elements:

1. *Sinoatrial node/SA node*: It is also called the *pacemaker* of the heart. It generates the impulses at the rate of about 70 per minute (normal healthy adult) to initiate the heartbeat. It is located in the upper end of the sulcus terminalis at the atriocaval junction. It is horseshoe shaped. The impulse then travels through the atrial wall to the AV node.
2. *Atrioventricular node/AV node*: It is smaller than the SA node. It is located in the posteroinferior part of the interatrial septum just above the orifice of the coronary sinus. It can generate impulse at the rate of 60 per minute.
3. *Atrioventricular bundle/Bundle of His*: It begins at the AV node and after crossing the atrioventricular ring descends along the membranous part of the interventricular septum. At the upper border of the muscular part of the interventricular septum, it divides into the right and left branches. The *right branch* passes on the right side of the interventricular septum. The major part of this passes along the septomarginal trabecula/moderator band to the anterior wall of the right ventricle. There it divides into the Purkinje fibres. The left branch of the bundle of His passes along the left side of the interventricular septum to be in the left ventricle where it divides into the Purkinje fibres.
4. *Purkinje fibres*: They form the subendothelial plexus. These fibres are large and are striated at their margins. Most of the conducting system is supplied by the right coronary artery except the left branch of the bundle of His, which is supplied by the left coronary artery. Vascular lesions involving coronaries may cause cardiac arrhythmias, that is, the normal rhythm of cardiac contraction is altered.

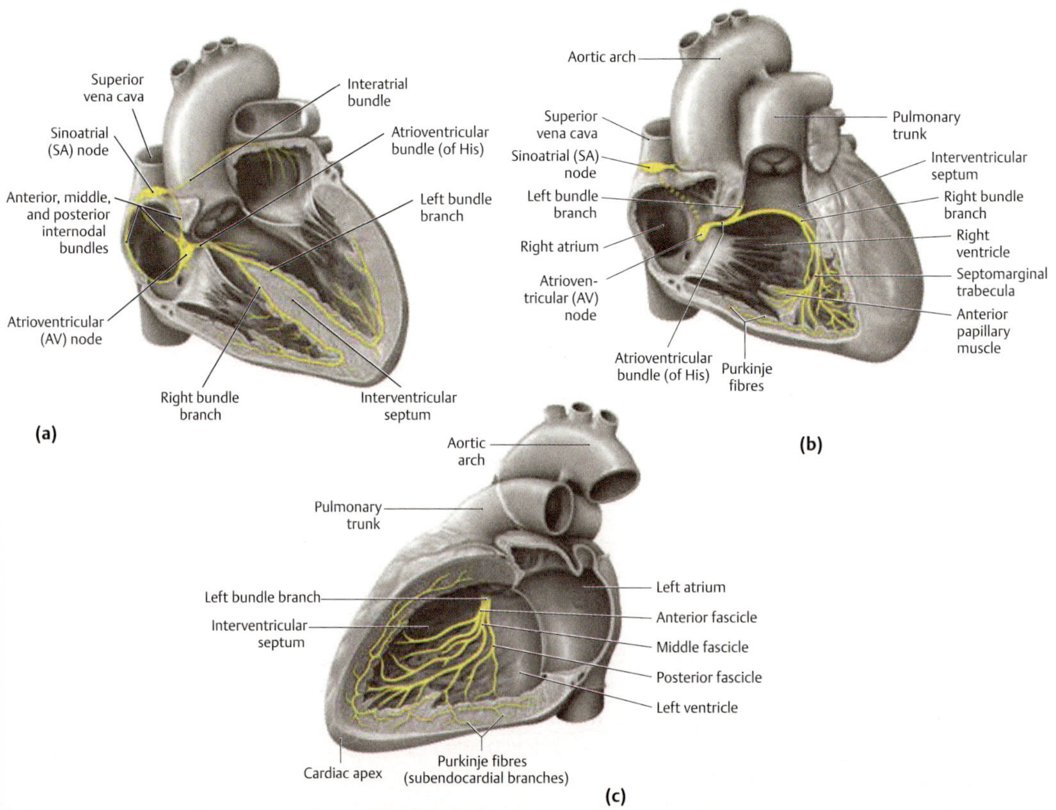

Fig. 14.22 Conduction system of the heart. **(a)** Anterior view. *Opened*: All four chambers. **(b)** Right lateral view. *Opened*: Right atrium and ventricle. **(c)** Left lateral view. *Opened*: Left atrium and ventricle.

Dissection and Identification

Left atrium:

1. To explore the internal features of the left atrium, examine the posterior surface of the heart. Note that the four pulmonary veins open into the left atrium.
2. Using a pair of scissors, make an inverted U-shaped cut on the posterior wall of the left atrium. Avoid cutting into the pulmonary veins. Design your cut between the pulmonary veins. Turn the flap downwards.
3. Remove the blood clots and rinse the chambers with water.
4. Note the interior of the left atrium which is smooth all over, except the left auricle which is rough.
5. Note the following:

   https://www.winkingskull.com/dissector/V1/video.aspx?vid=293

   - Site of the foramen ovale along the interatrial septum.
   - Opening that leads to the left auricle.
   - Opening of the left AV orifice with left atrioventricular valve guarding it.

Left Atrium

It is nearly quadrangular in shape and placed posteriorly. It has the left auricle as an appendage projecting anteriorly, overlapping the infundibulum of the right ventricle. The oblique pericardial sinus lies behind the left atrium. Two pulmonary veins open on each side of the posterior wall of the left atrium. The smooth part of the left atrium is derived by progressive absorption of the pulmonary veins. The small rough portion of the left atrium present in the auricle is derived from the primitive atrial chamber. The septal wall of the left atrium shows the *fossa lunata* corresponding to the fossa ovalis of the right atrium.

Superior Mediastinum

Introduction: It is bounded superiorly by the superior thoracic aperture, inferiorly by the plane at the sternal angle, anteriorly by the manubrium and posteriorly by the vertebrae T1-4. Laterally, it is limited by the mediastinal pleura on both sides. It contains structures that pass between the neck and thorax and the upper limb. It includes the trachea, oesophagus, thoracic duct, great blood vessels and their branches.

Dissection and Identification

1. If the upper limbs have been dissected already and the clavicles have been divided, then cut the first ribs anterior to the subclavian veins. Turn the manubrium sterni upwards. This exposes the contents of the superior mediastinum.
2. Identify the thymus. In a newborn, it can be visualized in the chest radiograph; however, in adults it is replaced by the connective tissue and is difficult to recognize.
3. After removing the thymus, identify the superior vena cava. Identify the *left brachiocephalic vein*. Clean it by blunt dissection.

   https://www.winkingskull.com/dissector/V1/video.aspx?vid=296

4. Identify the *right brachiocephalic vein*. Trace both the brachiocephalic veins as they unite to form the superior vena cava.
5. Trace the superior vena cava lower down as it passes anterior to the root of the right lung.
6. Observe the *azygos vein* on the right side of the mediastinum and trace it as it arches over the root of the right lung to terminate on the posterior side of the superior vena cava.
7. Cut the superior vena cava a little above the termination of the azygos vein. Turn the superior vena cava along with the brachiocephalic veins upwards.
8. Identify both the *phrenic nerves*. Each passes anterior to the root lung on the respective side. Each phrenic nerve is accompanied by the pericardiacophrenic vessels and enters the superior surface of the diaphragm.

9. Identify the *arch of the aorta*. It begins and ends at the level of the sternal angle. It has three branches arising from its superior side. These are the: (a) *brachiocephalic trunk*, (b) *left common carotid artery* and (c) *left subclavian artery*.

   https://www.winkingskull.com/dissector/V1/video.aspx?vid=297

10. Identify the *ligamentum arteriosum*, an obliterated remnant of the ductus arteriosus that connects the left pulmonary artery to the arch of the aorta. It is seen as a fibrous cord in the cadaver.
11. Identify the *left vagus* on the left side of the aortic arch and the *left recurrent laryngeal nerve* that takes a recurrent course, passes up behind the ligamentum arteriosum and then passes in the tracheaoesophageal gutter.

    https://www.winkingskull.com/dissector/V1/video.aspx?vid=298

12. Trace the left vagus downwards as it passes posterior to the root of the left lung.
13. Trace the right vagus down to the posterior side of root of the right lung. Note that the *right recurrent laryngeal nerve* loops around the proximal part of the right subclavian artery.
14. Identify the *trachea* and note that the *oesophagus* lies posterior to it.
15. Trace the trachea down to its bifurcation at the level of the sternal angle into the *right* and *left principal bronchus*. Note that the arch of azygos vein passes superior to the right principal bronchus, while the arch of the aorta passes superior to the left main bronchus.
16. Try to identify the *tracheobronchial lymph nodes* located at the bifurcation of the trachea.
17. Palpate the trachea and note that the tracheal rings (hyaline cartilage) are C-shaped with deficiency on the posterior side which is occupied by the *trachealis* muscle, offering soft cushion to the expanding oesophagus during swallowing.
18. Note the difference between the right and left principal bronchi. The right main bronchus is wider and more in line with the trachea than the left bronchus.
19. The inner side of the tracheal bifurcation shows a ridge of cartilage called the *carina* (L. carina = keel of boat). It serves as an important landmark during bronchoscopy.

Arch of the Aorta and Its Branches

The arch (**Fig. 14.23**) begins posterior to the right half of the sternal angle and then passes posteriorly with slight convexity to the left, arching under the lower half of the superior mediastinum. This convexity to the left is where the arch crosses the left side of the trachea and oesophagus. The arch of the aorta continues as the descending thoracic aorta at the level of the intervertebral disc between the T4 and T5 vertebrae.

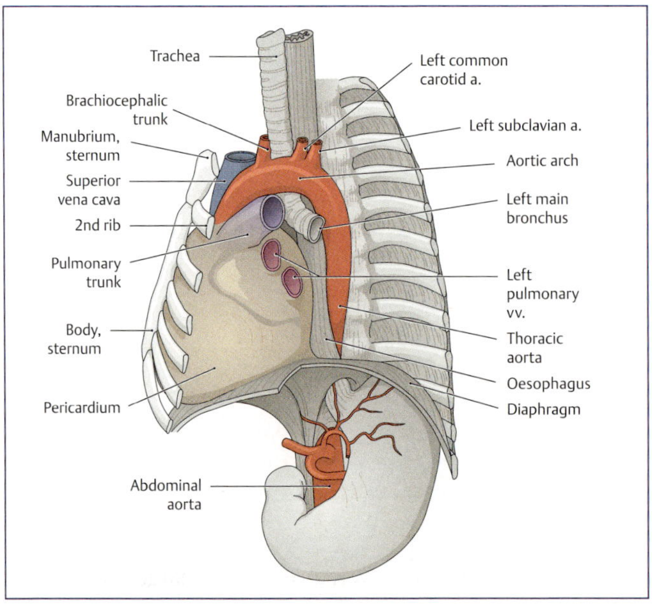

Fig. 14.23 Arch of aorta and its branches. (Left lateral view) *Removed*: Left thoracic wall and left lung.

Relations

Anterior and to the left:

1. The remains of the thymus
2. Left superior intercostal vein crossing the upper part of the arch
3. Phrenic nerve
4. Cervical cardiac branches of the left vagus nerve
5. Cervical cardiac branches of the left sympathetic trunk
6. Left vagus
7. Left pleura and lung

Inferior:

1. Bifurcation of the pulmonary trunk
2. Left pulmonary artery
3. Left principal bronchus
4. Ligamentum arteriosum
5. Left recurrent laryngeal nerve
6. Superficial cardiac plexus

Posterior and to the right:

1. The trachea, tracheobronchial nodes and deep cardiac plexus
2. Oesophagus
3. Left recurrent laryngeal nerve
4. Thoracic duct
5. Vertebral column

Superior:

1. Branches of the arch, namely (a) the brachiocephalic, (b) left common carotid and (c) left subclavian arteries
2. Left brachiocephalic vein

Branches of the Arch of the Aorta

1. *Brachiocephalic artery*: It is the largest branch. It arises behind the centre of the manubrium. It then passes superolaterally to the right side of the trachea and ends behind the right sternoclavicular joint by dividing into: (a) the right subclavian and (b) right common carotid arteries. It may give *thyroidea ima* artery to the isthmus of the thyroid gland.
2. *Left common carotid artery*: It arises from the arch immediately to the left of the brachiocephalic trunk and ascends superolaterally to the back of the left sternoclavicular joint. It is anterior to the left subclavian artery with the left phrenic and left vagus between them.
3. *Left subclavian artery*: It arises from the arch of the aorta posterior to the other two branches. Ascending ventrally in contact with the mediastinal pleura, it reaches to the left side of the trachea. It enters the neck a little posterior to the left sternoclavicular joint and then arches laterally to the left, grooving the cervical pleura and the apex of the lung.

Clinical Notes

1. *Patent ductus arteriosus*: It is a congenital malformation in which the ductus arteriosus remains patent instead of obliterating to form the ligamentum arteriosum. It can be surgically corrected.
2. *Aortic aneurysm*: It is localized dilatation of the aorta.
3. *Coarctation of the aorta*: Localized narrowing of the arch of the aorta. In relation to the ductus arteriosus, it may be (a) preductal, (b) ductal or (c) postductal coarctation. It is associated with the extensive collateral circulation between branches of the subclavian artery and the descending thoracic aorta evidenced by notching of the ribs due to large intercostal arteries and anastomosis between the anterior and posterior intercostals.
4. *Aortic knuckle*: It is a projection of the arch of the aorta beyond the left margin of the mediastinal shadow, seen in posteroanterior view of the radiograph of the chest.

Posterior Mediastinum

It lies behind the pericardium. It contains structures that pass between the thorax and the abdomen. In fact, these structures can be approached during dissection through the posterior wall of the pericardium.

Dissection and Identification

1. Observe/note the *boundaries* of the posterior mediastinum.
   - *Anterior*: Pericardium.
   - *Posterior*: Bodies of the thoracic vertebrae T5-12.
   - *Superior*: The plane of the sternal angle.
   - *Lateral*: The mediastinal pleura, that is, the right and left.
   - *Inferior*: The diaphragm.
2. Observe the inner surface of the posterior wall of the pericardium.
3. Move the heart into the pericardium and now review the relationship of the heart with the oesophagus. The left atrium is related to the oesophagus.

   ▶ https://www.winkingskull.com/dissector/V1/video.aspx?vid=208
4. Remove the pericardium in the region of the oblique pericardial sinus to expose the *oesophagus*. Slightly posterior to the oesophagus is the descending thoracic aorta.
5. Remove the rest of the pericardium by blunt dissection, except where it is adhered to the diaphragm.
6. Clean the oesophagus by blunt dissection. Note that the *oesophageal plexus* covers its surface.
7. Identify the *right vagus nerve* crossing anterior to the right subclavian artery. Trace it down to the posterior side of root of the right lung. Note its fibres spreading on the surface of the oesophagus.

   ▶ https://www.winkingskull.com/dissector/V1/video.aspx?vid=299
8. Identify the *left vagus nerve* crossing the left side of the aortic arch and follow it to the posterior side of root of the left lung. Note its contribution to the oesophageal plexus.
9. Note that the oesophageal plexus gives rise to the *anterior* and *posterior vagal trunks* on the respective sides of the oesophagus and innervates the large part of the gastrointestinal tract.
10. Find the *azygos vein* arching superior to the root of the right lung. Clean and trace it down to the level of the diaphragm. Note the *right posterior intercostal veins* ending in the azygos vein.
11. Identify the *thoracic duct*, retracting the oesophagus to the left and exploring the interval between the azygos vein and the thoracic aorta. The thoracic duct is posterior to the oesophagus and lies immediately to the left of the azygos vein. It is thin walled and may easily be torn.

    ▶ https://www.winkingskull.com/dissector/V1/video.aspx?vid=300
12. Using a probe, separate the thoracic duct from the neighbouring connective tissue. Inferiorly, it can be traced to the aortic orifice in the diaphragm. Superiorly, it ends at the junction of the left internal jugular vein with the left subclavian vein (jugulo-subclavian angle). Do not trace it to its termination in the neck at this stage.
13. Note that the thoracic duct crosses the anterior surface of the *right posterior intercostal arteries*, the *hemiazygos* and *accessory hemiazygos veins*.
14. Observe on the left side of the posterior mediastinum the *left posterior intercostal veins* terminating into the hemiazygos and accessory hemiazygos veins.
15. Note that the hemiazygos and accessory hemiazygos veins cross the bodies of the T8 and T9 vertebrae, respectively, to terminate into the azygos vein.
16. Note the *branches of the descending thoracic aorta*. These are the oesophageal arteries and the left bronchial arteries.
17. In one intercostal space, dissect a pair of posterior intercostal arteries and follow the intercostal space. Note that the right posterior intercostal arteries cross the midline passing anterior to the vertebral bodies.
18. Identify the *sympathetic trunk* on both sides. Note that the sympathetic trunk has one *sympathetic ganglion* at each thoracic vertebral level.
19. Identify the rami communicans, the white and grey rami connecting the intercostal nerve with the corresponding sympathetic ganglion.

20. Identify the *greater splanchnic nerve*. Note that it receives contribution from the T5 to T9 sympathetic ganglia.

https://www.winkingskull.com/dissector/V1/video.aspx?vid=301

21. The *lesser splanchnic nerve* arises from the tenth and eleventh thoracic sympathetic ganglia, while the twelfth thoracic sympathetic ganglion gives rise to the *lowest splanchnic nerve*.

Trachea

It is a 10- to 12-cm long, wide tube extending from the lower end of the larynx (lower border of C6 vertebra) to the tracheal bifurcation (lower border of T4 vertebra). It lies in the median plane, but near its lower end it deviates slightly to the right side (**Fig. 14.24**). The thoracic part of the trachea is related:

Anteriorly: The manubrium sterni, sternocleidomastoid muscles, remains of the thymus, aortic arch and its branches (i.e., the brachiocephalic trunk, left common carotid artery); the left brachiocephalic and inferior thyroid veins and the deep cardiac plexus.

Posteriorly: The oesophagus and vertebral column.

Left side: The aortic arch, left common carotid, left subclavian arteries and left recurrent laryngeal nerve.

Right side: The right vagus, azygos vein, right pleura and the lung.

Structure: The trachea is made up of fibroblastic wall duly supported by the C-shaped hyaline cartilages, about 16 to 20 in number. The posterior gap of the C-shaped cartilages is occupied by the *trachealis* muscle and fibroelastic tissue. The trachealis muscle provides a soft cushion for the oesophagus to dilate during swallowing. The muscle also controls (narrows) the calibre of the trachea compressing the air inside when the vocal cords are adducted (rima glottidis is closed), thus increasing the explosive force of the blast of compressed air as happens in sneezing or coughing.

1. The trachea is seen as a radiolucent column in front of the cervicothoracic part of the vertebral column in a plain radiograph.

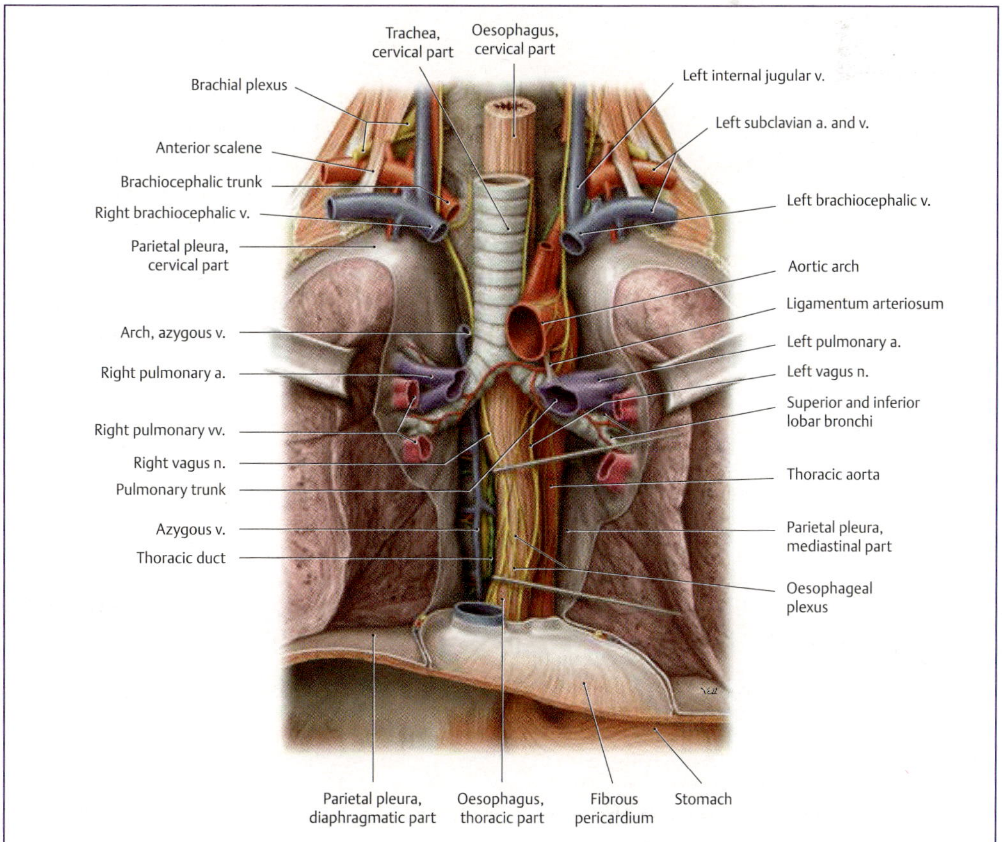

Fig. 14.24 Trachea and oesophagus in situ (anterior view).

2. The trachea can be palpated in the suprasternal notch in the midline. Any shift indicates a mediastinal shift.
3. *Tracheostomy*: It is an emergency operation done in laryngeal obstruction, such as diphtheria, foreign body airway obstruction, carcinoma. In this, a tracheostomy tube is inserted to facilitate breathing. It is usually done in the retrothyroid region, cutting the isthmus of the thyroid gland. It can be done in the suprahyoid region, but it carries menace of damaging vessels in front of the trachea.
4. Tracheal compression by enlargement of adjacent structures, such as the thyroid, thymus, aortic arch, can lead to *dyspnoea*.

Oesophagus

Oesophagus (**Fig. 14.25**) is a narrow muscular tube from the pharynx to the stomach, about 25 cm long. It extends from the neck (lower border of C6 vertebra) to the gastro-oesophageal junction in the upper part of the abdomen. It pierces the diaphragm at the level of T10 vertebra. It courses down the superior and posterior mediastinum in front of the vertebral column.

Curvatures and constrictions: Though the oesophagus is vertically oriented, along its passage it is slightly deviated to the left at the root of neck and at its lower end. It also exhibits an anteroposterior curvature conforming with the curve of the cervicothoracic region of the vertebral column. The oesophagus shows constrictions, which are important during instrumentation, for example, passing Ryle's tube or in endoscopy. These constrictions are as follows:

1. At its commencement: About 6 inches from the incisor teeth
2. Where it is crossed by the arch of the aorta: About 9 inches from the incisor teeth
3. Where it is crossed by the left principal bronchus: About 11 inches from the incisor teeth
4. Where it pierces the diaphragm: About 15 inches from the incisor teeth

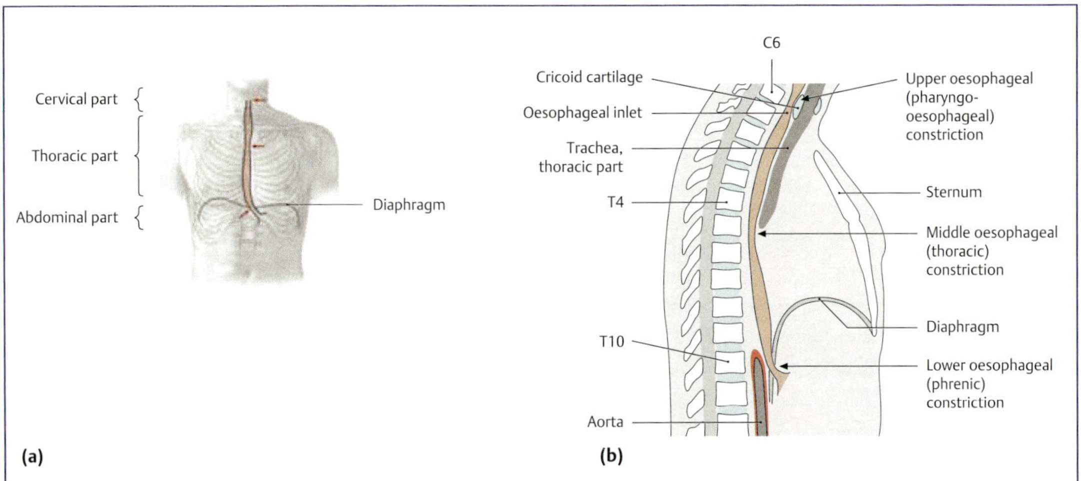

Fig. 14.25 Oesophagus: Location and constrictions. **(a)** Projection of oesophagus onto chest wall. Oesophageal constrictions are indicated with arrows. **(b)** Oesophageal constrictions, right lateral view.

Relations in the Thoracic Part

Anteriorly: It is related to the trachea, right pulmonary artery, left principal bronchus, left atrium, pericardium and diaphragm.

Posteriorly: It is related to the vertebral column, right posterior intercostal arteries, azygos vein, thoracic duct, thoracic aorta and right pleural recess.

Left side of the oesophagus is related to the aortic arch, left subclavian artery, thoracic duct, left pleura and lung.

Right side of the oesophagus is related to the right pleura and lung.

Blood supply: The *cervical part* is supplied by the inferior thyroid arteries, the *thoracic part* by the oesophageal branches of the thoracic aorta and the *abdominal part* by the oesophageal branches of the left gastric artery. Likewise, the venous drainage also follows the regional thoracic part drains into the azygos vein and abdominal part into the left gastric vein.

Innervation: Both the autonomic components, sympathetic and parasympathetic, supply the oesophagus. The *sympathetic nerves* are vasomotor and derived from the middle cervical ganglion and the upper four thoracic ganglia.

The *parasympathetic nerves* to the upper half are derived from the recurrent laryngeal nerves and to the lower half from the oesophageal plexus formed by the vagi.

Clinical Notes

1. In oesophagoscopy, one has to remember the normal sites of constrictions along the course of the oesophagus.
2. In portal hypertension, there is dilatation of the veins in the lower part of the oesophagus, leading to *oesophageal varices* which may cause *haematemesis*. On barium swallow, the oesophageal varices present worm-like appearance.
3. *Barium swallow*: It is a radiographic procedure to visualize the oesophagus by giving barium sulphate paste to the patient. In mitral stenosis, the left atrium is enlarged. This causes deeper indentation along the anterior wall of the barium-filled oesophagus.
4. *Dysphagia*: Difficulty in swallowing. It may be due to oesophageal compression, carcinoma of the oesophagus and mediastinal syndrome.
5. *Tracheo-oesophageal fistula*: It is a developmental defect due to defective development of the tracheo-oesophageal septum, separating the two tubes.

Descending Thoracic Aorta

It is a continuation of the arch of the aorta and so begins at the left side of the lower border of the T4 vertebra. It then descends in the posterior mediastinum with an inclination to the right and at the lower border of the T12 vertebra. Then it passes through the *aortic orifice* of the diaphragm into the abdomen to continue as the abdominal aorta.

It is related *anteriorly* to the root of the left lung, pericardium and heart; *posteriorly* to the vertebral column and hemiazygos veins; *on the right side* to the oesophagus, azygos vein, thoracic duct, right lung and pleura; *on the left side* to the left lung and pleura.

It has the following branches:

1. *Posterior intercostal arteries* on both sides in the third to eleventh intercostal spaces.
2. The pair of *subcostal arteries* (one on each side).
3. *Two left bronchial arteries*; among them, the upper left bronchial artery may give rise to the *right bronchial artery*.
4. *Pericardial branches* supplying the posterior surface of the pericardium.
5. *Mediastinal branches* supplying the lymph nodes and loose areolar tissue of the posterior mediastinum.
6. *Oesophageal branches* supplying the middle one-third of the oesophagus.
7. The *superior phrenic* arteries supplying the posterior part of the superior surface of the diaphragm.

Thoracic Duct

It is the largest lymphatic channel in the body and extends from the upper part of the abdomen to the neck. In the abdomen, it begins as a continuation of the *cisterna chyli* (an elongated lymphatic sac) against L1 and L2 vertebra and ascends through the posterior and superior mediastinum to the lower part of the neck. It is about 45 cm long and has beaded appearance due to the presence of numerous valves along its course.

It enters the thorax through the *aortic orifice* of the diaphragm at the level of T12 vertebra. In the posterior mediastinum, it ascends and crosses from the right to the left side at the level of T5 vertebra. It then runs upwards through the superior mediastinum along the left side of the oesophagus and reaches the neck.

In the neck, it arches rising about 3 to 4 cm above the clavicle to the left. Then passing in front of the subclavian artery, it terminates by opening into the left *jugulo-subclavian angle* formed by the left internal jugular vein and left subclavian vein.

The thoracic duct collects lymph from both halves of the body, below the diaphragm and the left half above the diaphragm. In the thorax, it receives lymphatics from the posterior mediastinal lymph nodes and some intercostal nodes also. In the neck, it receives *left jugular trunk* from the lymph nodes in the neck and *left subclavian trunk* from the axillary nodes. These trunks may open into the thoracic duct. The left mediastinal trunk draining the left half of the thorax usually opens into the left brachiocephalic vein, but may drain into the thoracic duct.

CHAPTER 15

Joints of the Thorax

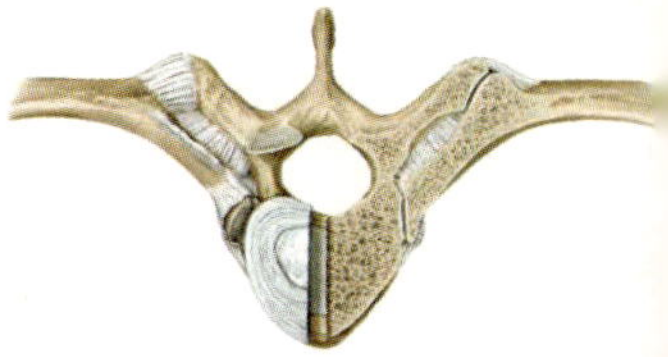

Learning Objectives

After reading this chapter, students should be able to identify the following:

- Joints and type of the joints of thorax.
- The role of joints of thorax in respiratory movements.
- Sternocostal, costochondral, interchondral, costovertebral and costotransverse joints.

Introduction

The joints of the thorax include the sternal, sternocostal, costochondral, interchondral, costovertebral, costotransverse and intervertebral joints. These joints allow the respiratory movements.

Sternal Joints

The sternal joints include the manubriosternal and xiphisternal joints.

1. *Manubriosternal joint*: This is a secondary cartilaginous joint. A *fibrous disc* is placed between the cartilage-covered ends of the manubrium and the body of the sternum. There may be a cavity in this disc. This joint moves during respiration. Rarely, it ossifies in old age.
2. *Xiphisternal joint*: It is also a cartilaginous type of joint and it ossifies around the middle age.

Sternocostal Joints/Sternochondral Joints (Fig. 15.1)

There are seven costal cartilages on each side that articulate with the lateral margin of the sternum. The first sternochondral joint is a primary cartilaginous joint; it does not permit any movement and the cartilage begins to ossify. Therefore, the first rib, costal cartilages and manubrium move as one unit on the costovertebral joints.

The second to seventh costal cartilages articulate with the sternum by synovial joints. They have a single cavity except the second sternochondral joint, which shows subdivision of the cavity into two parts by an intra-articular sternocostal ligament. Each joint has a fibrous capsule strengthened with the help of the *radiate sternocostal ligament*.

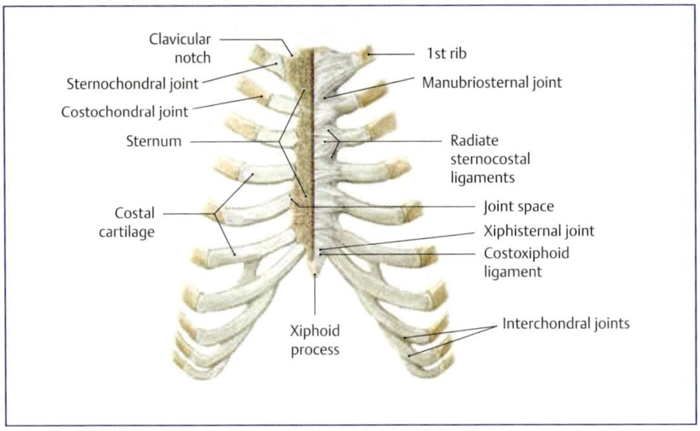

Fig. 15.1 Sternocostal joints.

Costochondral Joints (Fig. 15.1)

Anteriorly, each rib has a conical pit in which the cartilage fits forming the costochondral joint. It is primarily a cartilaginous joint and no movement occurs in it.

Interchondral Joints (Fig. 15.1)

These are placed between the adjacent margins of the costal cartilages of the sixth to ninth ribs. These are the synovial type of joints.

Costovertebral Joints

The head of the rib articulates with the corresponding vertebra and also with the vertebra above (**Fig. 15.2a**). Thus, it forms two plane synovial joints separated by an *intra-articular ligament*. This ligament is attached to the intervertebral disc and to the ridge on the head of the rib. In addition, there are other ligaments, such as, the *capsular ligament* and *triradiate ligament*.

Costotransverse Joints

The tubercle of the rib articulates with the transverse process of the corresponding vertebra, forming a synovial joint (**Fig. 15.2b**). Ligaments of this joint are as follows:

1. The *capsular ligament* is attached to the participating bones just peripheral to the articulating facets.
2. *Superior costotransverse ligament* having two laminae. It extends from the crest on the neck of the rib to the transverse process of the vertebra above.
3. *Inferior costotransverse ligament*: It extends from the posterior surface of the neck of the rib to the transverse process of the corresponding vertebra.
4. *Lateral costotransverse ligament*: It connects the non-articular part of the tubercle of the rib to the tip of the transverse process.

   The upper six ribs have convex articular facets on their tubercle, permitting rotation which occurs in the pump handle movement of the ribs, increasing anteroposterior dimension of the thoracic cavity. The articular facets on the tubercles of the seventh to tenth ribs are flat and permit gliding required in bucket handle movement of these ribs. This movement increases the transverse dimension of the thorax.

Interchondral Joints (Fig. 15.1)

The costal cartilages from the fifth to ninth articulate with one another to form synovial joints. However, the ninth costal cartilage articulates with the tenth by fibrous tissue.

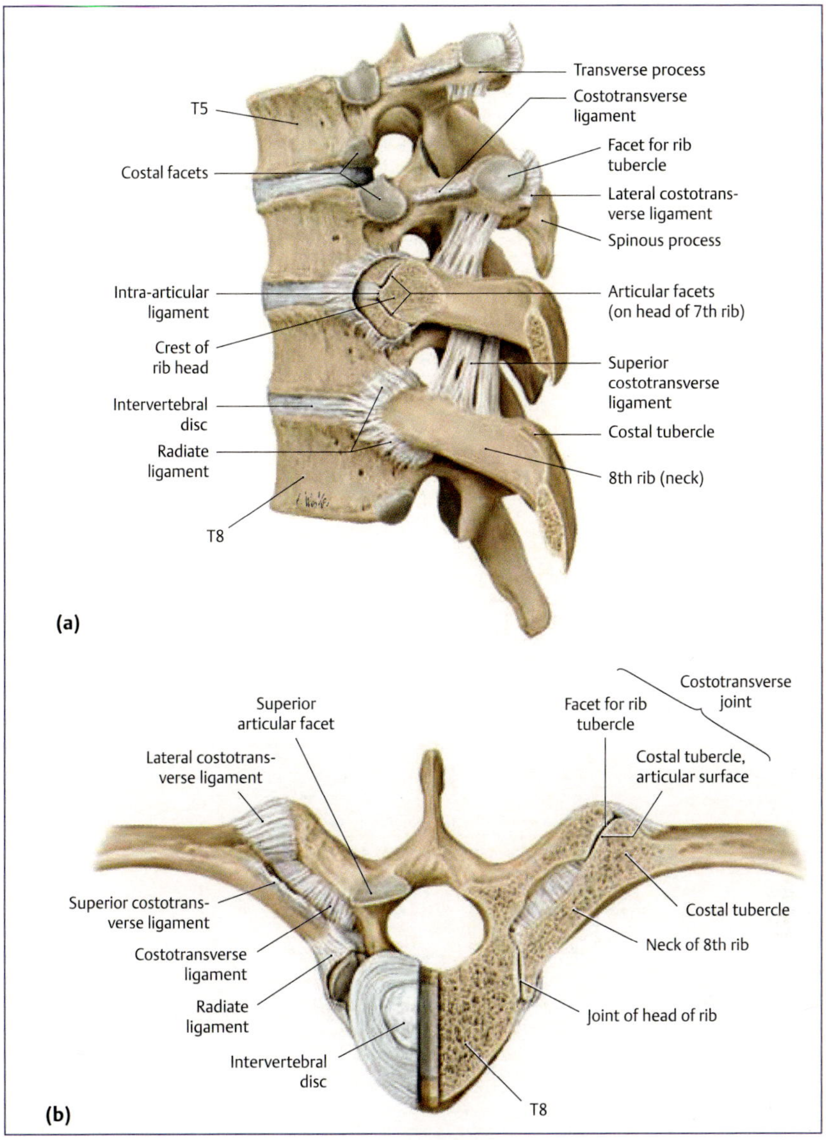

Fig. 15.2 **(a, b)** Costovertebral and costotransverse joints.

Respiratory Movements

The movements that occur at the joints described so far can be summed up as *respiratory movements* (**Figs. 15.3, 15.4, 15.5** and **15.6**). The expansion of the lungs during inspiration and retraction during expiration occurs due to the following factors:

1. Increment in the volume of the thorax creates negative intrathoracic pressure which draws air into the lungs. The volume of the thorax increases due to movement of the thoracic wall, chiefly involving the manubriosternal and costovertebral joints.
2. The elastic recoil of the lung alveoli and that of the thoracic wall expels the air during expiration.

Facts to Remember

1. The movements of rib cage during inspiration and expiration are shown in **Figs. 15.3** and **15.4**.
2. Assume that each rib is a lever with the fulcrum being at the tubercle of the rib. This essentially makes two unequal arms of the lever; therefore, a slight movement of the rib at its vertebral end is magnified to a great extent at the anterior end of the rib.
3. The anterior end of the rib lies at a lower level than its posterior or vertebral end. So, during elevation of the rib the anterior end moves forward. This holds true mostly for the vertebrosternal ribs

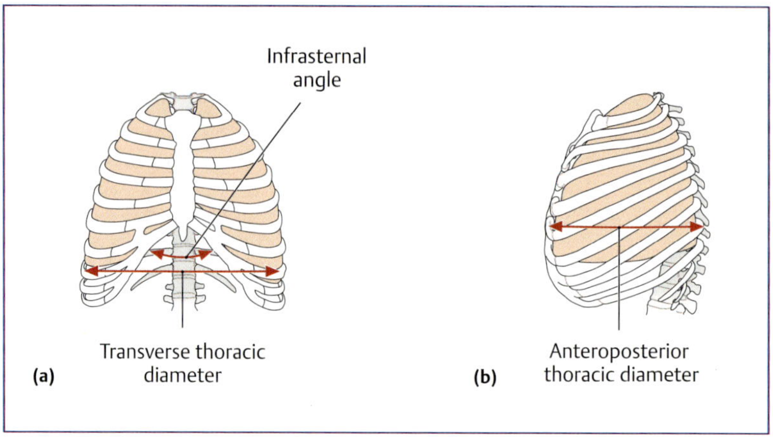

Fig. 15.3 Movements of rib cage and associated muscles during inspiration. **(a)** Increase in transverse thoracic diameter. **(b)** Increase in anteroposterior thoracic diameter.

(second to sixth ribs). The anterior end of these ribs moves up and down and is referred to as the *pump handle movement*. This movement increases the anteroposterior diameter of the thorax.

4. Considering the plane of the two ends of the rib, the mid portion of the shaft of the rib lies at the lower level. Therefore, when this part is elevated (by action of the intercostal muscles) it moves outwards, thus *increasing the transverse diameter of the thoracic cavity*. This movement is called the *bucket handle movement*.

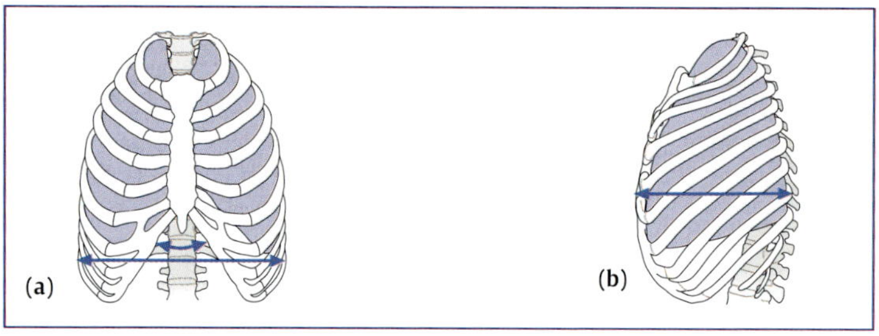

Fig. 15.4 **(a, b)** Movements of rib cage and associated muscles during expiration.

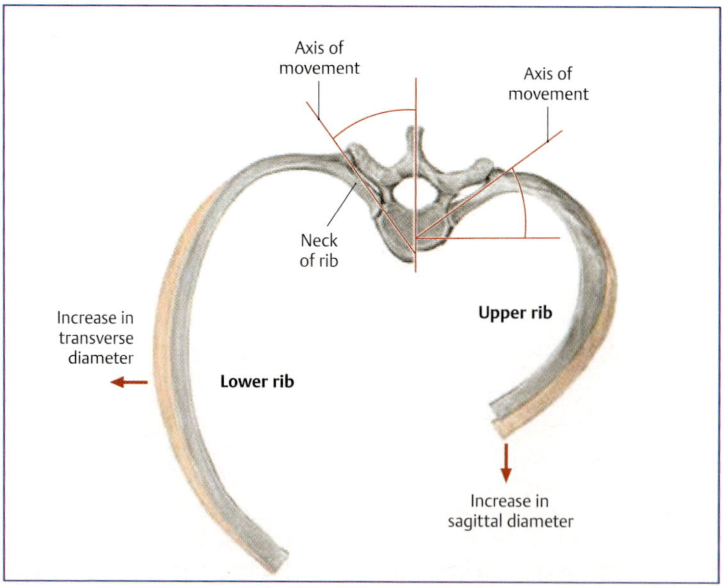

Fig. 15.5 Axes of rib movement (superior view).

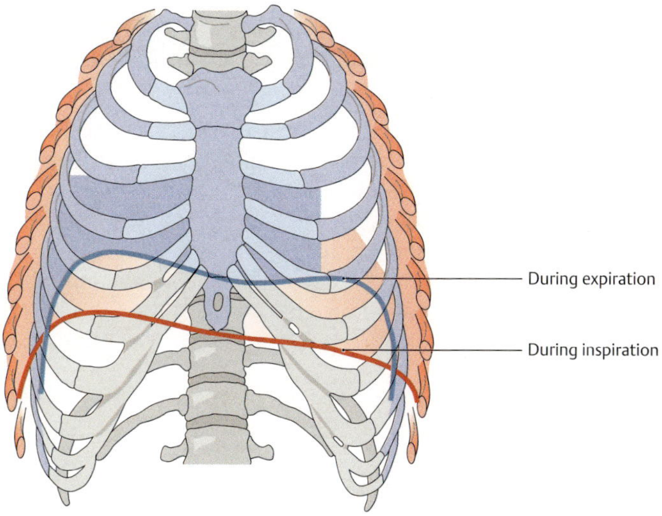

Fig. 15.6 Position of diaphragm during respiration.

The axes of rib movements during pump handle and bucket handle movements are shown in **Fig. 15.5**.

5. The *vertical diameter of the thorax is increased* by the contraction and subsequent depression of the diaphragm (**Fig. 15.6**).

During inspiration, the muscles involved in these respiratory movements, which have been described earlier, include the intercostal muscles, diaphragm, sternocleidomastoid, scalene, pectoralis minor and erector spinae. The abdominal muscles are involved during forced expiration.

Intervertebral Joints

The adjoining vertebrae form three joints, one between the vertebral bodies and two between their articular processes (refer to **Fig. 15.2a**). The joint between the vertebral bodies is a symphysis or secondary cartilaginous type of joint. The cartilage interposed is a fibrocartilage and is composed of the soft gelatinous core and the *nucleus pulposus* and outer fibrous element called the *annulus fibrosus*. Functionally, the intervertebral disc serves the following functions:

1. It serves as a buffer or shock absorber.
2. It helps in weight transmission.
3. It is responsible for curvatures (shape) of the vertebral column.
4. It permits movements of the vertebral column (evidenced in the cervical and lumbar regions).

The ligaments associated with the vertebral joints include:

1. Anterior longitudinal ligament
2. Posterior longitudinal ligament
3. Interspinous ligaments
4. Intertransverse ligaments
5. Supraspinous ligaments
6. Ligamentum flava (connecting laminae)

The movements that occur in the vertebral column involve several vertebrae. Individually, there is a slight movement between the vertebrae; however, the total range of movements occurring is considerable. This includes flexion, extension, lateral flexion and reasonable degree of rotation.

Clinical Notes

1. *Dyspnoea*: It is difficulty in breathing.
2. *Accessory rib*: It may be in the lumbar or cervical region. The cervical rib may compress the elements of the brachial plexus or subclavian artery leading to neurovascular symptoms.
3. *Spina bifida*: It is a congenital defect resulting from the failure of fusion of the two halves of the neural arch. The laminae and spine of the vertebra are missing. It may present in various forms, such as the spina bifida occulta and spina bifida cystica with meningocele or meningomyelocele.
4. *Hemivertebra*: It refers to the developmental defect due to failure of one of the chondrification centres and failure of formation of one-half of vertebra.

Index